Assisting With Patient Care

WORKBOOK

2nd Edition

Bernie Gorek, RNC, GNP, MA, NHA
Gerontology Consultant
Greeley, Colorado

Mosby
An Affiliate of Elsevier

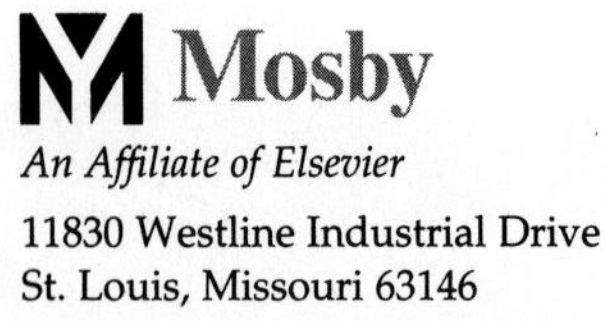

An Affiliate of Elsevier
11830 Westline Industrial Drive
St. Louis, Missouri 63146

ASSISTING WITH PATIENT CARE WORKBOOK

ISBN-13: 978-0-323-02658-1
ISBN-10: 0-323-02658-3

Executive Editor: Susan R. Epstein
Senior Developmental Editor: Maria Broeker
Publishing Services Manager: John Rogers
Senior Project Manager: Kathleen L. Teal
Senior Designer: Kathi Gosche

Printed in the United States of America

Last digit is the print number: 13 12 11 10

In memory of Ed and Betty.
You are missed.

Preface

Assisting With Patient Care Workbook, 2nd edition, is to be used with Mosby's textbook, *Assisting With Patient Care,* 2nd edition, by Sheila A. Sorrentino. All references to boxes, procedures, tables, and page numbers relate to this textbook. The student will not need other resources to complete the exercises in this workbook. Additional learning activities have been included to challenge students and to enhance their learning experience.

This workbook is designed to help students apply what they have learned in each chapter. Students are encouraged to use the workbook as a study guide. Various types of questions and learning exercises are included in each chapter to help students understand and apply the information in the textbook. The **Additional Learning Activities** encourage discussion and practical application of the information presented in each chapter. **Procedure Checklists** are provided, which correspond with the procedures in each chapter of *Assisting With Patient Care,* 2nd edition. These checklists are intended to help students become skilled at performing procedures that affect the quality of care they provide. Answers to the Workbook Questions are provided in the *Instructors' Guide and Test Bank for Assisting With Patient Care,* 2nd edition.

Assistive personnel are important members of the health and nursing teams. Completing the exercises in this workbook will increase the student's knowledge, skills, and confidence. The goal is to prepare students to provide the best possible care and to help them develop pride in the important work they do.

Bernie Gorek

Illustration Credits

Chapter 26, #31, page 165, from Thibodeau GA, Patton KT: *Structure and function of the body,* ed 11, St Louis, 2000, Mosby.

Chapter 26, #33, *A* and *B*, page 166, from Atwood S, Stanton C, Davenport J: *Introduction to basic cardiac dysrhythmias,* ed 3, St Louis, 2003, Mosby.

Chapter 26, #34, *A*, page 166, from Ignatavicius DD, Workman ML: *Medical-surgical nursing: Critical thinking for collaborative care,* ed 4, St Louis, 2002, Mosby.

Chapter 26, #34, *B*, page 166, from Atwood S, Stanton C, Davenport J: *Introduction to basic cardiac dysrhythmias,* ed 3, St Louis, 2003, Mosby.

Chapter 27, #35, page 172, from Bonewit-West K: *Clinical procedures for medical assistants,* ed 5, Philadelphia, 2003, Saunders.

Chapter 27, #36, page 172, from Bonewit-West K; *Clinical procedures for medical assistants,* ed 5, Philadelphia, 2003, Saunders.

Contents

1

Health Care Today

OBJECTIVES

The questions and student activities in this chapter will help you meet these objectives.

- Define the key terms listed in Chapter 1
- Explain the purposes and services of health care agencies
- Identify the members of the health team and the nursing team
- Describe the nursing service department
- Describe the nursing team members
- Describe four nursing care patterns
- Describe the programs that pay for health care
- Explain why standards are met

STUDY QUESTIONS

Matching

Match the terms with the correct definitions.

A. Case management
B. Primary nursing
C. Licensed practical nurse (LPN)
D. Terminal illness
E. Acute illness
F. Functional nursing
G. Health team
H. Team nursing
I. Hospice
J. Registered nurse (RN)
K. Chronic illness
L. Nursing team
M. Assistive personnel
N. Patient-focused care

1. e A sudden illness from which a person is expected to recover
2. m Individuals who give basic nursing care under the supervision of a licensed nurse
3. a A nursing care pattern; an RN coordinates a person's care from admission through discharge and into the home setting
4. K An ongoing illness, slow or gradual in onset, for which there is no known cure
5. f A nursing care pattern focusing on tasks and jobs

6. G Staff members who work together to provide health care

7. I A health care agency or program for persons who are dying

8. C A nurse who has completed a 1-year nursing program and passed a licensing test

9. L Individuals who provide nursing care—RNs, LPNs/LVNs, and assistive personnel

10. N A nursing care pattern; an RN is responsible for the person's total care.

11. B A nurse who has completed a 2-, 3-, or 4-year nursing program and has passed a licensing test

12. J A nursing care pattern; a team of nursing staff is led by an RN who decides the amount and kind of care each person needs

13. h An illness or injury for which there is no reasonable expectation of recovery

14. D Services are moved from the departments to the bed side

Fill in the Blanks

15. List 4 purposes of health care.

    A. ______

    B. ______

    C. ______

    D. ______

16. Rehabilitation starts when

    ______.

17. List and briefly describe 8 health care settings in which assistive personnel may work.

    A. ______

    B. ______

    C. ______

    D. ______

    E. ______

    F. ______

    G. ______

    H. ______

18. The governing body of a health care agency is called the ______.

19. The health team is also called

    ______.

20. The goal of the health team is to

    ______.

21. The ______ is responsible for the entire nursing staff and the care given.

22. You report to ______.

23. Nursing education staff do the following:

    A. ______

    B. ______

    C. ______

    D. ______

    E. ______

24. Medicare is ________________________________

____

________________________________.

25. ________________________________ limit the amounts paid by insurers, Medicare, and Medicaid. The amount paid for services is determined before the person receives care.

26. List 3 prospective payment systems.

A. ________________________________

B. ________________________________

C. ________________________________

27. Define the following terms.

A. Licensure

____

____

B. Certification

____

____

C. Accreditation

____

____

28. ________________________________ are done to see if the agency meets set standards.

29. What is your role in meeting standards and in the survey process?

A. ________________________________

B. ________________________________

C. ________________________________

D. ________________________________

E. ________________________________

F. ________________________________

G. ________________________________

H. ________________________________

Multiple Choice

Circle the BEST answer.

30. Managed care
    A. Is a health insurance plan sponsored by the federal government.
    B. Is a nursing care pattern.
    C. Deals with health care delivery and payment.
    D. Is required by OBRA.

31. Which provides health care for a prepaid fee?
    A. A health maintenance organization (HMO)
    B. Social Security
    C. Medicare part B
    D. A group insurance plan

32. Which is a group of doctors and hospitals that provide health care at a reduced rate?
    A. Private insurance plan
    B. Diagnostic related group (DRG)
    C. Preferred provider organization (PPO)
    D. Health care team

33. Which helps persons to return to their highest possible level of physical and psychological functioning?
    A. Health promotion
    B. Rehabilitation
    C. Disease prevention
    D. Detection of disease

34. This health team member fills drug orders written by the doctor.
    A. Physical therapist
    B. Pharmacist
    C. Nurse practitioner
    D. Respiratory therapist

35. This health team member diagnoses and treats diseases and injuries.
    A. Registered nurse
    B. Speech/language pathologist
    C. Radiographer
    D. Physician

ADDITIONAL LEARNING ACTIVITIES

1. Look in the yellow pages of the telephone book, and list the health care agencies in your community along with the services they provide.

2. Write about an experience you or a family member had with a health care agency. Answer these questions:
   A. What was the purpose of the contact?
   B. What type of agency was it?
   C. What members of the health care team were involved?
   D. What were the roles of each member of the team?

3. Provide the following information about RNS, LPNs/LVNs, and assistive personnel:
   A. Education requirements
   B. Licensure requirements
   C. Roles and responsibilities

4. Look at your health insurance policy. Do you know which services are covered and which are not? Does your policy limit where you can go for health care? Explain.

2

Roles and Functions of Assistive Personnel

OBJECTIVES

The questions and student activities in this chapter will help you meet these objectives.

- Define the key terms listed in Chapter 2
- Explain the history and current trends affecting assistive personnel
- Explain the laws that affect assistive personnel
- Explain what assistive personnel can do and their role limits
- Explain why you need a job description
- Describe the educational requirements for assistive personnel
- Describe the delegation process
- Explain how to accept or refuse a delegated task
- Explain how to prevent negligent acts
- Give examples of false imprisonment, defamation, assault, battery, and fraud
- Describe how to protect the right to privacy
- Explain the purpose of informed consent
- Describe child, elder, and domestic abuse

STUDY QUESTIONS

Complete the Crossword

Across

2. Negligence by a professional person
4. Intentionally attempting or threatening to touch a person's body without the person's consent
9. Touching a person's body without his or her consent
10. A function, procedure, activity, or work that does not require an RN's professional knowledge or judgment

Down

1. A rule of conduct made by a government body
3. A wrong committed against a person or the person's property
5. Making false statements orally
6. Making false statements in print, writing, or through pictures or drawings
7. Knowledge of what is right and wrong conduct
8. An act that violates a criminal law

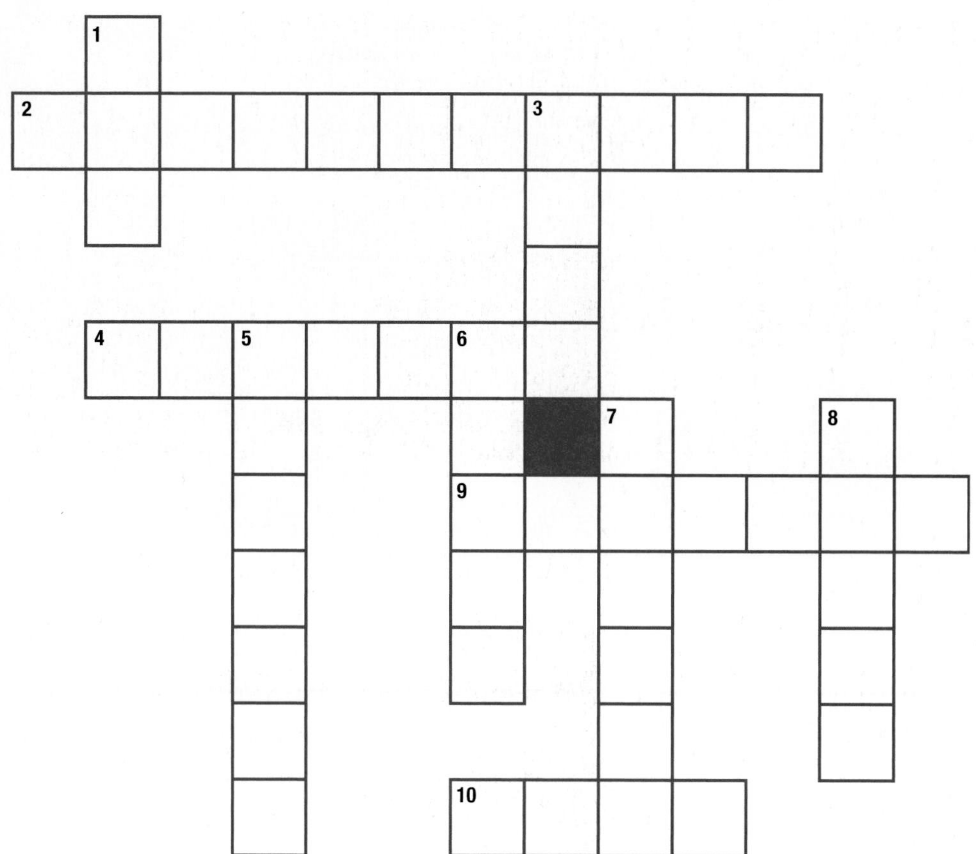

Matching

Match the following terms with the correct definitions.

1. D Violating a person's right not to have his or her name, photograph, or private affairs exposed or made public without giving consent
2. f Unlawful restraint or restriction of a person's movement
3. e Being responsible for one's actions and the actions of others who perform delegated tasks
4. G The law which sets the minimum training and competency evaluation for assistive personnel who work in nursing centers
5. J The duty or obligation to perform some act or function
6. H To authorize another person to perform a task
7. B Laws concerned with relationships between people
8. a The intentional mistreatment of another person
9. I The skills, care, and judgment required by a health team member under similar conditions
10. C A state law which regulates nursing practice in that state

A. Abuse
B. Civil laws
C. Nurse practice act
D. Invasion of privacy
E. Accountable
F. False imprisonment
G. The Omnibus Reconciliation Act of 1987 (OBRA)
H. Delegate
I. Standard of care
J. Responsibility

Fill in the Blanks

11. To protect patients and residents from harm, you need to know:

    A. ______________________________

    B. ______________________________

    C. ______________________________

12. List 6 measures used to reduce health care costs.

    A. ______________________________

    B. ______________________________

    C. ______________________________

    D. ______________________________

    E. ______________________________

    F. ______________________________

13. ______________________________ and ______________________________ provide direction for what you can do.

14. A state's nurse practice act is used to decide what assistive personnel can do. If you perform a task beyond the legal limits of your role, you could be ______________________________ ______________________________.

15. List 6 areas of study for assistive personnel training programs required by OBRA.

    A. ______________________________

    B. ______________________________

    C. ______________________________

    D. ______________________________

    E. ______________________________

    F. ______________________________

16. What information does the nursing assistant registry have about each nursing assistant?

    A. ______________________________

    B. ______________________________

    C. ______________________________

    D. ______________________________

    E. ______________________________

    F. ______________________________

    G. ______________________________

17. Before you perform a procedure, you must make sure that:

    A. ______________________________

    B. ______________________________

    C. ______________________________

    D. ______________________________

18. List 7 role limits for assistive personnel.

    A. ______________________________ ______________________________

    B. ______________________________ ______________________________

    C. ______________________________ ______________________________

    D. ______________________________ ______________________________

    E. ______________________________ ______________________________

    F. ______________________________ ______________________________

    G. ______________________________ ______________________________

19. The ______________________ lists the responsibilities and functions that the agency expects you to perform.

20. You should not take a job that requires you to:

    A. ______________________

    B. ______________________

    C. ______________________

21. Before the nurse delegates a task to you, the nurse must know:

    A. ______________________

    B. ______________________

    C. ______________________

    D. ______________________

    E. ______________________

    F. ______________________

22. List the 5 rights of delegation.

    A. ______________________

    B. ______________________

    C. ______________________

    D. ______________________

    E. ______________________

23. What are your choices when a task is delegated to you?

    ____

    ____

24. When should you refuse a task?

    A. ______________________

    B. ______________________

    C. ______________________

    D. ______________________

    E. ______________________

    F. ______________________

    G. ______________________

    H. ______________________

    I. ______________________

25. False imprisonment involves:

    A. ______________________

    B. ______________________

    C. ______________________

26. The person must consent to any

    ____

    ____

    ______________________.

27. List 5 elements of abuse.

    A. ______________________

    B. ______________________

    C. ______________________

    D. ______________________

    E. ______________________

Multiple Choice

Circle the BEST answer.

28. The nursing assistant registry is
    A. A skills evaluation.
    B. An official record of personnel who have completed a state approved training program.
    C. A list of rules and responsibilities for assistive personnel.
    D. A procedure book.

29. Retraining and a new competency evaluation program are required for nursing assistants who have not worked for
    A. 2 consecutive years.
    B. 3 consecutive years.
    C. 4 consecutive years.
    D. 5 consecutive years.

30. Assistive personnel
    A. Function under the supervision of RNs.
    B. Decide what should or should not be done for a person.
    C. Supervise other assistive personnel.
    D. Take telephone orders from the doctor.

31. You can refuse to do a delegated task for all of the following reasons *except*
    A. The task is not in your job description.
    B. You do not know how to use the equipment.
    C. You are busy and the task is unpleasant.
    D. The RN's direction is unclear.

32. You agree to perform a task. You must do all of the following *except*
    A. Complete the task safely.
    B. Ask for help when you are unsure.
    C. Report what you did and your observations to the nurse.
    D. Delegate the task to a co-worker.

33. Standards of care come from all of the following sources *except*
    A. The nursing assistant registry
    B. Textbooks
    C. Laws
    D. Job descriptions

34. Elder abuse takes many forms. Humiliation, harassment, ridicule, and threats of punishment is
    A. Sexual abuse
    B. False imprisonment
    C. Mental abuse
    D. Physical abuse

35. You suspect a person you are caring for is being abused. You must
    A. Call the police.
    B. Report your observations to the RN.
    C. Tell a co-worker.
    D. Tell the person's doctor.

36. Injuring a child on purpose is
    A. Physical abuse.
    B. Neglect.
    C. Mental abuse.
    D. Involuntary seclusion.

37. Abuse that occurs in relationships is called
    A. Neglect.
    B. Child abuse.
    C. Sexual abuse.
    D. Domestic abuse.

38. Nursing centers must thoroughly investigate all claims of abuse.
    A. True
    B. False

39. Which is *not* a sign of elder abuse?
    A. Weight gain
    B. Frequent injuries
    C. Poor personal hygiene
    D. Bleeding and bruising in the genital area

40. Which is *not* a sign of child abuse?
    A. Bruises on the face, back, buttocks, abdomen, chest, and inner thighs
    B. An abrasion on the knee
    C. Burns and scalds on the feet, hands, backs, or buttocks
    D. Bite marks

ADDITIONAL LEARNING ACTIVITIES

1. Read the rules of conduct for assistive personnel.
   A. Write down ways to apply these rules in a job setting.
   B. Discuss the importance of these rules with your classmates.

2. You are asked to do a task that you feel is unsafe.
   A. How would you handle the situation?
   B. What could you say?
   C. Who would you talk to about your concerns?

3. Are there any job functions that you are opposed to doing for moral or religious reasons? Explain.
   A. How will you advise your employer of your concerns?

4. Use the yellow pages of the phone book or the Internet to look up agencies in your community that deal with abuse.
   A. List the services each agency provides.

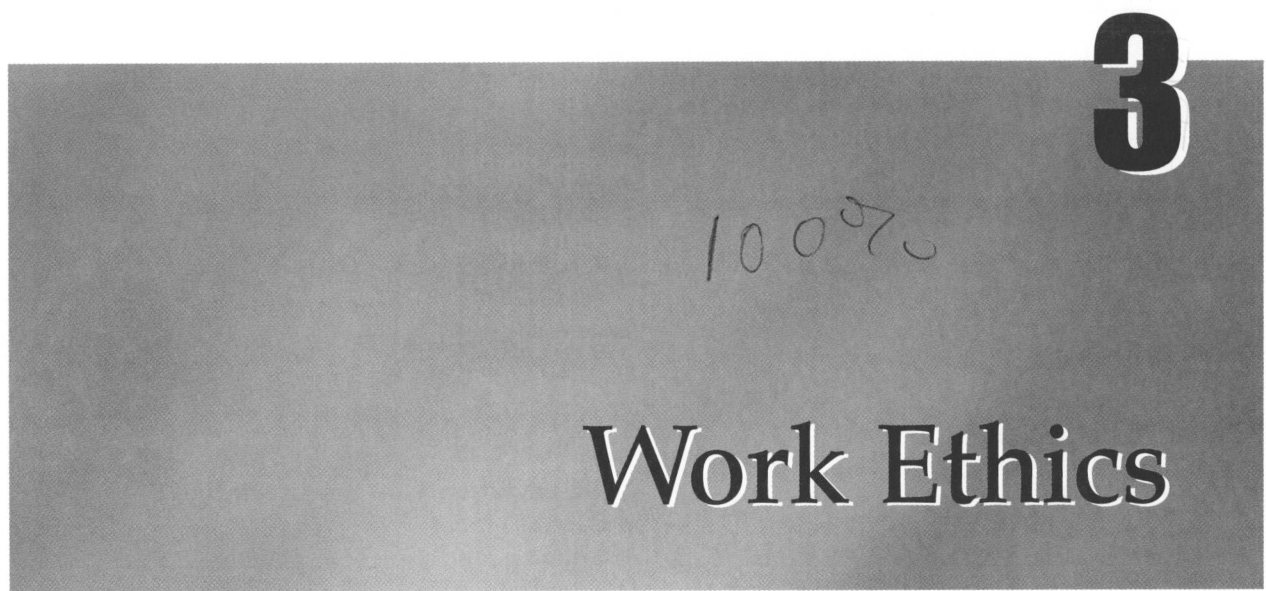

3 Work Ethics

OBJECTIVES

The questions and student activities in this chapter will help you meet these objectives.

- Define the key terms listed in Chapter 3
- Identify good health and personal hygiene practices
- Describe how to look professional
- Describe the qualities and traits of successful assistive personnel
- Explain how to get a job
- Explain how to plan for childcare and transportation
- Describe ethical behavior on the job
- Explain how to manage stress
- Explain the aspects of harassment
- Explain how to resign from a job
- Identify the common reasons for losing a job

STUDY QUESTIONS

Matching

Match the terms with the correct definitions.

A. Gossip
B. Harassment
C. Confidentiality
D. Stress
E. Self-awareness
F. Work ethics
G. Honesty
H. Courtesy
I. Preceptor
J. Stressor

1. C Trusting others with personal and private information
2. D The response or change in the body caused by any emotional, physical, social, or economic factor
3. h A polite, considerate, or helpful comment or act
4. a Spreading rumors or talking about the private matters of others
5. I A staff member who guides another staff member

6. B Troubling, tormenting, offending, or worrying a person by one's behavior or comments

7. f Behavior in the workplace

8. J The event or factor that causes stress

9. G Accurately reporting the care given, your observations, and any errors

10. e Knowing your feelings, strengths, and weaknesses

Fill in the Blanks

11. Work ethics involves:

A. ____________________

B. ____________________

C. ____________________

D. ____________________

E. ____________________

12. Your personal ____________________, ____________________, and ____________________ need careful attention.

13. List the ways you can find out about jobs.

A. ____________________

B. ____________________

C. ____________________

D. ____________________

E. ____________________

F. ____________________

G. ____________________

H. ____________________

14. Employers want employees who:

A. ____________________

B. ____________________

C. ____________________

D. ____________________

15. Nursing centers cannot hire persons who ____________________ ____________________.

16. Lying on a job application is ____________________.

17. You are writing a thank you note after a job interview. What should the note include?

A. ____________________

B. ____________________

C. ____________________

D. ____________________

E. ____________________

18. List 3 things you need to do when you accept a job.

A. ____________________

B. ____________________

C. ____________________

19. Some agencies have preceptor programs. What is the role of the preceptor?

A. ____

____

B. ____

____

C. ____

____

D. ____

____

E. ____

____

20. ____ and

____ are

common reasons for losing a job.

21. Many parts of your job are stressful.

Stress affects the person

____,

____,

____,

and ____.

22. You are resigning from a job. What information should you include in your written notice?

A. ____

B. ____

C. ____

Multiple Choice

Circle the BEST answer.

23. You want to make a good impression for a job interview. You must
   A. Look down or away from the interviewer.
   B. Give short "yes or no" answers.
   C. Dress in very casual and comfortable clothes.
   D. Be neat, clean, and well groomed.

24. Which of these statements reflects a negative attitude?
   A. "Can I help you?"
   B. "Please show me how this works."
   C. "I can't, I'm too busy."
   D. "Thank you for your help."

25. You can share information about a resident or patient with
   A. The person's family.
   B. The nurse supervising your work.
   C. Your co-worker during lunch.
   D. Your family and friends.

26. You feel that you are being harassed at work. You must
   A. Tell your co-worker.
   B. Ignore it. You don't want to cause trouble.
   C. Ask your family and friends for advice.
   D. Report it to your supervisor and the human resources officer.

27. You can protect your job by
   A. Always following good work ethics.
   B. Letting your friends visit you at work.
   C. Leaving early if your work is done.
   D. Discussing patient's information in the employee lounge.

28. Good work ethics involves all of the following *except*
   A. Working when scheduled
   B. Helping others
   C. Being cheerful and friendly
   D. Leaving work early to pick up your child at the mall

29. To avoid gossip, you must
   A. Avoid talking to co-workers
   B. Eat your meals alone
   C. Not make or repeat any comment that can hurt a person, family member, co-worker, or the agency
   D. Only talk to the nurse supervising your work

30. Which is *not* a practice for professional appearance?
    A. Wearing uniforms that fit well
    B. Wearing large, dangling earrings
    C. Wearing a wristwatch with a second hand
    D. Keeping fingernails clean, short, and neatly shaped

31. Which is a courtesy?
    A. Saying "please" and "thank you"
    B. Using slang
    C. Taking credit for another person's deed
    D. Entering elevators before visitors

32. Which action will keep personal matters out of the workplace?
    A. Borrowing money from co-workers
    B. Asking your friend to visit you on the unit
    C. Taking agency pens and pencils home
    D. Making personal phone calls during meals or breaks

33. Victims of sexual harassment are always women.
    A. True
    B. False

ADDITIONAL LEARNING ACTIVITIES

1. You are preparing for a job interview. How will you make a good impression? How will you show the employer that you have what he or she is looking for in these areas?
    A. Hygiene measures
    B. Professional appearance
    C. Skills and training
    D. Values and attitude

2. Make a list of at least 3 references on an index card to carry with you. Include name, address, and phone number. This will help you be prepared for a job interview.

3. You want to find the right job.
    A. What is important to you?
    B. What questions do you want to ask during the job interview?

4. You have succeeded in getting the job you want. Now, it is important to keep your job. How will you make sure that:
   A. You have dependable transportation?
   B. You have child care, if needed?
   C. You get to work on time?
   D. You are available to work at the times you are scheduled?
   E. You stay healthy so you can function at your best?

5. You will have stress on the job. List some measures that will help you reduce and cope with stress.

6. You are preparing for an interview with a home care agency. What questions should you ask the interviewer?

4

Communicating With the Health Team

OBJECTIVES

The questions and student activities in this chapter will help you meet these objectives.

- Define the key terms listed in Chapter 4
- Explain why health team members need to communicate
- Describe the rules for good communication
- Explain the purpose of the medical record
- Describe the parts and information in the medical record
- Describe the legal and ethical aspects of medical records
- Describe the purpose of the Kardex
- List the information you need to report to the nurse
- List the basic rules for recording
- Use the 24-hour clock, medical terminology, and abbreviations
- Explain how computers are used in health care
- Explain how to protect the right to privacy when using computers
- Describe the rules for answering phones
- Explain how to deal with conflict

STUDY QUESTIONS

Matching

Match the following terms with the correct definitions.

A. Prefix
B. Medical record
C. Kardex
D. Chart
E. Recording
F. Communication
G. Conflict
H. Root
I. Suffix
J. Abbreviation
K. Reporting
L. Word element

1. J A shortened form of a word or phrase
2. f The exchange of information
3. G A clash between opposing interests and ideas

4. C A type of file that summarizes information found in the medical record

5. B A written account of a person's condition and response to the treatment and care

6. D Another term for the medical record

7. a A word element placed at the beginning of a word to change the meaning of the word

8. e The written account of care and observations

9. K The oral account of care and observations

10. h A word element containing the basic meaning of the word

11. i A word element placed at the end of a root to change the meaning of the word

12. L A part of a word

Fill in the Blanks

13. The health team shares information about:

    A. ______

    B. ______

    C. ______

14. The ______ is a permanent, legal document.

15. Agency policies about the medical record address:

    A. ______

    B. ______

    C. ______

    D. ______

    E. ______

    F. ______

16. All information contained in the medical record is ______.

17. What parts of the medical record relate to your work?

    A. ______

    B. ______

    C. ______

    D. ______

    E. ______

18. Anyone who reads your charting should know:

    A. ______

    B. ______

    C. ______

19. Convert the following times from standard time to 24-hour clock time.

    A. 6:15 PM ______

    B. 8:00 AM ______

    C. 2:30 PM ______

    D. 5:02 PM ______

    E. 10:55 AM ______

F. 1:29 PM ______

G. 1:33 AM ______

H. 9:00 PM ______

20. Write the definition of each prefix:

A. ab ______

B. auto ______

C. dia ______

D. endo ______

E. hemi ______

F. intro ______

G. olig ______

H. post ______

I. sub ______

21. Write the meaning of each word root.

A. angi(o) ______

B. cephal(o) ______

C. colo ______

D. derma ______

E. gastr(o) ______

F. lith(o) ______

G. nephr(o) ______

H. orth(o) ______

I. stomat(o) ______

22. Write the meaning of each suffix.

A. algia ______

B. graph ______

C. pathy ______

D. plasty ______

E. stasis ______

23. Write the definition of these terms:

A. Splenectomy ______

B. Dysphagia ______

C. Bradycardia ______

24. List the four regions of the abdomen and the abbreviation for each.

A. ______

B. ______

C. ______

D. ______

25. Define these terms:

A. Anterior ______

______

B. Lateral ______

______

C. Medial ______

______

26. Write the meaning of each abbreviation.

A. CPR ______

B. FBS ______

C. GI ______

D. meds ______

27. You are taking a phone message. What information do you need to write down?

 A. ______________________________

 B. ______________________________

 C. ______________________________

28. You are caring for Mr. Lewis Smith in his home. You answer his telephone. How should you answer?

 ____

 ____

Multiple Choice

Circle the BEST answer.

29. For good communication, you should do all of the following *except*
 A. Use familiar words
 B. Be brief and concise
 C. Give unneeded but interesting information
 D. Give information in a logical and orderly manner

30. Who has access to a person's medical record?
 A. The person's family members
 B. Health team members involved in the person's care
 C. Laundry personnel
 D. Visitors

31. You are reporting patient care. Which is *incorrect?*
 A. Report your observations to the nurse.
 B. Report the care that was given by a co-worker.
 C. Reports must be prompt, thorough, and accurate.
 D. Any changes from normal are reported at once.

32. Daily recordings in the chart are not necessary in nursing centers. However, OBRA requires a written summary
 A. Weekly
 B. Monthly
 C. Every 3 months
 D. Twice a year

33. When recording, you should do all of the following *except*
 A. Use ink.
 B. Make sure writing is legible and neat.
 C. Use correct spelling and grammar.
 D. Use correcting fluid if you make a mistake.

34. Intake and output (I&O) are recorded on the
 A. Graphic sheet
 B. Kardex
 C. Admission sheet
 D. Nursing care plan

35. A person's blood pressure is taken every 2 hours. You record this on
 A. The Kardex.
 B. The progress notes.
 C. A flow sheet.
 D. The admission sheet.

36. Which abdominal region is the stomach located in?
 A. Right upper quadrant
 B. Left upper quadrant
 C. Right lower quadrant
 D. Left lower quadrant

37. Computers are often used in health care. Which is *false?*
 A. Computers save time.
 B. The right to privacy must be protected.
 C. Doctors can use computers to help diagnose.
 D. Computer passwords never change.

38. You have answered the phone at the nurses' station. You must put the caller on hold. Which is correct?
 A. Just say "I am putting you on hold."
 B. First ask who is calling and if the caller can hold.
 C. Lay the phone down on the desk.
 D. Cover the receiver with your hand until you can return to the caller.

39. Conflict can arise on the job over work schedules, absences, and amount and quality of work. Which will *not* help resolve conflict?
 A. Ask your supervisor to meet with you.
 B. Discuss the problem with co-workers during lunch break.
 C. Give facts and specific examples.
 D. Identify ways to solve the problem.

ADDITIONAL LEARNING ACTIVITIES

1. Practice answering the telephone and taking a message. You can do this with a classmate or with a family member.
   A. How would you answer the telephone in a professional, courteous manner?
   B. What information should you get when taking a message?
   C. What would you do before putting a person on hold?

2. Practice your observation, recording, and reporting skills. Ask a classmate or member of your family to help. Use Box 4-1 (page 55) in the textbook as a guide for recording your observations.
   A. Talk to the person for about 5 minutes. Then record the following information:
      (1) Color and length of hair
      (2) Color of eyes
      (3) Description of any jewelry the person is wearing
      (4) Description of clothing the person is wearing
      (5) Any special features (birth marks, scars, etc.)
      (6) Any information the person gave you about him or herself
   B. Use a note pad to record your observations.
   C. Use your notes to give a verbal report.
   D. Discuss the accuracy of what you recorded and reported about the person and the conversation.

3. Read the following vignette involving conflict in the work place. Then answer the questions at the end of the vignette.
   You are assigned to care for Mrs. Angie Gomez. When you return from your lunch break, Mrs. Gomez's signal light is on. When you answer her signal light, Mrs. Gomez tells you that her light has been on for 25 minutes. She also tells you that another nursing assistant walked in her room and told Mrs. Gomez that she would have to wait until you returned from lunch.
   A. How would you feel?
   B. What would you say to Mrs. Gomez?
   C. Who would you discuss the situation with?
   D. Where would you discuss the situation?
   E. What steps would you take to solve the problem?

4. Make flash cards of the prefixes, root words, and suffixes in Chapter 4. Write the meaning of each on the back of each flash card. Use the flash cards to help you study and learn medical terms. You can work alone or with a classmate.

5

Assisting With the Nursing Process

OBJECTIVES

The questions and student activities in this chapter will help you meet these objectives.

- Define the key terms listed in Chapter 5
- Explain the purpose of the nursing process
- Describe the steps of the nursing process
- Explain your role in each step of the nursing process
- Explain the difference between objective and subjective data
- Identify the observations you need to report to the nurse
- Explain the purpose of care conferences

STUDY QUESTIONS

Matching

Match the following terms with the correct definitions.

A. Nursing goal
B. Nursing care plan
C. Nursing intervention
D. Assessment
E. Evaluation
F. Symptoms
G. Objective data
H. Planning
I. Signs
J. Nursing diagnosis
K. Nursing process
L. Subjective data
M. Observation
N. Implementation
O. Medical diagnosis

1. __D__ Collecting information about the person
2. __e__ To measure if goals in the planning step of the nursing process were met
3. __a__ That which is desired in or by the person as a result of nursing care
4. __N__ To perform or carry out measures in the care plan
5. __O__ The identification of a disease or condition by a doctor
6. __B__ A written guide about the person's care

7. J Describes a health problem that can be treated by nursing measures

8. C An action or measure taken by the nursing team to help the person reach a goal

9. K The method RNs use to plan and deliver nursing care

10. G Information that is seen, heard, felt, or smelled

11. m Using the senses of sight, hearing, touch, and smell to collect information

12. h Setting priorities and goals

13. l Objective data

14. L Things a person tells you about that you cannot observe through your senses

15. f Subjective data

Fill in the Blanks

16. List the 5 steps of the nursing process.

 A. ______

 B. ______

 C. ______

 D. ______

 E. ______

17. Goals are aimed at the person's

______

______

______.

18. The ______

is a communication tool. It helps ensure that the nursing team gives the same care.

19. List and briefly define the two types of resident care conferences required by OBRA.

 A. ______

 ______

 ______

 B. ______

 ______

 ______

20. The following is a list of objective and subjective data. Mark O for objective data and S for subjective data.

 A. ______ A person is crying

 B. ______ Headache

 C. ______ Cold and moist skin

 D. ______ Drainage

 E. ______ Red eyes

 F. ______ Nausea

 G. ______ Abdominal pain

 H. ______ Rash

 I. ______ Numbness

 J. ______ Itching

 K. ______ Swollen finger

 L. ______ Bleeding

21. An assignment sheet is used to communicate delegated measures and tasks to you. The assignment sheet tells you about:

    A. ______________________

    B. ______________________

    C. ______________________

    D. ______________________

Multiple Choice

Circle the BEST answer.

22. The assessment tool required by OBRA for nursing center residents is
    A. The Kardex.
    B. The care plan.
    C. The minimum data set (MDS).
    D. The nursing diagnosis.

23. Resident assessment protocols (RAPS) are
    A. Problems on the care plan.
    B. Part of the nursing diagnosis.
    C. Actions to help a person meet goals.
    D. Guidelines used to develop the person's care plan.

24. The nurse has used the assignment sheet to delegate tasks and measures to you. What should you do if you do not understand the information on your assignment sheet?
    A. Ask a co-worker to explain.
    B. Do only the tasks and measures that you understand.
    C. Talk to the nurse.
    D. Discuss your concern with the director of nursing.

25. Which is a nursing diagnosis?
    A. Cancer
    B. Risk for falls
    C. Stroke
    D. Diabetes

26. Reporting and recording are done
    A. Whenever you have time.
    B. At the beginning of the shift.
    C. After giving care.
    D. Every hour.

27. Nursing diagnoses, goals, and the care plan may change as the person's needs change.
    A. True
    B. False

ADDITIONAL LEARNING ACTIVITIES

1. Mr. Adam Lewis is an 85-year-old nursing center resident. He is ambulatory with a walker. He needs assistance with dressing, hygiene, and grooming. You have been assigned to his care. Your assignment sheet gives you the following information:
   - Vital signs at 0800.
   - Morning tub bath.
   - Ambulate in the hallway bid.
   - Elevate both feet when sitting in the chair.

   Explain how you would use your senses to gather information when performing the tasks and measures on your assignment sheet.

2. Explain how RAPS and triggers are used in the care planning process.

3. Describe your role in each step of the nursing process.

6

The Whole Person and Basic Needs

OBJECTIVES

The questions and student activities in this chapter will help you meet these objectives.

- Define the key terms listed in Chapter 6
- Identify the parts that make up the whole person
- Describe Maslow's theory of basic needs
- Explain how culture and religion influence health and illness
- Describe the persons cared for in health care agencies
- Identify patients' and residents' rights
- Explain why family and visitors are important to the person
- Identify the courtesies given to patients, residents, and visitors
- Explain how to deal with behavior issue

STUDY QUESTIONS

Complete the Crossword

Across

5. The branch of medicine concerned with the care of women during pregnancy, labor, and childbirth
6. The characteristics of a group of people that are passed from one generation to the next
8. The branch of medicine concerned with the problems and diseases of old age and older persons

Down

1. A concept that considers the whole person
2. The branch of medicine concerned with mental health problems
3. The branch of medicine concerned with the growth, development, and care of children
4. The worth, value, or opinion one has of a person
7. Spiritual beliefs, needs, and practices

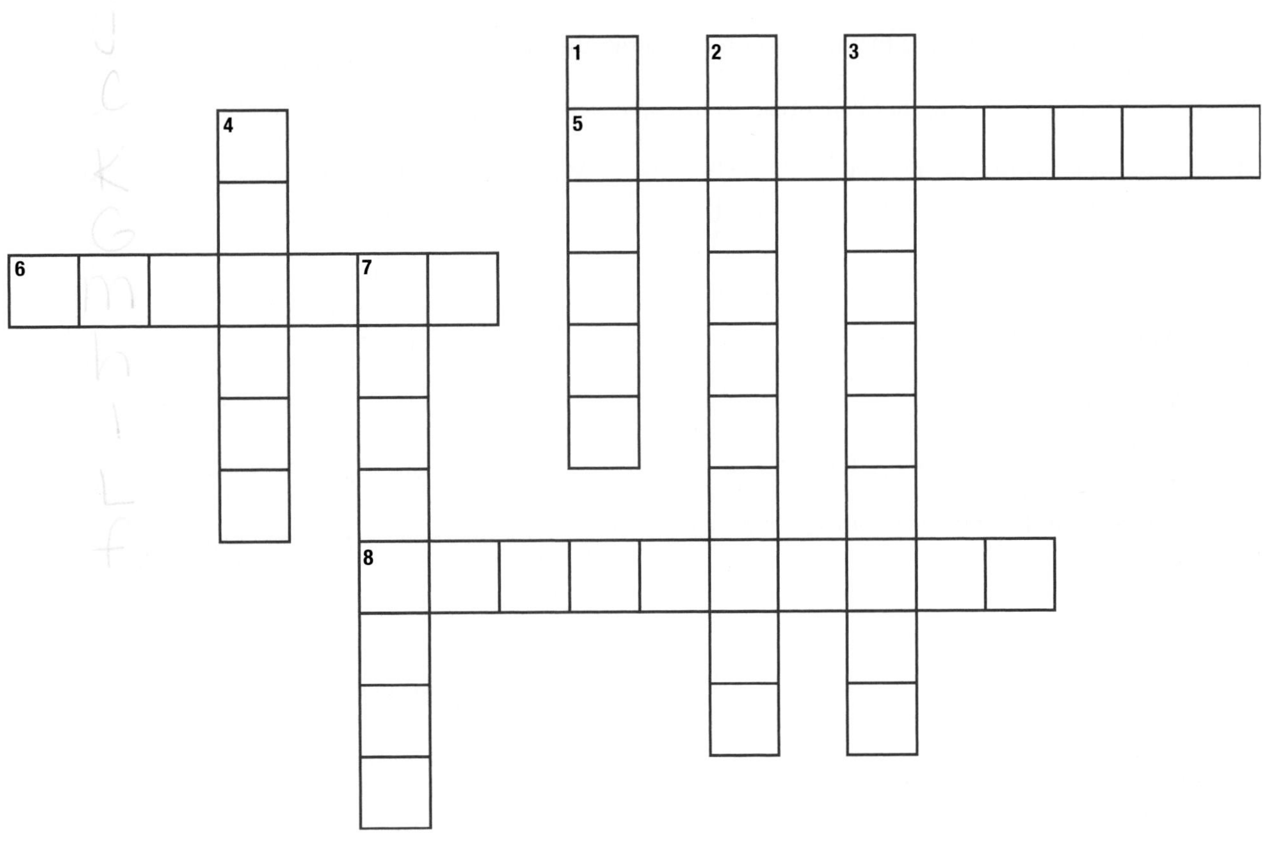

Matching

Match the following terms with the correct definitions.

A. Need
B. Self-actualization
C. Self-esteem
D. Disability

1. ______ A lost, absent, or impaired physical or mental function
2. ______ Something necessary or desired for maintaining life and mental well-being
3. ______ Experiencing one's potential
4. ______ Thinking well of oneself and seeing oneself as useful and having value

Match the following "resident rights" with the correct examples.

A. The right to disputes and grievances
B. The right to care and security of personal possessions
C. The right to quality of life
D. The right to information
E. The right to privacy and confidentiality
F. The right to personal choice
G. The right to refuse treatment

5. ______ The nurse explains a procedure to the resident before the resident signs the consent.
6. ______ A resident refuses to have blood drawn for a diagnostic test.
7. ______ The privacy curtain is pulled around a resident before helping the resident with the bedpan.
8. ______ A resident asks to speak to the Ombudsman about the food served at the center.

9. ______ A resident chooses to read in her room rather than play bingo.

10. ______ A resident brings her bedspread from home. The bedspread is marked with the resident's name.

11. ______ You address the resident by Mr., Mrs., Ms., or Miss. You do not use first names without the person's permission.

Fill in the Blanks

12. The ______________________ is the most important person in the agency.

13. You must treat the person as someone who can ______________________, ______________________, and ______________________.

14. A physical illness affects the person ______________________, ______________________, and ______________________.

15. List in order of importance and briefly describe the basic needs for life as described by Maslow.

    A. ______________________
    ____

    B. ______________________
    ____

    C. ______________________
    ____

    D. ______________________
    ____

    E. ______________________
    ____

16. People are grouped in health care agencies by their ______________________, ______________________, and ______________________.

17. List 8 groups of persons you may care for in health care agencies.

    A. ______________________

    B. ______________________

    C. ______________________

    D. ______________________

    E. ______________________

    F. ______________________

    G. ______________________

    H. ______________________

18. Some older persons need long-term care. List 7 types of persons needing long-term care.

    A. ______________________

    B. ______________________

    C. ______________________

    D. ______________________

    E. ______________________

    F. ______________________

    G. ______________________

19. List in the correct order the courtesies that you must extend before giving care.

    A. ______________________

    B. ______________________

    C. ______________________

20. Nursing centers must protect and promote

    ______________________.

21. How are nursing center residents informed of their rights?

    ____

22. Anger is a common emotion. List 5 possible causes of anger in persons you will care for.

    A. ______________________

    B. ______________________

    C. ______________________

    D. ______________________

    E. ______________________

23. What does self-centered behavior involve?

    A. ______________________

    B. ______________________

    C. ______________________

24. Mr. Edward Joel is a nursing center resident. He refuses IV therapy. What must the center do?

    ____

    ____

    ____

25. Nursing centers cannot employ persons who

    were convicted of ______________________

    ______________________.

26. Nursing centers must provide activities that

    allow personal choice and that promote

    ______________________.

Multiple Choice

Circle the BEST answer.

27. Which needs are the most important for survival?
    A. Self-esteem
    B. Safety and security
    C. Physical
    D. Love and belonging

28. Courteous and dignified care of residents includes all of the following *except*
    A. Using the resident's proper name and title.
    B. Listening carefully to what the resident is saying.
    C. Shouting to make sure the resident can hear you.
    D. Using good eye contact.

29. You observe that a visitor is upsetting a patient. You must
    A. Ask the visitor to leave.
    B. Report your observation to the nurse.
    C. Ask the patient if you can help.
    D. Not get involved.

30. A patient you are caring for asks to see a cleric (spiritual leader). Which is *false?*
    A. Report the request to the nurse.
    B. Stay with the patient during the visit.
    C. Make sure the room is neat and clean.
    D. Provide privacy during the visit.

31. Miss Sharon Spelling is a nursing center resident. She has the right to choose her doctor.
    A. True
    B. False

32. These statements are about a person's family and visitors. Which is *false?*
    A. They are treated with courtesy and respect.
    B. They often need support and understanding.
    C. They are allowed to visit in private.
    D. They are encouraged to stay in the patient or resident room when care is given.

33. You give visitors support by answering their questions about the person's condition.
    A. True
    B. False

ADDITIONAL LEARNING ACTIVITIES

1. Think of a time when you were sick or injured. Answer the following questions.
   A. What fears and anxieties did you have?
   B. What support systems did you have?
   C. How will your experience affect the care that you provide?

2. List some ways that knowing about a person's cultural and religious practices can help you give better care.

3. Do you have cultural or religious beliefs that are important to you? Explain. How do these beliefs influence your health practices?

4. Read the following vignette and then answer the questions that follow.
   Mrs. Jean Kramer is a 50-year-old hospital patient. She has been in the hospital for 2 days. She is scheduled for surgery in the morning. You answered her signal light. As soon as you enter her room, Mrs. Kramer shouts at you. She tells you that no one cares about her and she wants to go home. When you approach her she tries to hit you.
   A. What emotion is Mrs. Kramer expressing?
   B. What might be some reasons for her behavior?
   C. What measures can you take to deal with her behavior?
   D. How can you protect yourself and Mrs. Kramer from harm?

5. Read the following vignette and then answer the questions that follow.
   Mr. Brian is a 78-year-old nursing center resident. He has a doctoral degree in mathematics. He was the head of the mathematics department at the state university. He has poor vision and is very hard of hearing. He wears hearing aids in both ears. He needs some assistance with ADL. He uses a cane to walk. Mr. Brian has many visitors from the university. He likes to keep up with current events.
   A. What actions can you take to provide:
      (1) Courteous and dignified interactions?
      (2) Courteous and dignified care?
      (3) Privacy and self-determination?
      (4) Personal choice and independence?

7 Communicating With the Person

OBJECTIVES

The questions and student activities in this chapter will help you meet these objectives.

- Define the key terms listed in Chapter 7
- Identify the elements needed to communicate
- Describe how to use verbal and nonverbal communication
- Explain the methods and barriers to good communication
- Explain how to admit, transfer, and discharge persons

STUDY QUESTIONS

Matching

Match the following terms with the correct definitions.

A. Nonverbal communication
B. Verbal communication
C. Paraphrasing
D. Admission
E. Discharge
F. Transfer
G. Body language

1. D Official entry of a person into an agency
2. G Messages sent through facial expressions, gestures, posture, and hand and body movements, gait, eye contact, and appearance
3. e Official departure of a person from an agency
4. a Communication that does not use words
5. C Restating the person's message in your own words
6. f Moving a person from one room, or nursing unit to another
7. B Communication using written or spoken words

Fill in the Blanks

8. List the rules for verbal communication.

   A. ____________________

   B. ____________________

   C. ____________________

   D. ____________________

   E. ____________________

   F. ____________________

   G. ____________________

   H. ____________________

9. When writing messages, you must

   A. ____________________

   B. ____________________

   C. ____________________

10. The meaning of touch depends on

    ____________________,

    ____________________,

    ____________________,

    and ____________________.

11. To use touch, follow the ____________________

    ____________________.

12. Body language involves:

    A. ____________________

    B. ____________________

    C. ____________________

    D. ____________________

    E. ____________________

    F. ____________________

    G. ____________________

13. ____________________ means to focus on verbal and nonverbal communication. You focus on what the person is saying.

14. Paraphrasing does the following:

    A. ____________________

    B. ____________________

    C. ____________________

15. ____________________ focus on certain information. You ask the person something you need to know.

16. List 8 barriers to communication.

    A. ____________________

    B. ____________________

    C. ____________________

    D. ____________________

    E. ____________________

    F. ____________________

    G. ____________________

    H. ____________________

17. Opinions involve judging

    ____________________,

    ____________________,

    or ____________________.

Multiple Choice

Circle the BEST answer.

18. Nonverbal messages more accurately reflect a person's feelings than words do.
    A. True
    B. False

19. You want to show a person that you are listening. It is important to do all of the following *except*
    A. Give your opinions.
    B. Face the person.
    C. Have good eye contact.
    D. Ask questions.

20. You say to the patient, "Tell me about your pain." This is
    A. A direct question.
    B. Paraphrasing.
    C. An open-ended question.
    D. Clarifying

21. Which communication method is useful when a person rambles or wanders in thought?
    A. Focusing
    B. Clarifying
    C. Silence
    D. Paraphrasing

22. Silence is a useful way to communicate when
    A. A yes or no answer is needed.
    B. You do not understand the message.
    C. You want more information.
    D. The person is upset.

23. Touch is an important form of non-verbal communication. Which is *false?*
    A. Touch conveys comfort and caring.
    B. Everyone likes to be touched.
    C. Touch should be gentle.
    D. Touch means different things to different people.

24. Mr. Albert Farr is comatose. Which statement is *false?*
    A. Give care on the same schedule every day.
    B. Use touch to communicate.
    C. Assume he cannot hear you.
    D. He cannot respond to others.

25. You are admitting a patient to the unit. Your first action is to
    A. Ask the person his or her name.
    B. Greet the person by name.
    C. Tell the person that everything will be OK.
    D. Introduce the roommate.

26. You are admitting Mr. Grey to a hospital unit. Which is *false?*
    A. Ask him his name and what he wants to be called.
    B. Introduce yourself to Mr. Grey and his family.
    C. Provide for privacy.
    D. Orient Mr. Grey to furniture and equipment in the room.

27. Mr. Grey is being transferred to another unit. You can help him by
    A. Telling him not to worry.
    B. Changing the subject when Mr. Grey tells you that he is concerned about the transfer.
    C. Introducing him to new nursing team members.
    D. Talking and laughing a lot to cheer him up.

ADDITIONAL LEARNING ACTIVITIES

1. Observe the nonverbal communication in contacts with your family and friends.
   A. Write down your observations.
   B. Are you aware of how you communicate non-verbally? Explain.

2. Write down your thoughts about the meaning of touch. Answer the following questions:
   A. What does touch mean to you?
   B. Do you always like to be touched? Explain.
   C. Do you like everyone to touch you in the same way? Explain.
   D. Are you comfortable touching others? Explain.

3. Write down 2 examples of each of the following communication methods. Explain when you would use each method.
   A. Paraphrasing
   B. Direct questions
   C. Open-ended questions
   D. Clarifying
   E. Focusing

8

Body Structure and Function

OBJECTIVES

The questions and student activities in this chapter will help you meet these objectives.

- Define the key terms listed in Chapter 8
- Identify the basic structures of the cell
- Explain how cells divide
- Describe four types of tissue
- Identify the structures of each body system
- Describe the functions of each body system

STUDY QUESTIONS

Complete the Crossword

Across

5. The substance in red blood cells that carries oxygen and gives the blood its color
6. The process in which the lining of the uterus breaks up and is discharged from the body through the vagina
7. Groups of tissue with the same function
8. A blood vessel that carries blood away from the heart

Down

1. The process of physically and chemically breaking down food so that it can be absorbed for use by the cells
2. A blood vessel that carries blood back to the heart
3. A tiny blood vessel
4. Protection against a disease or condition
5. A chemical substance secreted by the endocrine glands into the bloodstream

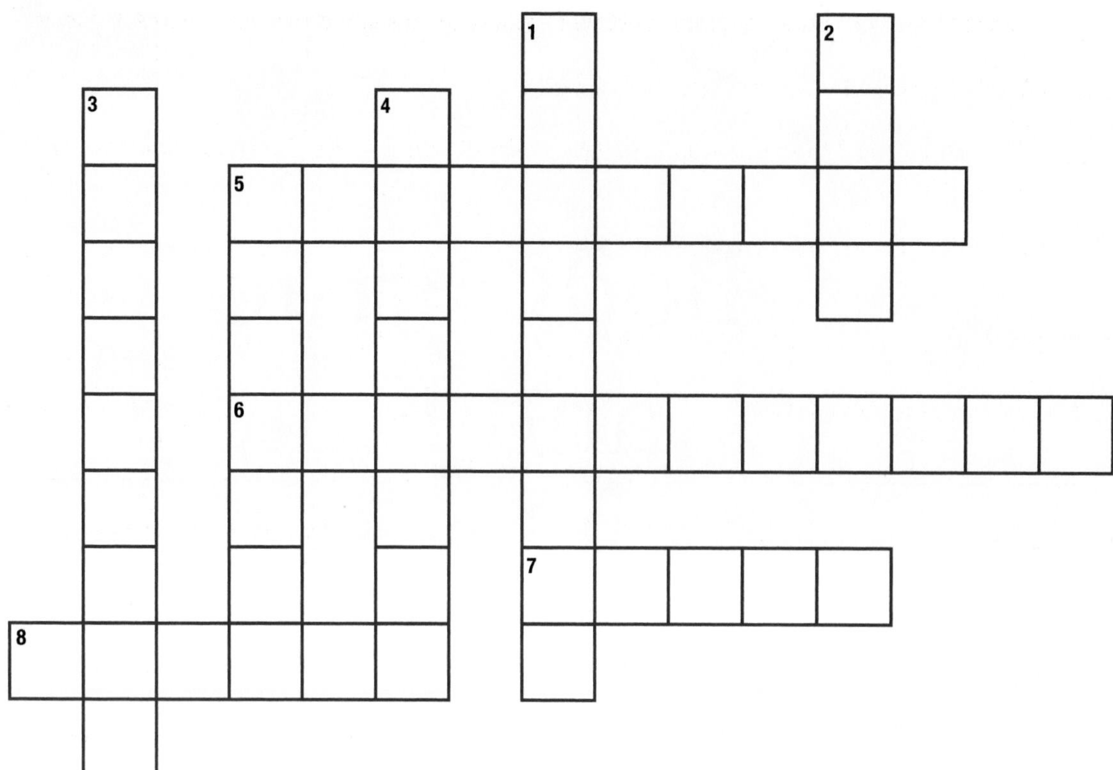

Matching

Match the following terms with the correct definitions.

A. Tissue
B. Peristalsis
C. Cell
D. Metabolism
E. Respiration
F. System

1. ___C___ The basic unit of body structure
2. ______ The process of supplying the cells with oxygen and removing carbon dioxide from them
3. ______ The burning of food for heat and energy by the cells
4. ______ Involuntary muscle contractions in the digestive system that move food through the alimentary canal
5. ______ Organs that work together to perform special functions
6. ______ A group of cells with the same function

Matching (Immune System)

Match the following terms pertaining to the immune system with the correct definitions.

A. Phagocytes
B. T lymphocytes (T cells)
C. Antibodies
D. Lymphocytes
E. B lymphocytes (B cells)
F. Antigens

7. ______ Normal body substances that recognize, attack, and destroy abnormal or unwanted substances
8. ______ Abnormal or unwanted substances

9. ______ White blood cells that digest and destroy microorganisms and other unwanted substances

10. ______ White blood cells that produce antibodies

11. ______ Cause the production of antibodies that circulate in the plasma; the antibodies react to specific antigens

12. ______ Cells that destroy invading cells

Fill in the Blanks

13. List and describe the basic structures of the cell.

    A. ______________________________

    B. ______________________________

    C. ______________________________

14. ______________________________ are threadlike structures in the nucleus of the cell. They contain genes.

15. Describe the following types of tissues.

    A. Epithelial tissue

    ____

    ____

    B. Connective tissue

    ____

    ____

    C. Muscle tissue

    ____

    ____

    D. Nerve tissue

    ____

    ____

16. The largest system is the ______________________________.

17. ______________________ gives skin its color.

18. The ______________________________ provides the framework for the body.

19. Name the types of bones and their functions.

    A. ______________________________

    ____

    B. ______________________________

    ____

    C. ______________________________

    ____

    D. ______________________________

    ____

20. A ______________________________ is the point at which two or more bones meet.

21. ______________________ is the connective tissue at the end of long bones. It cushions the joint so that bone ends do not rub together.

22. Describe the movement made by each type of joint.

    A. Ball and socket:

    ____

B. Hinge:

____

C. Pivot:

____

23. _______________ muscles can be consciously controlled.

24. List the three functions of muscles.

A. _______________

B. _______________

C. _______________

25. The nervous system _______________, _______________, and _______________ body functions.

26. The central nervous system consists of _______________.

27. _______________ carry messages or impulses to and from the brain.

28. The three main parts of the brain are:

A. _______________

B. _______________

C. _______________

29. The brainstem contains the _______________, _______________, and _______________.

30. _______________ circulates around the brain and spinal cord. It protects the central nervous system.

31. The peripheral nervous system has 12 pairs of _______________ and 31 pairs of _______________.

32. The _______________ nervous system speeds up functions.

33. Name the five senses.

A. _______________

B. _______________

C. _______________

D. _______________

E. _______________

34. List and briefly describe the three layers of the eye.

A. _______________

____

B. _______________

____

C. _______________

____

35. The ear functions in _______________ _______________.

36. List the three parts of the ear.

A. _______________

B. _______________

C. _______________

37. The circulatory system is made up of the _______________, _______________, and _______________.

38. List four functions of the circulatory system.

A. ______________________________

____

B. ______________________________

____

C. ______________________________

____

D. ______________________________

____

39. Red blood cells are called ______________

______________________________.

40. White blood cells are called ______________

______________________________.

41. List and describe the three layers of the heart.

A. ______________________________

____

B. ______________________________

____

C. ______________________________

____

42. Name and define the two phases of heart action.

A. ______________________________

B. ______________________________

43. Arterial blood is rich in ______________

______________________________.

44. Veins connect to the capillaries by ______________

______________________________.

45. The ______________________ carries blood from the head and arms.

46. The respiratory system brings ______________________ into the lungs and removes ______________.

47. Oxygen and carbon dioxide are exchanged between the ______________________ and ______________________.

48. Each lung is covered by a two-layered sac called the ______________________.

49. The accessory organs of digestion are the

______________________________,

______________________________,

______________________________,

______________________________,

______________________________,

and ______________________________.

50. ______________________ moistens food particles to ease swallowing and begin digestion.

51. ______________________ is a greenish liquid made in the liver.

52. The waste products of digestion are a semisolid material called ______________.

53. What are the two functions of the urinary system?

A. ______________________________

B. ______________________________

54. The ______________________________ carry urine from the kidneys to the bladder.

55. Urine passes from the bladder through the ______________________________.

56. The male sex glands are called ______________ or ______________________________.

57. ______________________________ is the male hormone.

58. The female sex glands are called ______________________________.

59. The female hormones secreted by the ovaries are ______________________________ and ______________________________.

60. The neck or narrow section of the uterus is the ______________________________.

61. ______________________ regulate the activities of other organs and glands in the body.

62. How do these hormones secreted by the anterior pituitary lobe affect the body?

A. Growth hormone

____

____

B. Thyroid-stimulating hormone (TSH)

____

____

C. Adrenocorticotropic hormone (ACTH)

____

____

63. ______________________________ causes uterine muscles to contract during childbirth.

64. The thyroid gland regulates ______________ ______________________________.

65. The parathyroid gland secretes parathormone, which regulates the body's use of ______________________________.

66. List and describe the three groups of hormones secreted by the adrenal cortex.

A. ______________________________

____

B. ______________________________

____

C. ______________________________

____

67. The ______________________________ protects the body from disease and infection.

Multiple Choice

Circle the BEST answer.

68. The process of cell division is called
A. Digestion.
B. Dermis.
C. Mitosis.
D. Aqueous.

69. What type of tissue lines the nose and mouth?
A. Epithelial
B. Connective
C. Muscle
D. Nerve

70. The outer layer of the skin is the
A. Pigment.
B. Dermis.
C. Integument.
D. Epidermis.

71. What types of muscles work automatically and cannot be consciously controlled?
    A. Voluntary muscles
    B. Involuntary muscles
    C. Cardiac muscles
    D. Striated muscles

72. Which part of the brain regulates and coordinates body movements?
    A. Cerebellum
    B. Pons
    C. Midbrain
    D. Cerebrum

73. This part of the brain is the center of thought and intelligence.
    A. Spinal column
    B. Brainstem
    C. Cerebrum
    D. Medulla

74. Where does digestion begin?
    A. In the esophagus
    B. In the stomach
    C. In the large intestine
    D. In the mouth

75. Male sex cells are called
    A. Sperm.
    B. Semen.
    C. Prostate.
    D. Testosterone.

76. The female sex cells are called
    A. Progesterone.
    B. Cervix.
    C. Ova.
    D. Vagina.

77. The uniting of the sperm and ovum into one cell is called
    A. Ovulation.
    B. Menstruation.
    C. Endometrium.
    D. Fertilization.

78. Which gland is called the "master gland"?
    A. Pituitary
    B. Thyroid
    C. Adrenal
    D. Parathyroid

79. Which gland secretes insulin?
    A. Thyroid
    B. Pancreas
    C. Gonads
    D. Pituitary

Labeling

80. Label the three types of joints.

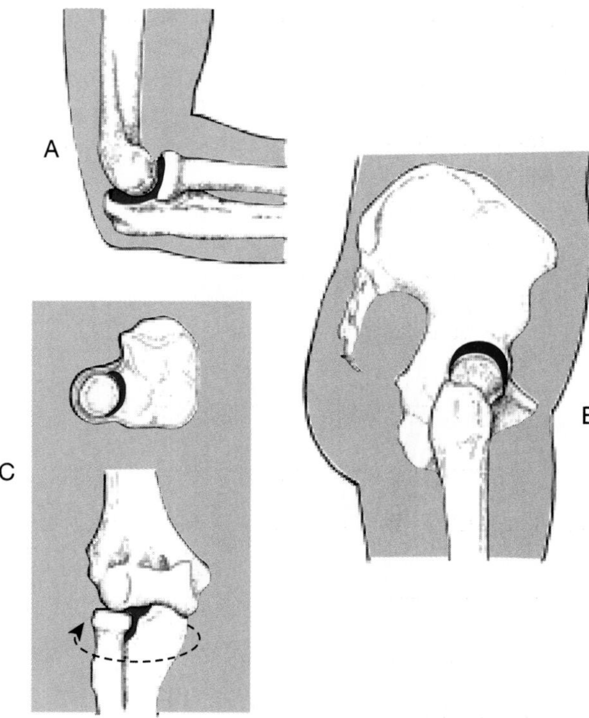

A. ______________________

B. ______________________

C. ______________________

81. Label the major parts of the central nervous system.

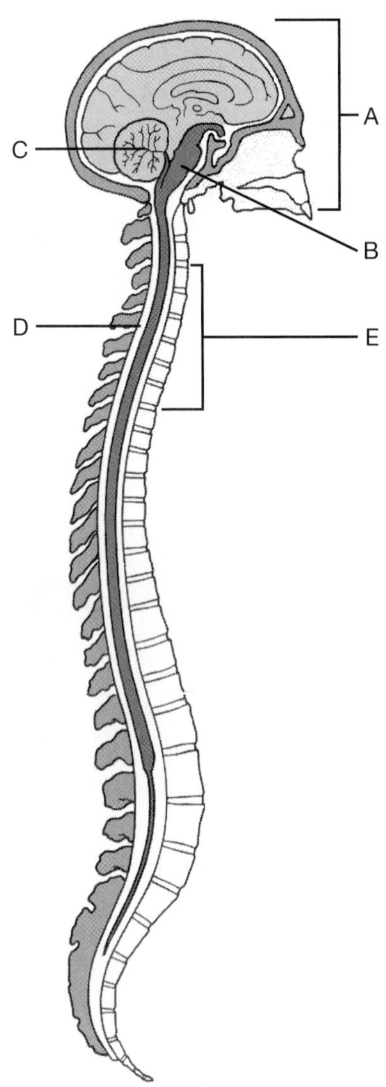

A. ______________________

B. ______________________

C. ______________________

D. ______________________

E. ______________________

82. Label the structures of the heart.

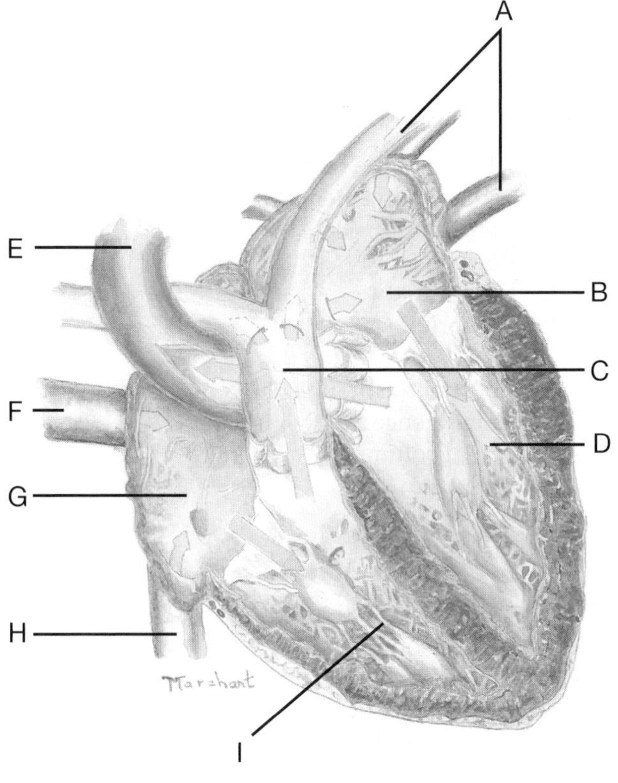

A. ______________________

B. ______________________

C. ______________________

D. ______________________

E. ______________________

F. ______________________

G. ______________________

H. ______________________

I. ______________________

83. Label the structures of the male reproductive system.

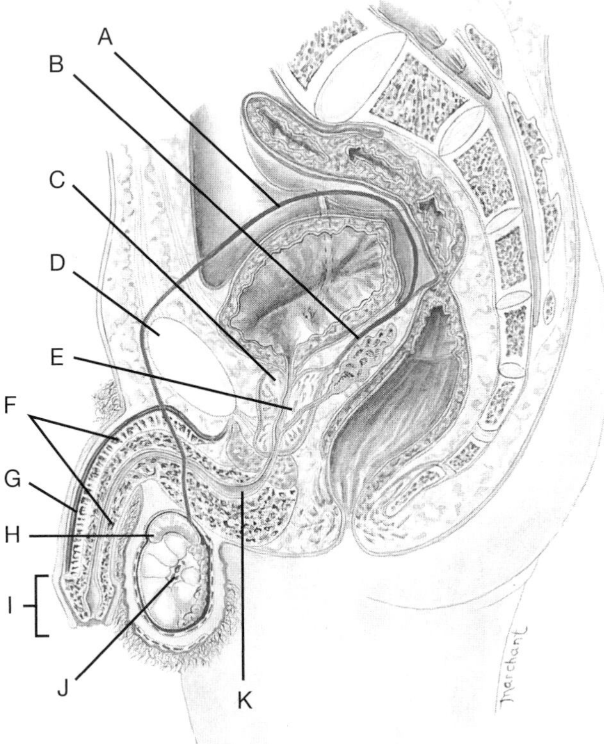

A. ______________________

B. ______________________

C. ______________________

D. ______________________

E. ______________________

F. ______________________

G. ______________________

H. ______________________

I. ______________________

J. ______________________

K. ______________________

84. Label the structures of the female external genitalia.

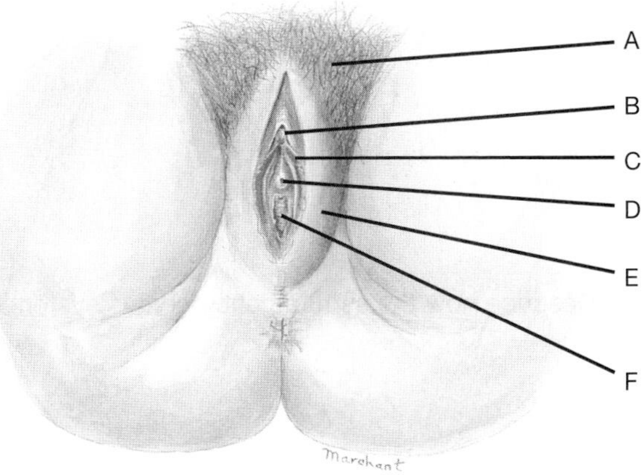

A. ______________________

B. ______________________

C. ______________________

D. ______________________

E. ______________________

F. ______________________

ADDITIONAL LEARNING ACTIVITIES

1. List and define the three layers of connective tissue that line the brain and spinal cord.

2. Describe how the sympathetic nervous system and the parasympathetic nervous system balance each other.

3. Explain how the eye uses light to see.

4. Outline how the blood flows through the circulatory system.

5. Outline the process of respiration.

6. Outline the process of digestion.

7. Explain how urine is formed and how it passes through the urinary system.

8. Outline the process of menstruation.

9. Outline the process of fertilization.

10. If available in your school or class site, use anatomical models to practice identifying body structures. You can also practice locating the body structures on your own body.

11. If a microscope is available, look at slides of the various types of cells, tissues, and blood.
    NOTE: Some of these learning aids may also be available at the public library. Where available, the library at the community college or university is also a good resource.

9

Growth and Development

OBJECTIVES

The questions and student activities in this chapter will help you meet these objectives.

- Define the key terms listed in Chapter 9
- Explain the principles of growth and development
- Identify the stages of growth and development
- Identify the developmental tasks for each age-group
- Describe the normal growth and development for each age-group

STUDY QUESTIONS

Matching

Match the following terms with the correct definitions.

A. Development
B. Growth
C. Puberty
D. Adolescence
E. Menarche
F. Developmental task
G. Gerontology
H. Primary caregiver
I. Ejaculation
J. Reflex
K. Geriatrics
L. Menopause

1. ______ The time between puberty and adulthood; a time of rapid growth and physical and social maturity

2. ______ Changes in mental, emotional, and social function

3. ______ A skill that must be completed during a stage of development

4. ______ The release of semen

5. ______ The care of aging people

6. ______ The study of the aging process

7. ______ The physical changes that are measured and that occur in a steady, orderly manner

8. ______ The first menstruation and the start of menstrual cycles

9. ______ The time when menstruation stops

10. ______ The person mainly responsible for providing or assisting with the child's basic needs

11. ______ The period when reproductive organs begin to function and secondary sex characteristics appear

12. ______ An involuntary movement

Fill in the Blanks

13. Although they differ, growth and development have these characteristics.

    A. ______________________

    B. ______________________

    C. ______________________

14. List the basic principles of growth and development.

    A. ______________________

    ____

    B. ______________________

    ____

    C. ______________________

    ____

    D. ______________________

    ____

    E. ______________________

    ____

    F. ______________________

    ____

15. List the developmental tasks of infancy (birth to 1 year).

    A. ______________________

    B. ______________________

    C. ______________________

    D. ______________________

    E. ______________________

16. The ______________________ of infancy is from birth to 1 month.

17. In newborns, movements are ______________________ and ______________________.

18. Describe the following reflexes that are present in newborns.

    A. Moro reflex (startle reflex)

    ____

    ____

    B. Sucking reflex

    ____

    ____

    C. Step reflex

    ____

    ____

19. List the developmental tasks of toddlerhood (1-3 years).

    A. ______________________

    B. ______________________

C. ______________________

D. ______________________

20. Bowel and bladder control is related to

______________________.

21. Children must be ______________________

and ______________________

ready for toilet training.

22. List the developmental tasks of the preschool years (3-6 years).

A. ______________________

B. ______________________

C. ______________________

D. ______________________

E. ______________________

F. ______________________

23. List the developmental tasks of the school-age years (6-9 or 6-10 years).

A. ______________________

____

B. ______________________

____

C. ______________________

____

D. ______________________

____

E. ______________________

____

F. ______________________

____

24. School-age children are concerned about being well liked. Being part of a peer group is important for ______________________,

______________________,

and ______________________ needs.

25. A person in late childhood (preadolescence) is expected to show more refinement and maturity in achieving these developmental tasks.

A. ______________________

____

B. ______________________

____

C. ______________________

____

D. ______________________

____

E. ______________________

____

F. ______________________

____

26. List the developmental tasks of adolescence (12-18 years).

A. ______________________

____

B. ______________________

____

C. ______________________

____

D. ______________________

____

E. ______________________________

____

27. ______________________________ marks the onset of puberty in girls.

28. ______________________________ signals the onset of puberty in boys.

29. Boys usually stop growing between the ages of

______________________________.

30. List the developmental tasks of young adulthood (18-40 years).

A. ______________________________

B. ______________________________

C. ______________________________

D. ______________________________

E. ______________________________

31. Many factors affect the selection of a partner.

They include ______________________________,

______________________________,

______________________________,

______________________________,

______________________________,

______________________________,

and ______________________________.

32. List the developmental tasks of middle adulthood (40-65 years).

A. ______________________________

B. ______________________________

C. ______________________________

D. ______________________________

33. Menstruation stops between the ages of

______________ and ______________.

34. Most older people live in

______________________________.

35. Define the following terms.

A. Young-old

____

____

B. Old

____

____

C. Old-old

____

____

36. List the developmental tasks of late adulthood (65 years and older).

A. ______________________________

B. ______________________________

C. ______________________________

D. ______________________________

E. ______________________________

37. Older persons are at greater risk for

______________________________,

______________________________,

and ______________________________.

38. Retirement usually means reduced income. Give examples of how reduced income may force lifestyle changes.

A. ______________________________

B. ______________________________

C. ______________________________

D. ______________________________

E. ______________________________

F. ______________________________

39. As couples age, the chances increase that a partner will die. Death of a partner results in the loss of a ______________________________, ______________________________, ______________________________, and ______________________________.

Multiple Choice

Circle the BEST answer.

40. Which is *not* characteristic of a newborn?
    A. The skin is smooth.
    B. The head is large compared to the rest of the body.
    C. The abdomen is large and round.
    D. The eyes are deep blue.

41. At what age can infants roll from front to back?
    A. 1 week
    B. 1 month
    C. 2 months
    D. 4 to 5 months

42. You would expect all of the following from a 6-month-old infant *except*
    A. Sits with support
    B. Smiles at himself or herself in the mirror
    C. Responds to his or her name
    D. Walks with help

43. Solid foods are given at what age?
    A. 2 to 3 months
    B. 1 year
    C. 4 to 6 months
    D. 10 months

44. A toddler can do all of the following *except*
    A. Walk up and down stairs
    B. Print his or her name
    C. Drink from a cup
    D. Turn book pages

45. Three-year-olds enjoy
    A. Coloring books and crayons
    B. Jumping rope
    C. Word games
    D. Riding a bicycle

46. At what age do children begin to lose baby teeth?
    A. 3 years
    B. 4 years
    C. 8 years
    D. 6 years

47. It is important to begin giving children factual sex education during
    A. Toddlerhood.
    B. Late childhood.
    C. Adolescence.
    D. Young adulthood.

48. During late childhood
    A. Arguments are common between boys and girls.
    B. Peer groups are not important.
    C. Boys show more signs of maturing sexually than girls.
    D. Children accept adult rules without question.

49. The process of growth and development occurs from the center of the body outward.
    A. True
    B. False

50. Which statement about newborns is *false?*
    A. They see in color.
    B. They prefer male voices.
    C. Loud sounds startle them.
    D. They react to touch and can feel pain.

51. Toddlers express anger and frustration by kicking and screaming.
    A. True
    B. False

52. Teenagers prefer spending time with family to being with peers.
    A. True
    B. False

ADDITIONAL LEARNING ACTIVITIES

1. Observe infants and children at various stages of growth and development.
   A. Can you identify physical differences related to age? Explain.
   B. Can you identify differences in social behaviors related to age? Explain.
   C. How might these age-related differences affect the way you provide care for children of various ages?

2. Review the developmental tasks of your own age-group.
   A. Describe the tasks that have meaning to you.
   B. What are some ways you are involved in completing each task?
   C. What developmental tasks are other members of your family involved in completing?

3. Interview a person who has recently retired. Ask the person to discuss any changes in life-style as a result of retirement.

4. Write down how you are preparing for retirement financially, socially, and physically.

5. Spend time with persons in late adulthood (parents, grandparents, uncles, aunts, or friends).
   A. Notice the physical changes.
   B. Ask the person to share some positive and negative aspects of aging.
   C. What brings joy and meaning to the person's life?

10

Sexuality

OBJECTIVES

The questions and student activities in this chapter will help you meet these objectives.

- Define the key terms listed in Chapter 10
- Describe sex and sexuality
- Explain why sexuality is important throughout life
- Describe five types of sexual relationships
- Explain how injury, illness, and aging can affect sexuality
- Explain how the nursing team can promote sexuality
- Describe how to deal with sexually aggressive persons

STUDY QUESTIONS

Matching

Match the following terms with the correct definitions.

A. Homosexual
B. Transsexual
C. Sex
D. Bisexual
E. Erectile dysfunction
F. Heterosexual
G. Sexuality
H. Transvestite
I. Impotence

1. ______ A person who is attracted to both sexes

2. ______ A person who is attracted to members of the other sex

3. ______ A person who is attracted to members of the same sex

4. ______ The inability of the male to have an erection

5. ______ Another term for impotence

6. ______ The physical activities involving the organs of reproduction

7. ______ The physical, psychological, social, cultural, and spiritual factors that affect a person's feelings and attitudes about his or her sex

8. ______ A person who believes that he or she is really a member of the other sex

9. ______ A person who becomes sexually excited by dressing in the clothes of the other sex

Fill in the Blanks

10. When does sexuality develop?

____

____

____

11. Attitudes and sex needs are affected by life events. These include ______________________,

______________________________,

______________________________,

and ______________________________.

12. ______________________________ and ______________________________ are great risks for sexually active teenagers.

13. List 7 causes of impotence.

A. ______________________________

B. ______________________________

C. ______________________________

D. ______________________________

E. ______________________________

F. ______________________________

G. ______________________________

14. ______________________________,

______________________________,

______________________________,

and ______________________________ are common responses to changes in a person's sexual functioning.

15. As men age, the hormone

____

decreases. This hormone affects

______________________________,

______________________________,

and ______________________________.

16. When menopause occurs, the female hormones ______________________________ and ______________________________ decrease.

17. List 4 nonsexual causes of sexually aggressive behaviors.

A. ______________________________

B. ______________________________

C. ______________________________

D. ______________________________

18. What should you do if a patient or resident acts in a sexually aggressive way toward you?

A. ______________________________

____

B. ______________________________

____

C. ______________________________

____

D. ______________________________

____

E. ______________________________

____

Multiple Choice

Circle the BEST answer.

19. As men age, the hormone testosterone decreases. This causes the following changes in sexual activity *except*
    A. Erection takes longer.
    B. The phase between erection and orgasm is longer.
    C. Orgasm is more forceful.
    D. Erections are lost quickly.

20. After menopause female hormones decrease. This causes the uterus, vagina, and genitalia to atrophy.
    A. True
    B. False

21. A married couple is living in a nursing center. Which is *false?*
    A. They are allowed to share the same room.
    B. They have the right to be sexual.
    C. They cannot share a bed.
    D. They are allowed privacy.

22. Two single residents living in a nursing center are attracted to one another. You must help keep them apart.
    A. True
    B. False

23. Which statement about sexuality is *false?*
    A. Sexuality involves the mind and the body.
    B. Sexuality can be affected by illness and injury.
    C. Attitudes about sex change as a person ages.
    D. Sexuality is not important for the very young and the old.

24. Mr. Jones is masturbating in the dining room. You should
    A. Get the nurse at once.
    B. Scold him for his bad behavior.
    C. Take him to a private area.
    D. Refuse to take care of him.

25. Mrs. Adams is a 75-year-old nursing center resident. Which action does *not* promote her sexuality?
    A. Helping her apply makeup and nail polish
    B. Knocking before entering her room
    C. Letting her choose what clothes to wear
    D. Telling her she has to wear a hospital gown to bed

26. Masturbation is always a sexually aggressive behavior.
    A. True
    B. False

27. Love, affection, and intimacy are needed throughout life.
    A. True
    B. False

ADDITIONAL LEARNING ACTIVITIES

1. You will care for persons with sexual attitudes and practices different from yours.
   A. How do you feel about this?
      (1) Write down any questions or concerns you have and discuss them with your instructor.
      (2) Discuss constructive ways of dealing with your feelings.
   B. Discuss how your feelings can affect the care you give.

2. You may have to deal with persons who are sexually aggressive towards you.
   A. How do you feel about this?
      (1) Write down any questions or concerns you have and discuss them with your instructor.
   B. Discuss how you would handle these uncomfortable situations. What would you say, and who would you talk to?

3. List some ways that you can help patients and residents express their sexuality.

4. List the ways you express your sexuality. Think of how it might feel if you were not allowed to do the things that help you express your sexuality.

11

Safety

OBJECTIVES

The questions and student activities in this chapter will help you meet these objectives.

- Define the key terms listed in Chapter 11
- Describe accident risk factors
- Identify safety measures for infants and children
- Explain why you identify a person before giving care
- Explain how to accurately identify a person
- Describe the safety measures to prevent falls, burns, poisoning, and suffocation
- Explain how the call system is used
- Explain how to prevent equipment accidents
- Explain how to handle hazardous substances
- Describe safety measures for fire prevention and oxygen use
- Explain what to do during a fire
- Give examples of natural and human-made disasters
- Explain how to protect yourself from workplace violence
- Describe your role in risk management
- Perform the procedure described in Chapter 11

STUDY QUESTIONS

Complete the Crossword

Across

3. When breathing stops from lack of oxygen
4. Paralysis from the neck down
5. Paralysis from the waist down

Down

1. That which carries leaking electricity to the earth and away from an electrical item
2. Paralysis on one side of the body

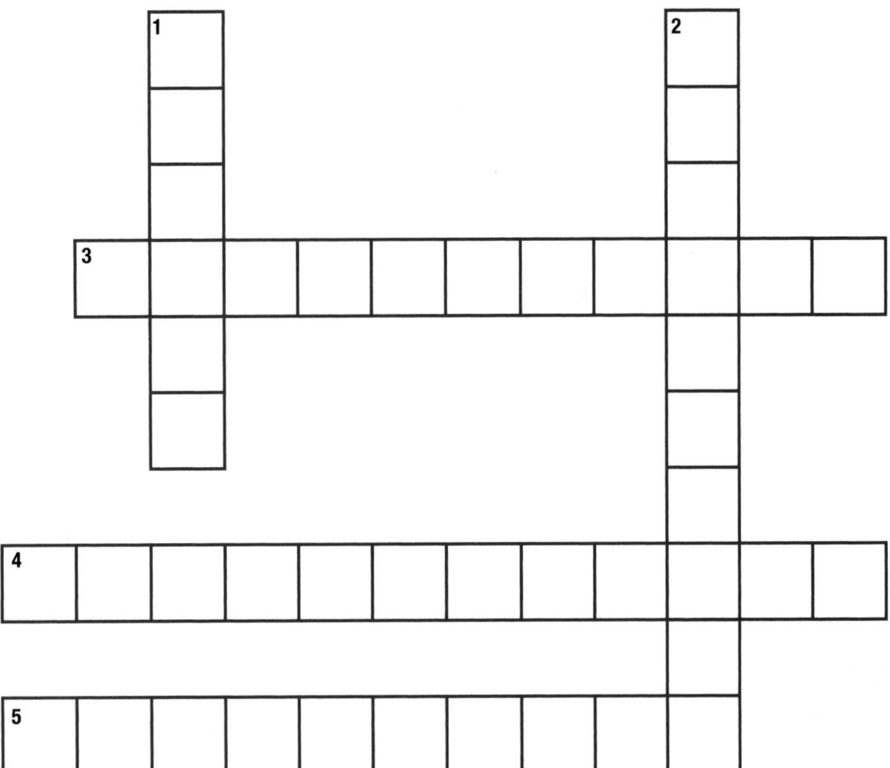

Matching

Match the following terms with the correct definitions.

1. ______ When electrical current passes through the body
2. ______ A state of being unaware of one's surroundings and being unable to react or respond to people, places, or things
3. ______ A sudden catastrophic event in which many people are injured and killed, and property is destroyed
4. ______ Any chemical in the workplace that can cause harm
5. ______ Violent acts directed toward persons at work or while on duty

A. Coma
B. Workplace violence
C. Hazardous substance
D. Electric shock
E. Disaster

Fill in the Blanks

6. List 7 factors that increase a person's risk for accidents

   A. ______________________________

   B. ______________________________

   C. ______________________________

   D. ______________________________

   E. ______________________________

   F. ______________________________

   G. ______________________________

7. In a safe setting, a person has little risk of ______________________________ or ______________________________.

8. You must give the right care to the right person. To identify the person before giving care, you must:

   A. ______________________________

   ____

   ____

   B. ______________________________

   ____

   ____

   ____

9. Most falls occur in ______________________________ and ______________________________.

10. When are falls most likely to occur?

    ____

    ____

11. List 3 safety measures to help prevent falls in bathrooms.

    A. ______________________________

    ____

    B. ______________________________

    ____

    C. ______________________________

    ____

12. The ______________________________ and ______________________________ tell you when to raise bed rails.

13. Bed rails present hazards. Entrapment is a risk from bed rail gaps. Where can bed rail gaps occur?

    A. ______________________________

    B. ______________________________

    C. ______________________________

14. Bed rails cannot be used unless they are needed to ______________________________ ______________________________.

15. When caring for children, crib safety is important. The space between crib rail slats must be no more than ______________________________.

16. What are the purposes of hand rails and grab bars?

    ____

    ____

    ____

    ____

17. Bed legs have wheels. When are bed wheels locked?

    ____

    ____

18. You must always ______________________________ on beds, wheelchairs, and stretchers before you transfer a person.

19. List 5 emergency numbers that should be kept by the telephone.

    A. ______________________________

    B. ______________________________

    C. ______________________________

D. ______________________

E. ______________________

20. Common causes of suffocation include

______________________,

______________________,

______________________,

______________________,

and ______________________.

21. The call system lets the person signal for help. To meet the person's needs, you must:

A. ______________________

B. ______________________

C. ______________________

D. ______________________

E. ______________________

22. When is equipment unsafe?

A. ______________________

B. ______________________

C. ______________________

23. Frayed cords and overloaded electrical outlets can cause ______________________ and ______________________.

24. The ______________________ requires that agencies report equipment-related illnesses, injuries, and deaths.

25. You are transporting Mr. Lewis in a wheelchair. Which direction should the casters point and why?

____

____

26. Exposure to hazardous substances can occur in the workplace. List 7 hazardous substances found in health care agencies.

A. ______________________

B. ______________________

C. ______________________

D. ______________________

E. ______________________

F. ______________________

G. ______________________

27. To protect employees, OSHA requires a hazard communication program. The program includes

______________________,

______________________,

and ______________________.

28. Every hazardous substance has a material safety data sheet (MSDS). When must you check the MSDS?

____

____

29. List three things needed for a fire.

A. ______________________

B. ______________________

C. ______________________

30. The word RACE will help you remember what to do first if a fire occurs. What do the letters R-A-C-E stand for?

A. R ______________________

B. A ______________________

C. C ______________________

D. E ______________________

31. The goal of violence prevention programs is to

____

______________________________________.

32. Your responsibilities in workplace violence prevention programs include:

A. ______________________________________

____

B. ______________________________________

____

C. ______________________________________

____

D. ______________________________________

____

E. ______________________________________

____

F. ______________________________________

____

33. Risk management involves

____

______________________________________.

34. Accidents and errors are reported at once. What do accidents and errors include?

A. ______________________________________

B. ______________________________________

C. ______________________________________

D. ______________________________________

E. ______________________________________

F. ______________________________________

Multiple Choice

Circle the BEST answer.

35. Infants and children have increased risk for accidents because
    A. They have not learned the difference between safety and danger.
    B. They have poor hearing.
    C. They are confused and disoriented.
    D. They have a reduced sense of touch.

36. Infants and young children need supervision
    A. In strollers.
    B. In bathtubs.
    C. When playing outside.
    D. At all times.

37. Which statement about bed rails is *false?*
    A. Bed rails prevent persons from getting out of bed.
    B. Bed rails are necessary for all residents and patients.
    C. A person can get caught or entangled in bed rails.
    D. Bed rails can cause serious injury and death.

38. Which action will *not* help prevent burns in children?
    A. Storing matches and lighters where children cannot reach them
    B. Allowing children to help you cook at the stove
    C. Teaching children fire safety and fire prevention measures
    D. Covering car seats with towels if you park in the sun

39. Which action will help prevent burns while cooking?
    A. Turning pot and pan handles so they point outward
    B. Wearing clothing with long, loose sleeves
    C. Putting wet food into frying pans and deep fryers
    D. Using dry oven mitts and pot holders

40. Floor coverings with bold designs help prevent falls in older persons.
    A. True
    B. False

41. Which is a safety measure to help prevent poisoning?
    A. Mixing cleaning products
    B. Storing cleaning products near food
    C. Discarding harmful substances that are outdated
    D. Keeping drugs in purses and backpacks

42. Which action will help prevent suffocation in children?
    A. Placing safety plugs in outlets
    B. Positioning infants on their stomachs for sleep
    C. Using pillows to position infants
    D. Using latex balloons for children

43. Carbon monoxide is a colorless, odorless, and tasteless gas. It is harmless.
    A. True
    B. False

44. Which action will help prevent equipment accidents?
    A. Turning off equipment before unplugging it
    B. Using electrical items near water
    C. Running electrical cords under rugs
    D. Trying to repair broken items yourself

45. Which is a wheelchair safety measure?
    A. Letting the person's feet drag on the floor when the chair is moving
    B. Pulling the chair backwards
    C. Letting the person stand on the footrests when repositioning
    D. Locking both brakes before you transfer a person to or from the wheelchair

46. You find a bottle of liquid in the tub room without a label. You should:
    A. Open it to see what is inside.
    B. Leave the container and get the nurse.
    C. Take the container to the nurse and explain the problem.
    D. Ask a co-worker what is in the container.

47. Special safety precautions are practiced where oxygen is used and stored.
    A. True
    B. False

48. The first thing you must do when a fire occurs is to
    A. Pull the fire alarm.
    B. Rescue persons in immediate danger.
    C. Get the fire extinguisher.
    D. Turn off electrical equipment.

49. Which is a fire prevention measure?
    A. Emptying ash trays into wastebaskets
    B. Smoking in patient homes
    C. Leaving food unattended on stoves and barbeques
    D. Storing flammable liquids in their original containers

50. A person's clothing is on fire. You should do all of the following *except*
    A. Get the person to the floor.
    B. Roll the person.
    C. Cover the person with a blanket or coat.
    D. Remove the person's clothing as quickly as possible.

51. You are caring for Mrs. Kramer in her home. She is using an electric space heater in her living room. Which action will *not* promote safety?
    A. Keeping the heater at least 3 feet away from items that will burn
    B. Following the manufacturer's instructions for use
    C. Keeping the heater away from water
    D. Leaving the heater unattended while you give Mrs. Kramer a bath

52. When dealing with an agitated or aggressive person, you should
    A. Use touch to calm the person.
    B. Keep your hands free.
    C. Tell the person to calm down.
    D. Stand close to the person.

53. You are providing care for Mr. Grange in his home. You should report all of the following to the nurse *except*
    A. You think that Mr. Grange has a girlfriend.
    B. You see mice in the kitchen.
    C. Mr. Grange tells you that he keeps a loaded gun under his pillow.
    D. Mr. Grange uses obscene language and verbal threats when he is angry.

54. What should you do if you feel an immediate threat to your health or well-being while in Mr. Grange's home?
    A. Document your concerns.
    B. Call your agency and ask the nurse what to do.
    C. Leave the home and call your supervisor.
    D. Tell Mr. Grange how you feel.

55. Accidents and errors in care are reported only if someone is injured.
    A. True
    B. False

ADDITIONAL LEARNING ACTIVITIES

1. Carefully review the safety measures to prevent falls, burns, poisoning, and suffocation.
   A. List the safety measures you practice related to falls, burns, poisoning, and suffocation in your home.
   B. List the safety measures you practice related to each in your workplace.
   C. Is your home safe and free from safety hazards? Explain.
   D. Do you have a fire safety plan in your home? Explain.
   E. If you don't already have one, develop an evacuation plan for your home. Make sure that there are at least 2 possible exits from each room. Have regular fire drills with your family.

2. Make a list of emergency phone numbers (poison control, police, ambulance, hospital, and doctor). Keep the list by each phone in your home. Make sure all family members know where the list is.

3. Carefully review the personal safety practices in Box 11-12 on page 165 in the textbook.
   A. List the personal safety practices that you use in your daily activities.
   B. List the ways that you can improve your personal safety practices.

4. Describe what you would do if threatened or attacked. Answer these questions:
   A. What would your first action be?
   B. What would you shout?
   C. What items should you carry, and how can you use each item as a weapon?
   D. How can you use your body to defend yourself?
   E. What areas of the person's body should you attack?

5. Read the vignette. Then answer the questions that follow.

You are caring for Miss Rita Kelly in her home. She has a moderate hearing loss and has fair vision with eye-glasses. She uses a cane for ambulation. You assist her with bathing, grooming, and laundry twice a week. You also do her grocery shopping weekly.

Miss Kelly lives in a small two-bedroom home. She collects newspapers and old books. She has smoke alarms in her kitchen and in her bedroom. She tells you that she is not sure the smoke alarms work, as the batteries have not been changed for over a year. She does not have a fire extinguisher. The back entrance to the house is partially blocked with boxes of books. The lock on that door has been broken. There are scatter rugs in the bathroom and kitchen. Miss Kelly braided them herself and is very proud of them. There is one telephone. It has a very long cord, which allows Miss Kelly to take it from room to room.

Miss Kelly prepares her own meals. The kitchen stove is a gas range.

Miss Kelly tells you that she always leaves her bedroom window open at night because she likes the cool air and she sleeps better. You notice that she usually wears flowing comfortable gowns and comfortable slippers.

A. What are the risk factors:
   (1) For falls?
   (2) For burns?
   (3) For suffocation?
   (4) For fires?
   (5) Related to personal safety?

B. What do you need to report to the nurse?

C. What are the care planning challenges?

12

Restraint Alternatives and Safe Restraint Use

OBJECTIVES

The questions and student activities in this chapter will help you meet these objectives.

- Define the key terms listed in Chapter 12
- Describe the purpose and complications of restraints
- Identify restraint alternatives
- Explain how to use restraints safely
- Perform the procedure described in Chapter 12

STUDY QUESTIONS

Matching

Match the following terms with the correct definitions.

1. __C__ A restraint attached to the person's body and to a fixed (non-movable) object
2. __B__ A restraint near but not directly attached to the person's body
3. __A__ Any item, object, device, garment, material, or drug that limits or restricts a person's freedom of movement or access to one's body

A. Restraint

B. Passive physical restraint

C. Active physical restraint

Fill in the Blanks

4. ____________________, ____________________, and ____________________ have guidelines about restraint use in hospitals and nursing centers. So do ____________________ and ____________________.

5. List 7 risks of restraint use.

   A. ______________________________

   B. ______________________________

   C. ______________________________

   D. ______________________________

   E. ______________________________

   F. ______________________________

   G. ______________________________

6. Restraints are not used to ______________ a person. They are not used for staff ______________________________.

7. ______________________ is any action that punishes or penalizes a person.

8. Convenience is any action that:

   A. ______________________________

   B. ______________________________

   C. ______________________________

9. The nurse restrains Mr. Gomez to the chair in his room so she can make rounds without being interrupted. This action is ______________________________.

10. Restraints are used only when necessary to ______________________________.

11. Drugs are restraints if they:

    A. ______________________________

    B. ______________________________

12. The doctor may order drugs to help persons who are confused or agitated. What is the goal?

    ____

    ____

    ____

13. What must you remember about using restraints?

    A. ______________________________

    ____

    B. ______________________________

    ____

    C. ______________________________

    ____

    D. ______________________________

    ____

    E. ______________________________

    ____

    F. ______________________________

    ____

    G. ______________________________

    ____

    H. ______________________________

    ____

    I. ______________________________

    ____

    J. ______________________________

    ____

    K. ______________________________

    ____

L. ______________________________

____

M. ______________________________

____

14. Mrs. Monroe's doctor writes an order for a restraint. What must the doctor's order include?

A. ______________________________

B. ______________________________

C. ______________________________

D. ______________________________

15. The nurse tells you to apply a wrist restraint to Mr. Clark's right wrist. You do not understand why the restraint is being used. What should you do and why?

____

____

____

____

16. Before you apply any restraint, what information do you need from the nurse and the care plan?

A. ______________________________

____

B. ______________________________

____

C. ______________________________

____

D. ______________________________

____

E. ______________________________

____

F. ______________________________

____

G. ______________________________

____

H. ______________________________

____

I. ______________________________

____

J. ______________________________

____

K. ______________________________

____

17. You apply a belt restraint to Mrs. Monroe when she is in her wheelchair. What information must you report to the nurse?

A. ______________________________

B. ______________________________

C. ______________________________

D. ______________________________

E. ______________________________

F. ______________________________

G. ______________________________

H. ______________________________

I. ______________________________

J. ______________________________

18. Mr. Clark has a wrist restraint on his right wrist. You are checking the circulation in his right wrist. What signs and symptoms must you report to the nurse at once?

A. ______________________________

B. ______________________________

C. ______________________

D. ______________________

19. Why are persons restrained in the supine position monitored constantly?

____

____

20. What is the purpose of bed rail covers and gap protectors?

____

____

Multiple Choice

Circle the BEST answer.

21. Physical restraints
    A. Restrict freedom of movement or access to one's body.
    B. Should be used to control a person's behavior.
    C. Are effective in preventing falls.
    D. Should never be used.

22. The most serious risk from restraints is:
    A. Loss of dignity.
    B. Fractured hip.
    C. Increased agitation.
    D. Death from strangulation.

23. Which is *not* a restraint alternative?
    A. An exercise program is provided.
    B. A floor cushion is placed next to the person's bed.
    C. The person's chair is placed so close to the wall that the person cannot move.
    D. Extra time is spent with the person who is restless.

24. You may need to apply restraints or care for persons who are restrained. Which is an unsafe action?
    A. Using the restraint noted in the person's care plan
    B. Using only restraints that have manufacturer instructions and warning labels
    C. Using a sheet to position a person on a toilet
    D. Padding bony areas and skin

25. Back cushions are used when a person is restrained in a chair.
    A. True
    B. False

26. How often do you need to check the person's circulation if mitt, wrist, or ankle restraints are used?
    A. At least every 15 minutes
    B. At least every 30 minutes
    C. Every hour
    D. Every 2 hours

27. Which restraints limit arm movements?
    A. Wrist restraints
    B. Mitt restraints
    C. Belt restraints
    D. Vest restraints

28. Which type of restraint is the most restrictive?
    A. A wrist restraint
    B. A mitt restraint
    C. A belt restraint
    D. A vest restraint

29. You are applying a wrist restraint. The person is in bed. Where do you tie the straps?
    A. To the headboard
    B. To the bedrail out of the person's reach
    C. To the footboard
    D. To the moveable part of the bed frame out of the person's reach

ADDITIONAL LEARNING ACTIVITIES

1. Read the vignette. Then answer the questions that follow.
   Mrs. Ann Bert is a patient on the orthopedic unit in Valley View Hospital. She fell and fractured her right hip. She broke her glasses in the fall. The fracture was repaired surgically. This is her second day after surgery.
   Mrs. Bert is very restless. She tries to get out of bed. She pulled her IV catheter out this morning. She keeps calling for her daughter. She says "I need to go home" over and over. She is receiving drugs for pain management every 4 hours. She has a urinary catheter.
   Before Mrs. Bert fell, she lived in her own home. She drove her car and enjoyed visiting her friends. Her daughter called her every day and visited weekly. Mrs. Bert has 2 cats. She has not been in a hospital for more than 30 years.
   A. What are some of Mrs. Bert's safety needs?
   B. What might be some of the causes for Mrs. Bert's behaviors?
   C. How can the RN use the nursing process to decide how to meet Mrs. Bert's safety needs?
   D. What questions might the RN ask to find out the causes of Mrs. Bert's behaviors?
   E. What restraint alternatives might be tried?
   F. How might family and friends help prevent the need for restraints?

2. You are caring for a person who is restrained. List some things you can do to protect the person's quality of life. Think of how you would want to be treated.

3. Under the supervision of your instructor, practice the procedures for applying restraints with a classmate.
   A. Use the procedure checklists to evaluate your technique. Remember that restraints can cause serious injury and even death. They must always be applied correctly.

4. Under the supervision of your instructor, allow a classmate to practice applying restraints to you. Discuss how it feels to be restrained. Answer these questions.
   A. Did you feel safe? Explain.
   B. Did you feel comfortable? Explain.
   C. Did you feel in control? Explain.
   D. What fears did you have?

5. Imagine that you are in the hospital. You are having a lot of pain. You do not know the staff. The medication you are taking makes you drowsy. You are not sure what day it is. You have an IV in your right arm and a tube in your nose. You are frightened.
   A. What behaviors might you have?
   B. What could be some reasons for your behavior?
   C. Might the staff believe that you are confused? Explain.
   D. Would you feel safer and less fearful if you were restrained?
   E. What measures would make you feel safe and less fearful?

.2

13

Preventing Infection

OBJECTIVES

The questions and student activities in this chapter will help you meet these objectives.

- Define the key terms listed in Chapter 13
- Identify what microbes need to live and grow
- List the signs and symptoms of infection
- Explain the chain of infection
- Describe nosocomial infection and the persons at risk
- Describe the practices of medical asepsis
- Describe disinfection and sterilization methods
- Explain how to care for equipment and supplies
- Explain Standard Precautions, Transmission-Based Precautions, and the Bloodborne Pathogen Standard
- Explain the principles and practices of surgical asepsis
- Perform the procedures described in Chapter 13

STUDY QUESTIONS

Complete the Crossword

Across

1. Being free of disease-producing microbes
4. The process of becoming unclean
5. A bacterium protected by a hard shell
6. The absence of all microbes
7. A microorganism

Down

2. A microbe that is harmful and can cause an infection
3. A disease resulting from the invasion and growth of microbes in the body

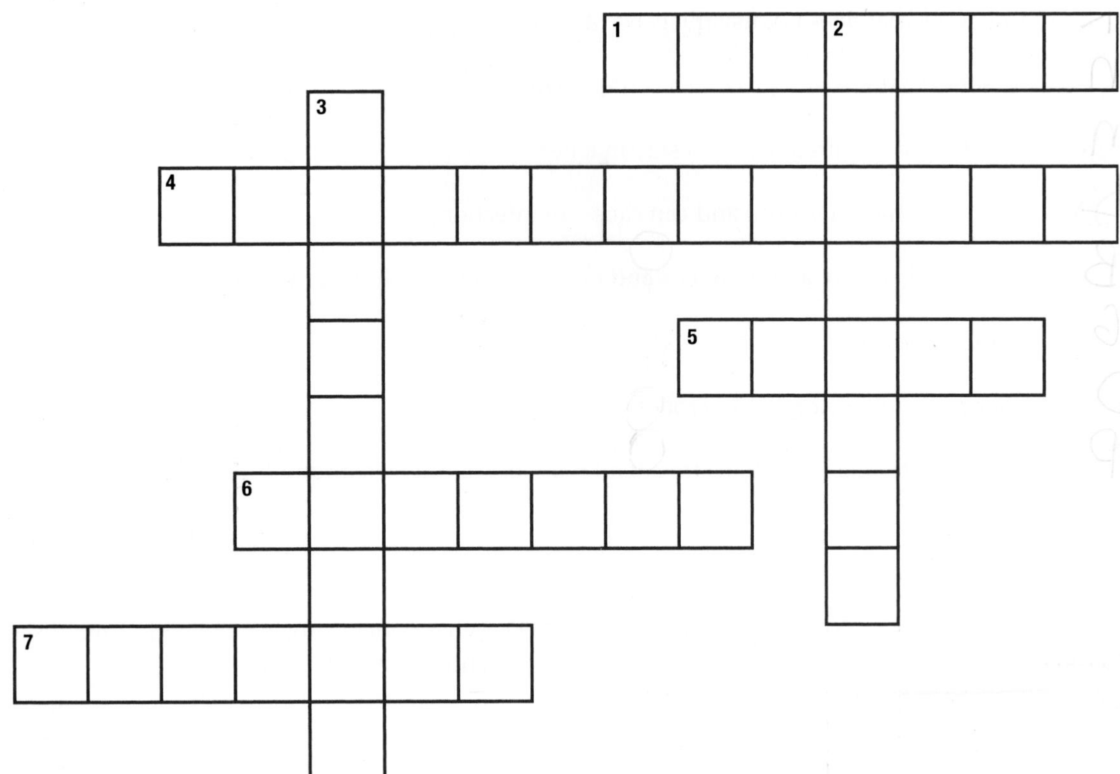

Matching

Match the following terms with the correct definitions.

A. Carrier
B. Sterile field
C. Microorganism
D. Sterilization
E. Biohazardous waste
F. Disinfection
G. Sterile technique
H. Normal flora
I. Medical asepsis
J. Clean technique
K. Non-pathogen
L. Pathogen
M. Nosocomial infection
N. Germicide
O. Communicable disease
P. Surgical asepsis
Q. Immunity

1. e Items contaminated with blood, body fluids, secretions, and excretions and that may be harmful to others
2. a A human or animal that is a reservoir for microbes but does not have signs and symptoms of infection
3. J Medical asepsis
4. O A disease caused by pathogens that spread easily; a contagious disease
5. f The process of destroying pathogens
6. n A disinfectant applied to skin, tissues, or nonliving objects
7. Q Protection against a certain disease
8. i Practices used to remove or destroy pathogens and to prevent their spread from one person or place to another person or place
9. C A small living plant or animal seen only with a microscope

10. K A microbe that does not usually cause an infection

11. h Microbes that live and grow in a certain area

12. m An infection acquired during a stay in a health agency

13. L A microbe that is harmful and can cause an infection

14. B A work area free of all pathogens and nonpathogens (including spores)

15. G Surgical asepsis

16. D The process of destroying microbes

17. P The practices that keep items free of all microbes; sterile technique

Fill in the Blanks

18. List and briefly describe the five types of microbes.

    A. ____________________

    B. ____________________

    C. ____________________

    D. ____________________

    E. ____________________

19. What is required for microbes to live and grow?

    A. ____________________

    B. ____________________

    C. ____________________

    D. ____________________

20. *E. coli* is a microbe that normally lives in the large intestine. What happens if it enters the urinary system?

    ____

    ____

21. A ____________________ is in a body part. A ____________________ involves the whole body.

22. What system protects the body from disease and infection?

    ____

23. The chain of infection is a process involving:

    A. ____________________

    B. ____________________

    C. ____________________

    D. ____________________

    E. ____________________

    F. ____________________

24. List 8 factors that affect the ability to resist infection.

    A. ____________________

    B. ____________________

    C. ____________________

    D. ____________________

    E. ____________________

    F. ____________________

    G. ____________________

    H. ____________________

25. How are nosocomial infections prevented?

A. ______________________

B. ______________________

C. ______________________

D. ______________________

26. When must you wash your hands?

A. ______________________

____

B. ______________________

____

C. ______________________

____

D. ______________________

____

E. ______________________

____

27. Mrs. Mary Martin has dementia. She does not understand aseptic practices. When should you assist her with handwashing?

A. ______________________

B. ______________________

C. ______________________

D. ______________________

28. Why is lotion or cream applied to hands after hand hygiene?

____

____

29. ______________________ prevent the spread of communicable or contagious diseases.

30. Isolation Precautions are based on ______________________.

31. Standard Precautions are used for ______________________.

32. Standard Precautions prevent the spread of infection from:

A. ______________________

B. ______________________

C. ______________________

D. ______________________

33. Describe when each type of Transmission-Based Precaution is used.

A. Airborne Precautions

____

____

____

B. Droplet Precautions

____

____

____

C. Contact Precautions

____

____

____

34. The nurse practices surgical asepsis when changing Mr. Bradley's abdominal dressing.

    A. Why are drafts prevented during the dressing change?

    ____

    ____

    B. Why are wet items held down during the dressing change?

    ____

    ____

    C. Why are sterile gloves used to handle the sterile dressings?

    ____

    ____

35. When are gloves worn?

    ____

    ____

36. After you remove your latex gloves, you notice a red, raised rash on your hands. What should you do?

    ____

37. Masks prevent the spread of infection from the

    ______________________________.

38. You are wearing a gown to protect your clothes, wrists, and arms from splashes. What parts of the gown are clean?

    ____

39. How should you bag and transport contaminated linens?

    ____

40. When is double bagging needed?

    ____

    ____

41. You are caring for Anna Franks. Anna is 6 years old. She is on Droplet Precautions. What can you do to promote her safety and security?

    ____

    ____

    ____

    ____

    ____

42. What is the purpose of the Bloodborne Pathogen Standard?

    ____

    ____

43. ______________________________ and ______________________________ reduce employee exposure risks in the workplace.

44. How is the hepatitis B virus spread?

    ____

    ____

45. List 4 measures required by OSHA to safely handle and use personal protective equipment.

    A. ______________________________

    ____

    B. ______________________________

    ____

    C. ______________________________

    ____

    D. ______________________________

    ____

46. When are work surfaces decontaminated?

A. ______________________________

____

B. ______________________________

____

C. ______________________________

____

D. ______________________________

____

47. What does "regulated waste" include?

A. ______________________________

B. ______________________________

C. ______________________________

D. ______________________________

48. What precautions does OSHA require for contaminated laundry?

A. ______________________________

____

B. ______________________________

____

C. ______________________________

____

D. ______________________________

____

E. ______________________________

____

49. An exposure incident is ______________________________

____

______________________________.

50. ______________________________ means piercing the mucous membranes or the skin barrier.

51. The ______________________________ is the person whose blood or body fluids are the source of an exposure incident.

52. Do not perform a sterile procedure unless:

A. ______________________________

B. ______________________________

C. ______________________________

D. ______________________________

E. ______________________________

53. Before opening a sterile package, you must make sure that it is ______________________________

______________________________.

54. You must inspect sterile solution containers before using the solution. You should not use the solution if:

A. ______________________________

B. ______________________________

55. After sterile gloves are on, you can handle items

______________________________.

56. What should you do if you contaminate sterile gloves while assisting with a sterile procedure?

____

____

57. What parts of sterile gloves are *not* considered sterile?

____

____

Multiple Choice

Circle the BEST answer.

58. The most important measure to prevent the spread of infection is
   A. Sterilization of equipment.
   B. Practicing hand hygiene.
   C. Surgical asepsis.
   D. Isolation Precautions.

59. The environment where microbes live and grow is the
   A. Infection.
   B. Portal of entry.
   C. Reservoir or host.
   D. Source.

60. These statements are about handwashing. Which is *false?*
   A. Stand away from the sink. Your hands, body, and uniform should not touch the sink.
   B. Keep your hands and forearms higher than your elbows.
   C. Clean fingernails by rubbing the tips against your palms.
   D. Wash your hands for at least 15 seconds.

61. To prevent foodborne illnesses, do all of the following *except*
   A. Buy meat products first when shopping.
   B. Open egg cartons before buying them.
   C. Store fresh and frozen foods promptly.
   D. Wash your hands before preparing food.

62. Disposable gloves are worn when using chemical disinfectants.
   A. True
   B. False

63. All non-pathogens and pathogens are destroyed by
   A. Disinfection.
   B. Cleaning.
   C. Sterilization.
   D. Handwashing.

64. You are controlling portals of exit by
   A. Using leakproof plastic bags for soiled linens.
   B. Holding equipment and linens away from your uniform.
   C. Covering your nose and mouth when coughing or sneezing.
   D. Washing contaminated areas with soap and water.

65. You are controlling transmission by
   A. Wearing personal protective equipment.
   B. Assisting the person with handwashing.
   C. Making sure linens are dry and wrinkle free.
   D. Following the care plan to meet nutrition and fluid needs.

66. You help prevent the spread of infection by
   A. Cleaning toward your body.
   B. Using leakproof plastic bags for soiled linens.
   C. Holding equipment and linens against your uniform.
   D. Cleaning from the dirtiest area to the cleanest area.

67. Isolation Precautions involve
   A. Wearing gloves, gowns, and a mask.
   B. Special procedures for removing trash from the room.
   C. Special measures to collect specimens.
   D. All of the above.

68. Which is *not* a rule for Isolation Precautions?
   A. Collect all needed items before entering the room.
   B. Remove items from the room in leakproof plastic bags.
   C. Use paper towels to turn faucets on and off.
   D. Shake linens to remove wrinkles.

69. Which statement about wearing gloves is *false?*
   A. Gloves are easier to put on when your hands are dry.
   B. Remove and discard torn, cut, and punctured gloves at once.
   C. The same pair of gloves is used to care for persons in the same room.
   D. Wear gloves once. Discard them after use.

70. Protective gowns
   A. Are contaminated when wet.
   B. Open in the front.
   C. Are used more than once.
   D. Are clean on the outside.

71. Surgical asepsis is required
   A. When caring for persons on Isolation Precautions.
   B. When handling contaminated laundry.
   C. When the skin or sterile tissues are penetrated.
   D. When collecting urine specimens.

72. Which statement about surgical asepsis is *false?*
   A. Hold wet items up.
   B. Use sterile gloves or sterile forceps to handle sterile items.
   C. If you cannot see an item, it is contaminated.
   D. Do not reach over a sterile field.

73. Before opening a sterile package, do all of the following *except*
   A. Wash your hands.
   B. Put on sterile gloves.
   C. Make sure that the package is intact.
   D. Make sure that the package is dry.

74. Sterile solutions are poured into clean containers.
   A. True
   B. False

75. The Bloodborne Pathogen Standard is
   A. A regulation of the Occupational Safety and Health Organization (OSHA).
   B. An OBRA guideline.
   C. A recommendation from Medicare and Medicaid.
   D. The same as Standard Precautions.

76. When caring for persons on Transmission-Based Precautions, do all of the following *except*
   A. Provide hobby materials if possible.
   B. Say hello from the doorway often.
   C. Spend as little time in the person's room as possible.
   D. Treat the person with respect, kindness, and dignity.

77. All agencies must have an exposure control plan which identifies staff at risk for exposure to blood and other potentially infectious material (OPIM).
   A. True
   B. False

78. Personal protective equipment is free to employees.
   A. True
   B. False

79. OSHA requires these work practice controls *except*
   A. Do not store food or drinks where blood or OPIM are kept.
   B. Practice hand hygiene after removing gloves.
   C. Recap, bend, or remove needles by hand.
   D. Never shear or break contaminated needles.

80. Which statement about exposure incidents is *false?*
   A. Report an exposure incident at the end of your shift.
   B. Medical evaluation and follow-up are free.
   C. Your blood is tested for HBV and HIV.
   D. If you refuse testing, the blood is kept for 90 days. Testing is done later if you change your mind.

81. Do not open a sterile package while wearing sterile gloves. You will contaminate your gloves.
   A. True
   B. False

82. Once a sterile field is set up you cannot add other sterile items to the field.
   A. True
   B. False

83. Sterile forceps are used to transfer sterile items to a sterile field. Which is correct when using sterile forceps?
   A. Hold sterile forceps below your waist.
   B. Keep the tips of wet forceps higher than your wrist.
   C. Keep sterile forceps within your sight.
   D. Lay the forceps down carefully outside the sterile field.

ADDITIONAL LEARNING ACTIVITIES

1. List the measures you practice in your personal life to prevent infection.

2. List the special care needs of persons on Transmission-Based Precautions. How can you help meet their needs?

3. Carefully review the procedures in Chapter 13.
   A. Practice the procedures for handwashing, removing gloves, wearing a mask, donning and removing a gown, and double bagging.
      (1) Use the procedure checklists provided on pages 257 through 261.
   B. Practice the procedures for opening sterile packages, opening and pouring a sterile solution, setting up a sterile field, and donning and removing sterile gloves.
      (1) Use the procedure checklists provided on pages 262 through 267.
      Remember, some states and agencies do not allow assistive personnel to perform some of the procedures in Chapter 13.

14

Body Mechanics

OBJECTIVES

The questions and student activities in this chapter will help you meet these objectives.

- Define the key terms listed in Chapter 14
- Explain the purpose and rules of body mechanics
- Explain how ergonomics can prevent workplace accidents
- Identify the causes, signs, and symptoms of back injuries
- Identify comfort and safety measures for lifting, turning, and moving persons in bed
- Know the basic bed positions
- Explain how to safely perform transfers
- Explain why body alignment and position changes are important
- Identify the comfort and safety measures for positioning a person
- Position persons in the basic bed positions and in a chair
- Perform the procedures described in Chapter 14

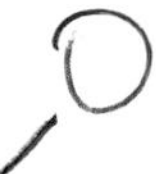

STUDY QUESTIONS

Matching

Match the following terms with the correct definitions.

A. Body mechanics
B. Friction
C. Logrolling
D. Reverse Trendelenburg's position
E. Shearing
F. Supine position
G. Base of support
H. Sim's position
I. Trendelenburg's position
J. Body alignment
K. Dorsal recumbent position
L. Fowler's position
M. Ergonomics
N. Semi-Fowler's position
O. Transfer belt
P. Prone position
Q. Lateral position

1. ______ The area on which an object rests
2. ______ The way the head, trunk, arms, and legs are aligned with one another; posture
3. ______ Using the body in an efficient and careful way
4. ______ The back-lying or supine position

5. m The science of designing a job to fit the worker
6. L A semi-sitting position; the head of the bed is raised between 45 and 90 degrees
7. B The rubbing of one surface against another
8. Q The side-lying position
9. C Turning the person as a unit, in alignment, with one motion
10. P Lying on the abdomen with the head turned to one side
11. D The head of the bed is raised and the foot of the bed is lowered
12. n The head of the bed is raised 30 degrees and the knee portion is raised 15 degrees; or the head of the bed is raised 30 degrees and the knee portion is raised 15 degrees
13. e When skin sticks to a surface and muscles slide in the direction the body is moving
14. H A left side-lying position in which the upper leg is sharply flexed so it is not on the lower leg and the lower arm is behind the person
15. f The back-lying or dorsal recumbent position
16. O A belt used to support persons who are unsteady or disabled; a gait belt
17. I The head of the bed is lowered, and the foot of the bed is raised

Fill in the Blanks

18. Your largest and strongest muscles are in the ______________________, ______________________, ______________________, and ______________________. Use these muscles to lift and move heavy objects.

19. Why should you stand with your feet apart?
____
____

20. How should you pick a heavy object up off the floor?
____

21. Why should you hold items close to your body?
____
____

22. ______________________, ______________________, or ______________________ heavy objects whenever you can, rather than lifting them.

23. Do not lift heavy objects higher than ______________________.

24. Use ______________________ to protect yourself and others from injury.

25. Some beds have manual cranks at the foot of the bed. Describe the purpose of each crank.

   A. Left crank

   ____

   ____

   B. Right crank

   ____

   ____

   C. Center crank

   ____

   ____

26. When is the flat bed position used?

   ____

   ____

27. You are providing home care for Mr. Adams. He has a regular bed. How can you position him in Fowler's position?

   ____

   ____

   ____

28. When are bed wheels locked?

   ____

   ____

29. When are bed rails used?

   ____

   ____

30. You reduce friction and shearing by

   ______________________________.

31. Friction and shearing can cause

   ______________ and ______________.

32. What information do you need from the nurse and the care plan before lifting or moving a person in bed?

   A. ______________________________

   B. ______________________________

   C. ______________________________

   D. ______________________________

   E. ______________________________

   F. ______________________________

   G. ______________________________

   H. ______________________________

   I. ______________________________

33. When should you decide how you will move a person and how much help you will need?

   ____

34. At least two workers are needed to move

   ______________________________,

   ______________________________,

   and ______________________________

   persons up in bed.

35. What measures promote quality of life before starting any procedure?

   A. ______________________________

   B. ______________________________

   C. ______________________________

36. When are lift sheets used to move persons up in bed?

   A. ______________________________

   B. ______________________________

   C. ______________________________

   D. ______________________________

37. Why is the person moved to the side of the bed before turning?

____

____

38. Using a lift sheet to turn a person helps prevent

_______________,

_______________,

and _______________.

39. Why is it important to position persons in good alignment?

____

____

40. Logrolling is used to turn:

A. _______________

B. _______________

C. _______________

D. _______________

41. List four reasons that persons sit on the side of the bed (dangle).

A. _______________

B. _______________

C. _______________

D. _______________

42. To transfer a person means

____

_______________.

43. How many staff members are needed for chair or wheelchair transfers?

____

____

44. What factors does the nurse consider when deciding to transfer a person to a chair or wheelchair with assistance?

A. _______________

B. _______________

C. _______________

D. _______________

45. The agency has a "no lift" policy. What does this mean?

____

____

____

46. You will use a mechanical lift to transfer some persons. Before using a lift you must:

A. _______________

____

B. _______________

____

C. _______________

____

D. _______________

____

47. Why are elevated toilet seats used for wheelchair to toilet transfers?

____

____

48. Stretchers are used to transport persons who:

A. _______________

B. _______________

C. _______________

49. List 4 reasons why the person must be properly positioned at all times.

A. ______________________________

B. ______________________________

C. ______________________________

D. ______________________________

50. What guidelines are followed to safely position a person?

A. ______________________________

B. ______________________________

C. ______________________________

D. ______________________________

E. ______________________________

F. ______________________________

G. ______________________________

51. Why must you check with the nurse before positioning an older person in the prone or Sim's position?

____

____

____

Multiple Choice

Circle the BEST answer.

52. Which is *not* involved in good body mechanics?
   A. Keeping objects close to your body
   B. Pushing, sliding, or pulling heavy objects
   C. Working with sudden motions
   D. Facing your work area

53. To pick up a box using good body mechanics, you must
   A. Use the muscles of the lower back.
   B. Bend your knees and squat.
   C. Hold items away from your body.
   D. Stand with your feet very close together.

54. According to the U.S. Department of Labor, nursing assistants are at great risk for work-related musculoskeletal disorders (MSD).
   A. True
   B. False

55. Which action leads to back disorders?
   A. Avoiding unnecessary bending and reaching
   B. Staying in one position too long
   C. Turning your whole body when changing the direction of your movement
   D. Working with smooth and even movements

56. Persons with heart and respiratory disorders usually breathe more easily in which position?
   A. Fowler's position
   B. Supine
   C. Prone position
   D. Lateral position

57. Lift sheets are often used to move persons up in bed. Which is *false?*
   A. Shearing and friction are reduced.
   B. Place the sheet under the person from the waist to the knees.
   C. Lift sheets are used to move older persons.
   D. The person is lifted more easily.

58. To apply a transfer belt correctly, you do all of the following *except*
   A. Apply the belt around the person's waist under clothing.
   B. Tighten the belt so it is snug but does not cause discomfort or impair breathing.
   C. Make sure a woman's breasts are not caught under the belt.
   D. Make sure the buckle is not over the person's spine.

59. When helping a person transfer from a bed to a chair
   A. The person is helped out of bed on his or her weak side.
   B. The bed is kept in the high position.
   C. Two workers are always needed.
   D. The person wears nonskid footwear.

60. To safely transfer a person to a stretcher
   A. Ask a co-worker to help you.
   B. Position the bed in Fowler's position.
   C. Make sure the bed and stretcher wheels are locked.
   D. Have the bed in the lowest horizontal position.

Labeling

Label the positions shown.

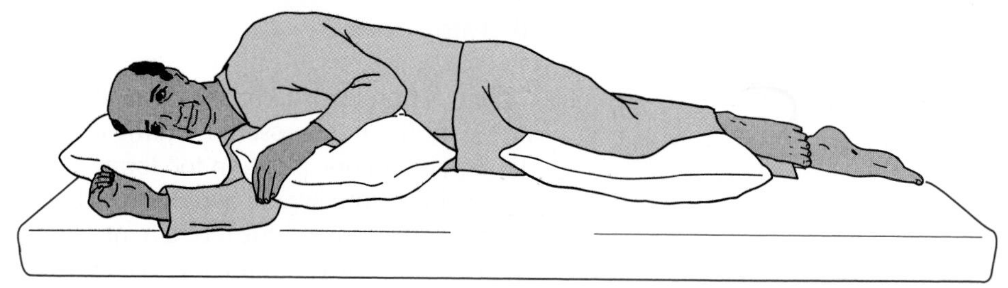

61. ______________________________

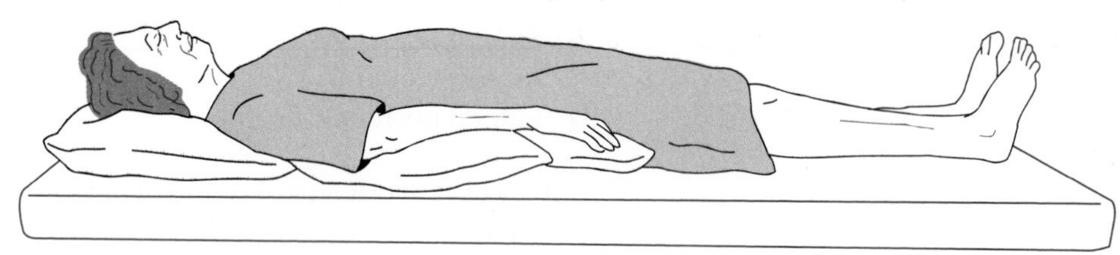

62. ______________________________

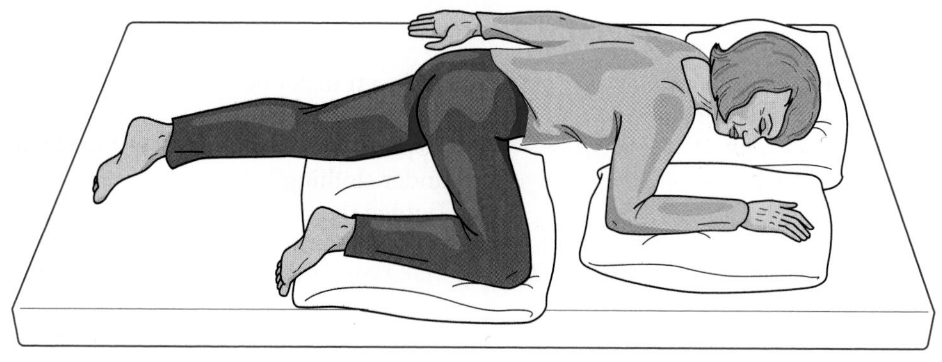

63. ______________________________

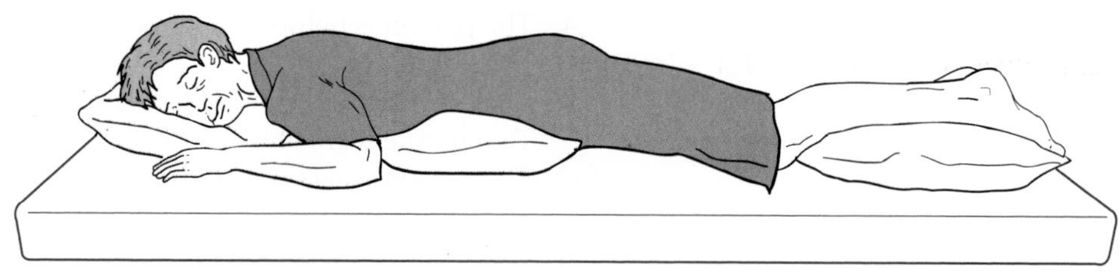

64. ______________________________

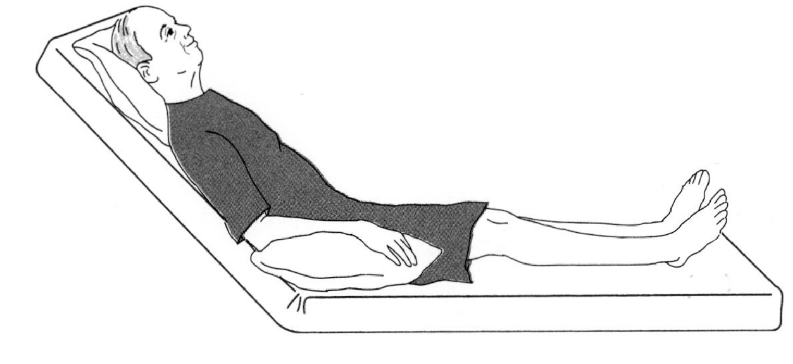

65. ______________________________

ADDITIONAL LEARNING ACTIVITIES

1. Review the rules for good body mechanics. Answer the following questions.
   A. Do you practice these rules in your daily activities? Explain.
   B. Do you practice these rules in your work activities? Explain.
   C. How can you change the way you move, lift, and work to decrease your risk for injury?

2. List the factors that lead to back injuries. Identify which factors relate to you. List the actions you can take to reduce your risk for back disorders.

3. List special considerations for lifting and moving older persons in bed.

4. Review the rules for stretcher safety listed in Chapter 11.

5. List the measures needed for good alignment for each of the following positions:
   A. Fowler's position
   B. Supine position
   C. Lateral position
   D. Sim's position
   E. Chair position

6. Describe how you would reposition a person in the chair or wheelchair:
   A. If the person is alert, cooperative, can follow instructions, and has the strength to help.
   B. If the person cannot assist with repositioning.

7. Review the procedures in Chapter 14.
   A. Under the supervision of your instructor, practice each procedure.
      (1) Use the procedure checklists provided on pages 268 through 293.
      (2) Take your turn being the patient or resident.
      (3) Discuss the experience with your classmates and instructor. Answer these questions.
         a. Did you feel safe? Explain.
         b. Did you feel comfortable? Explain.

8. Practice proper positioning (Fowler's, supine, prone, lateral, and Sim's) with a classmate or family member. Use pillows to promote comfort and good body alignment. Take your turn as the person being positioned.

15

Bedmaking

OBJECTIVES

The questions and student activities in this chapter will help you meet these objectives.

- Define the key terms listed in Chapter 15
- Describe open, closed, occupied, and surgical beds
- Explain how to use drawsheets
- Handle linens following the rules of medical asepsis
- Perform the procedures described in Chapter 15

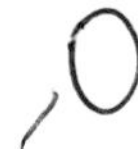

STUDY QUESTIONS

Matching

Match the following terms with the correct definitions.

A. Surgical bed
B. Drawsheet
C. Occupied bed
D. Closed bed
E. Plastic drawsheet
F. Open bed

1. B A small sheet placed over the middle of the bottom sheet; it helps keep the mattress and bottom linens clean and dry.
2. e A waterproof drawsheet placed between the bottom sheet and the cotton drawsheet to keep the mattress and bottom linens clean and dry.
3. D A bed that is not in use. The bed is ready for a new patient or resident.
4. f A bed that is in use. Top linens are folded back so the person can get into bed.
5. C A bed made with the person in it.
6. A The bed is made to transfer a person from a stretcher to the bed. Also called a postoperative bed or recovery bed.

Fill in the Blanks

7. What must you do to keep beds neat and clean?

   A. ______________________________

   B. ______________________________

   C. ______________________________

   D. ______________________________

   E. ______________________________

   F. ______________________________

8. When handling linen and making beds, practice ______________________________.

9. When removing dirty linen, roll the linen ______________________________ from you.

10. A closed bed becomes an open bed by ______________________________.

11. In hospitals which linens are changed daily?

    ____

12. Linens are changed right away if ______________________________.

13. Why is it important to never mix ammonia with bleach or other chemicals?

    ____

14. You brought an extra bottom sheet into a patient's room. What should you do with it?

    ____

15. List 5 safety measures for crib bumper pads.

    A. ______________________________

    B. ______________________________

    C. ______________________________

    D. ______________________________

    E. ______________________________

16. Why is it important to know the person's treatment, therapy, and activity schedule before making the person's bed?

    ____

17. In long-term care and home care, what type of bed is made for persons who are up for most or all of the day?

    ____

18. Why are gloves worn when removing soiled linens from a bed?

    ____

19. List 5 safety measures to practice when making an occupied bed.

    A. ______________________

    B. ______________________

    C. ______________________

    D. ______________________

    E. ______________________

20. When are surgical beds made?

    A. ______________________

    B. ______________________

    C. ______________________

    D. ______________________

21. What should you do after you transfer a person to a surgical bed?

____

____

____

22. Why should you make as much of one side of the bed as possible before going to the other side?

____

23. How is the pillow placed on the bed?

____

____

Multiple Choice

Circle the BEST answer.

24. Linens are changed
    A. Once a week.
    B. When you have time.
    C. Whenever they become wet, soiled, or damp.
    D. Whenever they are loose or wrinkled.

25. When handling linens and making beds, which is *incorrect?*
    A. Hold linens away from your body and uniform.
    B. Clean linens are placed on clean surfaces.
    C. Never shake linens in the air.
    D. Place soiled linens on the floor.

26. You bring extra linens to a room. The extra linens are
    A. Used for another person.
    B. Considered contaminated.
    C. Returned to the linen closet.
    D. Placed on the floor.

27. A plastic drawsheet
    A. Protects the mattress and bottom linen from dampness and soiling.
    B. Is placed on all beds.
    C. Can be placed on the bed without a cotton drawsheet.
    D. Is changed every day.

28. In the home, you can use plastic trash bags or dry cleaning bags in place of a plastic draw-sheet.
    A. True
    B. False

29. Cribs and crib linens present safety hazards. Which statement is *false?*
    A. The crib mattress must be soft.
    B. The mattress must fit snuggly to the crib frame.
    C. Bumper pads are secured in place with at least six ties.
    D. Pillows are not used for babies.

ADDITIONAL LEARNING ACTIVITIES

1. Carefully review the procedures in Chapter 15.
   A. Use the procedure checklists on pages 294 through 301 as a guide.
   B. Use good body mechanics.
   C. Take a turn being the patient or resident when an occupied bed is made.
      (1) Discuss the experience. Did you feel safe and comfortable?

2. Practice gathering linen in the correct order.

3. List the correct order for gathering linen on an index card. Carry the card with you until you have the order memorized.

16

-2

Personal Hygiene

OBJECTIVES

The questions and student activities in this chapter will help you meet these objectives.

- Define the key terms listed in Chapter 16
- Explain why personal hygiene is important
- Describe the care given before and after breakfast, after lunch, and in the evening
- Describe the rules for bathing
- Identify the safety measures for tub baths and showers
- Explain the purposes of a back massage
- Explain the purposes of perineal care
- Identify the observations to make while assisting with hygiene
- Perform the procedures described in Chapter16

STUDY QUESTIONS

Complete the Crossword

Across

3. Breathing fluid or an object into the lungs
5. Hardened plaque on teeth

Down

1. Cleansing the genital and anal areas
2. A thin film that sticks to the teeth
4. Evening or PM care

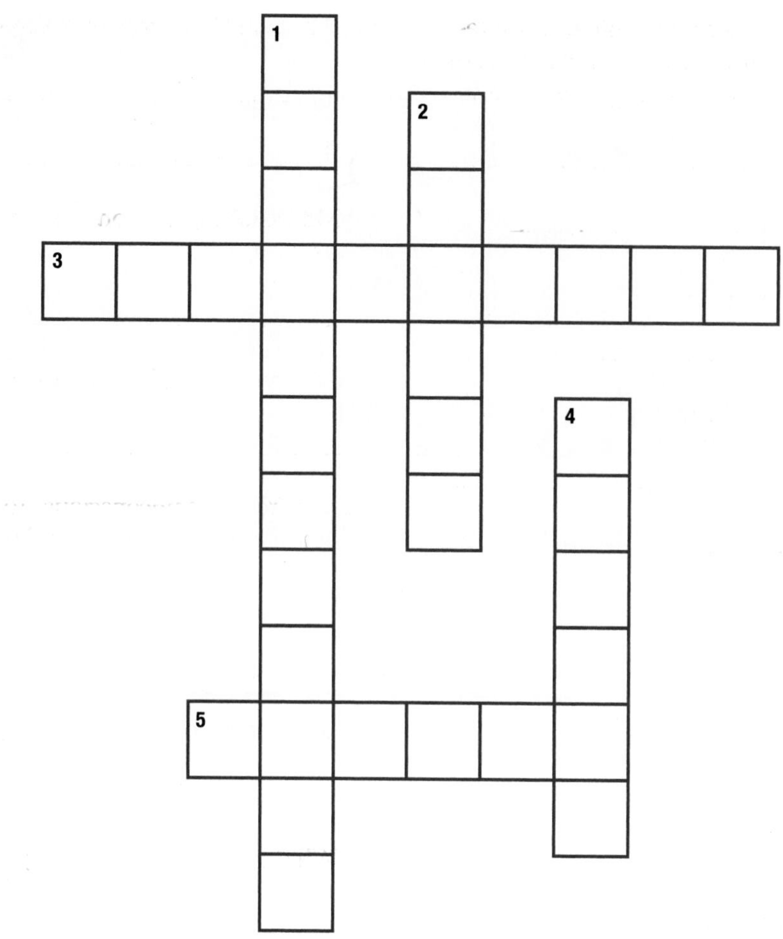

Matching

Match the following terms with the correct definitions.

1. e Routine care before breakfast
2. C Care given at bedtime
3. B Care given after breakfast; hygiene measures are more thorough at this time
4. D Mouth care
5. a Perineal care

A. Pericare
B. Morning care
C. Evening care
D. Oral hygiene
E. Early morning care (AM care)

Fill in the Blanks

6. Hygiene promotes ______________________, ______________________, and ______________________.

7. Intact skin prevents ______________________ from entering the body.

8. To meet the person's hygiene needs, you must follow ______________________ and ______________________.

9. Miss Peters is a nursing center resident. She resists your efforts to assist with washing her face and hands. List 4 reasons she might resist care.

   A. ______________________

   B. ______________________

   C. ______________________

   D. ______________________

10. Oral hygiene does the following:

    A. ______________________

    B. ______________________

    C. ______________________

    D. ______________________

    E. ______________________

11. ______________________ is an inflammation of the tissues around the teeth caused by tartar buildup.

12. What information do you need from the nurse and the care plan before you assist with oral hygiene?

    A. ______________________

    B. ______________________

    C. ______________________

    D. ______________________

    E. ______________________

    F. ______________________

    G. ______________________

13. List 3 reasons to follow Standard Precautions and the Bloodborne Pathogen Standard when giving oral hygiene.

    A. ______________________

    B. ______________________

    C. ______________________

14. What are the purposes of flossing teeth?

    A. ______________________

    B. ______________________

15. Mr. Watson flosses once a day. What is the best time for him to floss?

    ____

16. At what age should flossing begin?

    ____

17. Mrs. Young is unconscious. To prevent aspiration when assisting with her oral hygiene, you must:

    A. ______________________

    ____

    B. ______________________

    ____

18. What should you use to keep Mrs. Young's mouth open while giving oral hygiene?

    ____

    ____

19. List 6 reasons that bathing is important.

    A. ______________________

    B. ______________________

    C. ______________________

    D. ______________________

    E. ______________________

    F. ______________________

20. Bathing method depends on

    ______________________,

    ______________________,

    and ______________________.

21. The purpose of bath oils is to

____

______________________________.

22. What safety precautions are needed when using bath oils?

____

____

23. Powders are used to

____

______________________________.

24. Excessive amounts of powder cause

____

______________________________.

25. Mrs. Vance has dementia. Bathing frightens her. What measures might be part of her care plan to help her through the bathing procedure?

A. ______________________________

B. ______________________________

C. ______________________________

D. ______________________________

E. ______________________________

F. ______________________________

G. ______________________________

26. You have finished giving Mrs. Vance a bath. What observations do you report and record?

A. ______________________________

B. ______________________________

C. ______________________________

D. ______________________________

E. ______________________________

F. ______________________________

G. ______________________________

H. ______________________________

I. ______________________________

J. ______________________________

27. Water temperature for a complete bed bath is usually ______________________________ ______________________________ for adults.

28. The partial bath involves bathing the

______________________________,

______________________________,

______________________________,

______________________________,

______________________________,

and ______________________________.

29. What are the risks when taking tub baths and showers?

A. ______________________________

B. ______________________________

C. ______________________________

30. How long does a tub bath last?

____

31. What is the usual water temperature for tub baths and showers?

____

32. You observe the skin when giving a back massage. What should you look for?

A. ______________________

B. ______________________

C. ______________________

D. ______________________

33. Lotion is warmed before being applied. List 3 ways to warm lotion before applying it.

A. ______________________

B. ______________________

C. ______________________

34. Back massages are dangerous for persons with

______________________,

______________________,

______________________,

______________________,

and ______________________.

35. Perineal care involves cleaning the genital and anal areas. Why is this important?

____

____

36. ______________________,

______________________,

and ______________________ are followed when giving perineal care.

37. When giving perineal care, you work from the cleanest area to the dirtiest. This means that you clean from the ______________________ to the ______________________.

38. You have finished giving perineal care to Mrs. Ruiz. What observations do you need to report and record?

A. ______________________

B. ______________________

C. ______________________

D. ______________________

39. Why is it important to report and record the care you give?

____

____

____

40. List 2 Hindu beliefs about bathing.

A. ______________________

____

B. ______________________

____

Multiple Choice

Circle the BEST answer.

41. When providing mouth care to the unconscious person
    A. Use your fingers to hold the mouth open.
    B. Position the person on his or her back.
    C. Explain what you are doing step by step.
    D. Use a hard bristle toothbrush.

42. How often is mouth care given to unconscious persons?
    A. At least every 2 hours
    B. Twice a day
    C. Every 4 hours
    D. Every 6 hours

43. You should always use a hard bristle toothbrush when brushing teeth.
    A. True
    B. False

44. When cleaning dentures
   A. Use hot water.
   B. Firmly hold them over a basin of water lined with a towel.
   C. Store them dry in a container with a lid.
   D. Clean the dentures at the bedside.

45. Which statement about bathing an older person is *true?*
   A. A complete bath is needed twice a week.
   B. Always use soap.
   C. Thorough rinsing is needed when using soap.
   D. Briskly rub the skin dry.

46. You are giving Mr. Jones a complete bed bath. Do all of the following *except*
   A. Expose only the body part needed.
   B. Change the water if it is soapy or cool.
   C. Provide for privacy.
   D. Keep the bed in the lowest horizontal position.

47. Lower water temperatures are used when bathing infants and older persons.
   A. True
   B. False

48. You are giving Mrs. Smith a tub bath. Which is *true?*
   A. The bath should last 30 minutes.
   B. Burns and falls are a risk.
   C. Use bath oils in the water.
   D. Drain the tub after Mrs. Smith gets out of the tub.

49. When assisting the person with a bath, you must do all of the following *except*
   A. Provide for privacy.
   B. Reduce drafts by closing doors and windows.
   C. Protect the person from falling.
   D. Do everything for the person.

50. Which action will *not* promote safety when giving tub baths or showers?
   A. Cleaning the tub or shower before and after use
   B. Placing a bath mat in the tub or on the shower floor
   C. Turning hot water on first, then cold water
   D. Placing the signal light within the person's reach

51. Towel bars can be used for support when the person gets in and out of the tub.
   A. True
   B. False

52. Powder is not used near persons with respiratory difficulties.
   A. True
   B. False

53. When giving a back massage
   A. Keep your hands in contact with the person's skin.
   B. Use circular strokes over the back.
   C. Massage bony areas.
   D. Use short, gentle strokes.

54. A back massage is safe for all persons.
   A. True
   B. False

55. Which position is best for a back massage?
   A. Sim's position
   B. The left side-lying
   C. The prone position
   D. The horizontal position

ADDITIONAL LEARNING ACTIVITIES

1. Discuss the importance of hygiene and cleanliness in your personal life. Answer these questions.
   A. How important is it for you to feel clean and free from unpleasant odors when you are around other people? Explain.
   B. What care routines do you practice daily to promote your cleanliness?

2. Have illnesses ever prevented you from carrying out your personal daily hygiene routines? Explain.
   A. Discuss how this affected your personal comfort.
   B. Discuss how your experiences will help you meet the hygiene needs of the persons you care for.

3. The procedures in this chapter require you to provide personal care to another person. They must be performed in a way that respects the person's privacy and dignity. It will help you to understand how the person feels if you practice the procedures with a classmate. Take your turn being the patient or resident. Under the supervision of your instructor, use the procedure checklist provided on pages 302 through 326 to practice the procedures in Chapter 16. Use a simulator to practice female and male perineal care.
   A. After practicing each procedure, discuss your experience.
   B. Discuss how your experience will help you provide better care.

4. Read the vignette. Then answer the questions that follow.
   Mr. Sanchez is a patient on the medical unit in Valley View Hospital. He is on bed rest with bathroom privileges. He is weak and tires easily. He has heart disease and becomes short of breath with too much exertion. You have been assigned to care for him.

   Mr. Sanchez needs assistance with a bed bath and oral hygiene. He has his own teeth.The nurse tells you that Mr. Sanchez is a very quiet and shy person. He has never been in the hospital before. When at home, he is used to taking a shower every day.
   A. What additional information do you need from the nurse and the care plan before you begin?
   B. Will you give Mr. Sanchez a back massage? Explain.
   C. What fears and concerns might Mr. Sanchez have?
   D. Do you think that Mr. Sanchez will be comfortable with you giving him a bed bath? Explain.
   E. What will you do to promote his comfort and safety?
      (1) How will you promote his right to privacy?
      (2) How will you promote his right to personal choice?
   F. What items do you need to collect to assist Mr. Sanchez with oral hygiene?
   G. What items do you need to collect to assist Mr. Sanchez with his bed bath?
   H. What observations will you report to the nurse after assisting Mr. Sanchez with oral hygiene?
   I. What observations will you report to the nurse after assisting Mr. Sanchez with his bed bath?
   J. Why are good skin care, good body alignment, and frequent position changes important for Mr. Sanchez?

17

Grooming

OBJECTIVES

The questions and student activities in this chapter will help you meet these objectives.

- Define the key terms listed in Chapter 17
- Explain why grooming is important
- Identify the factors that affect hair care
- Explain how to care for matted and tangled hair
- Describe how to shampoo hair
- Describe the measures practiced when shaving a person
- Explain why nail and foot care are important
- Describe the rules for changing gowns and clothing
- Perform the procedures described in Chapter 17

STUDY QUESTIONS

Matching

Match the following terms with the correct definitions.

1. __C__ Hair loss
2. __G__ The excessive amount of dry, white flakes from the scalp
3. __B__ Excessive body hair in women and children
4. __f__ The infestation with lice
5. __D__ The infestation of the scalp with lice
6. __a__ The infestation of the body with lice
7. __e__ The infestation of the pubic hair with lice

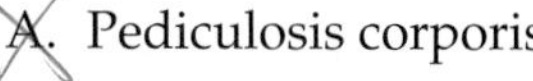
A. Pediculosis corporis

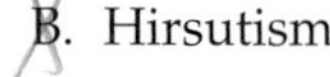
B. Hirsutism

C. Alopecia

D. Pediculosis capitis

E. Pediculosis pubis

F. Pediculosis

G. Dandruff

Fill in the Blanks

8. Grooming measures prevent

_______________ and

promote _______________.

They also affect _______________,

_______________, and

_______________ needs.

9. The nurse tells you what hair care is needed for each person. The nursing process reflects the person's _______________,

_______________,

_______________,

_______________,

and _______________.

10. List 8 causes of alopecia.

A. _______________

B. _______________

C. _______________

D. _______________

E. _______________

F. _______________

G. _______________

H. _______________

11. Hirsutism results from _______________

and _______________.

12. How do lice spread to others?

____

____

____

13. When is hair care done?

____

____

14. When brushing and combing hair, start at the

_______________.

15. What are the steps involved in combing through matted or tangled hair?

A. _______________

B. _______________

C. _______________

D. _______________

E. _______________

16. How would you comb curly hair?

____

____

____

____

17. How do you protect the person's garments when giving hair care?

____

____

18. You are assisting Mr. Crane with hair care. What observations do you need to report and record?

A. _______________

B. _______________

C. _______________

D. _______________

E. _______________

19. List 4 shampooing methods.

A. ______

B. ______

C. ______

D. ______

20. You are shampooing Miss Martin's hair. What observations do you need to report and record?

A. ______

B. ______

C. ______

D. ______

21. You used a medicated shampoo for Miss Martin. What should you do with the shampoo when you are finished shampooing Miss Martin's hair?

______

22. Why are safety razors *not* used for persons with dementia?

______

______

______

23. Discard razor blades and disposable shavers in the ______.

24. Nail and foot care prevents

______,

______,

and ______.

25. You are giving foot care to Miss Martin. What observations do you need to report and record?

A. ______

B. ______

C. ______

D. ______

E. ______

26. You do *not* cut or trim toenails if a person:

A. ______

B. ______

C. ______

D. ______

27. List the rules to follow when helping a person change gowns and clothing.

A. ______

______

B. ______

______

C. ______

______

D. ______

______

E. ______

______

F. ______

______

28. What information do you need from the nurse and the care plan before changing a person's clothing?

A. ______

B. ______

C. ______

Multiple Choice

Circle the BEST answer.

29. Brushing and combing hair is:
   A. Part of AM care.
   B. Done when you have time.
   C. Not your responsibility.
   D. Always done by the patient or resident.

30. Which statement about assisting with hair care is *true?*
   A. You decide how to style the person's hair.
   B. You can cut matted and tangled hair.
   C. Braid long hair to keep it neat.
   D. The person chooses how to brush, comb, and style hair.

31. Dandruff can occur in the eyebrows and ear canals.
   A. True
   B. False

32. The shampooing method used depends on all of the following *except*
   A. Personal choice.
   B. Safety factors.
   C. The person's condition.
   D. How busy you are.

33. You must ask the nurse before shampooing a person's hair.
   A. True
   B. False

34. These statements are about shaving a person. Which is *false?*
   A. Follow Standard Precautions and the Bloodborne Pathogen Standard.
   B. Use electric shavers for persons taking anticoagulant drugs.
   C. Hold the skin taut as needed.
   D. Shave against hair growth when shaving the face and underarms.

35. You have nicked Mr. Jay's face while shaving him. What should you do?
   A. Put a Band-Aid on the area.
   B. Apply a small piece of tissue to the area.
   C. Apply direct pressure to the nick.
   D. Call the nurse at once.

36. Mr. White has a beard. Do all of the following *except*
   A. Wash and comb the beard daily.
   B. Trim the beard once a week.
   C. Ask Mr. White how to groom his beard.
   D. Wash the beard whenever mouth or nose drainage is present.

37. When trimming fingernails
   A. Let the fingernails soak for 30 minutes before starting.
   B. Clip the fingernails in a curved shape.
   C. Be careful not to damage surrounding tissue.
   D. Use a scissors.

38. Mr. Juarez has an IV pump. The IV is in his left arm. You are putting on a standard gown. Which is *correct?*
   A. Disconnect the IV pump while changing his gown.
   B. His left arm is not put through the sleeve.
   C. Put the gown on the right arm first.
   D. Put the gown on the left arm first.

ADDITIONAL LEARNING ACTIVITIES

1. List the grooming activities you perform every day. Answer these questions.
   A. How important are your grooming routines?
   B. How important is personal choice when you are performing your grooming activities?
   C. How important is privacy when you are performing your grooming activities?
   D. How would you feel if you were unable to perform your grooming activities?
      (1) How would you want to be treated?

2. Read the vignette. Then answer the questions that follow.
   Mr. Benson is a nursing center resident. He has weakness on his left side. He is taking an anticoagulant drug. You have been assigned to shave him. You will also remove his gown and dress him for the day. He is able to follow directions and assist with his care.
   A. What type of razor will you use? Why?
   B. What items do you need to collect to shave Mr. Benson?
   C. What safety measures will you practice when shaving Mr. Benson?
   D. How will you provide for Mr. Benson's privacy?
   E. What will you do when you finish the procedure?
   F. What information do you need from the nurse and the care plan before you dress Mr. Benson?
   G. How will you remove Mr. Benson's gown?
   H. How will you promote Mr. Benson's right to personal choice?
   I. Mr. Benson has chosen a shirt that buttons in the front. How will you put on the shirt?
   J. How will you put on Mr. Benson's pants?
   K. What will you do when you finish the procedure?

3. Read the vignette. Then answer the questions that follow.
   Mrs. Dunn is an 80-year-old patient. You will be shampooing her hair during her tub bath. She wants to use the shampoo she brought from home. The nurse tells you that Mrs. Dunn has an open area the size of a dime on top of her head.
   Mrs. Dunn has arthritis and is unable to tip her head back.
   A. What additional information do you need from the nurse and the care plan before you shampoo Mrs. Dunn's hair?
   B. Can you use the shampoo that Mrs. Dunn brought from home? Explain.
   C. How can you promote Mrs. Dunn's right to personal choice?
   D. What safety measures will you practice when shampooing Mrs. Dunn's hair?
   E. How will you keep shampoo out of Mrs. Dunn's eyes?
   F. How will you promote Mrs. Dunn's right to privacy?
   G. How will you shampoo Mrs. Dunn's hair?
   H. What observations do you need to report and record?

4. Carefully review the procedures in Chapter 17. Under the supervision of your instructor, use the procedure checklists on pages 327 through 342 to practice each procedure.
   A. Practice dressing and undressing procedures with classmates or family members.
      (1) Use different types of clothing. (For example: clothes that open in front and clothes that open in back, button and pullover shirts, pants with zippers and buttons and pants that pull on.)
      (2) Role-play weakness on one side of the body.
      (3) Role-play that the person is not able to help.
      (4) Take your turn being the patient or resident.
   B. Discuss the experience.
      (1) How will your experience affect how you help others with grooming and dressing activities?

18 Comfort, Rest, and Sleep

OBJECTIVES

The questions and student activities in this chapter will help you meet these objectives.

- Define the key terms listed in Chapter 18
- Explain why comfort, rest, and sleep are important
- Explain how to promote comfort
- Describe four types of pain and the factors that affect pain
- List the signs and symptoms of pain
- List the nursing measures that relieve pain
- Explain why meeting basic needs is important for rest
- Identify when rest is needed
- Describe the factors that affect sleep and the common sleep disorders
- Explain how circadian rhythm affects sleep
- Describe the stages of sleep
- Know the sleep requirements for each age-group
- List the nursing measures that promote rest and sleep

STUDY QUESTIONS

Matching

Match the following terms with the correct definitions.

A. Comfort
B. REM sleep
C. Insomnia
D. Pain
E. Acute pain
F. Enuresis
G. Relaxation
H. Sleep
I. Chronic pain
J. NREM sleep
K. Radiating pain
L. Rest
M. Phantom pain
N. Guided imagery
O. Circadian rhythm
P. Distraction

1. ______ Pain that is felt suddenly from injury, disease, trauma, or surgery
2. ______ Pain lasting longer than 6 months; it is constant or occurs off and on

3. O A daily rhythm pattern based on a 24-hour cycle

4. d A state of well-being; the person has no physical or emotional pain and is calm and at peace

5. D To ache, hurt, or be sore; discomfort

6. P To change the person's center of attention

7. f Urinary incontinence in bed at night

8. n Creating and focusing on an image

9. C A chronic condition in which the person cannot sleep or stay asleep all night

10. J The phase of sleep when there is no rapid eye movement; non-REM sleep

11. m Pain felt in a body part that is no longer there

12. K Pain felt at the site of tissue damage and in nearby areas

13. G To be free from mental and physical stress

14. B The phase of sleep when there is rapid eye movement

15. L To be calm, at ease, and relaxed; no anxiety and stress

16. H A state of unconsciousness, reduced voluntary muscle activity, and lowered metabolism

Fill in the Blanks

17. How do comfort, rest, and sleep problems affect the person?

____

____

18. Rest and sleep restore _______________ and _______________.

19. _______________ and _______________ increase the need for rest and sleep.

20. List the OBRA room requirements that promote comfort, rest, and sleep.

A. _______________

B. _______________

C. _______________

D. _______________

E. _______________

F. _______________

G. _______________

H. _______________

I. _______________

J. _______________

K. _______________

21. List 8 factors that affect comfort.

A. _______________

B. _______________

C. _______________

D. _______________

E. ______________________________

F. ______________________________

G. ______________________________

H. ______________________________

22. What can you do to protect infants, older persons, and those who are ill from drafts?

A. ______________________________

B. ______________________________

C. ______________________________

D. ______________________________

23. Why are older persons sensitive to cold?

____

____

24. ______________________________,

______________________________, and

______________________________ help

prevent odors.

25. If you smoke, you must ____________________

______________________________ after handling

smoking materials and before giving care.

26. You decrease noise in health care agencies by:

A. ______________________________

B. ______________________________

C. ______________________________

D. ______________________________

27. Good lighting is needed for ____________________

and ______________________________.

28. Comfort and discomfort are subjective. What does this mean?

____

____

29. In the Philippines, pain is viewed as

______________________________.

30. In China, showing emotion is

______________________________.

Therefore pain is often ____________________.

31. Gallbladder disease can cause pain in the right upper abdomen, the back, and the right shoulder. What kind of pain is this?

____

32. Mr. Smith's right arm was amputated a year ago. He still senses pain in his right arm. What kind if pain is this?

____

33. List 9 factors that affect a person's reaction to pain.

A. ______________________________

B. ______________________________

C. ______________________________

D. ______________________________

E. ______________________________

F. ______________________________

G. ______________________________

H. ______________________________

I. ______________________________

34. How are pain and anxiety related?

____

____

35. Why does pain often seem worse at night?

____

____

____

36. Dealing with pain is often easier when family and friends offer ______________________________.

37. Miss Ryan has dementia. What might signal that she has pain?

____

38. What information does the nurse need to assess the person's pain?

A. ______________________________

B. ______________________________

C. ______________________________

D. ______________________________

E. ______________________________

F. ______________________________

G. ______________________________

39. Factors causing pain are called

______________________________.

40. List 5 body responses to pain.

A. ______________________________

B. ______________________________

C. ______________________________

D. ______________________________

E. ______________________________

41. Drugs given to relieve pain can cause

______________________________,

______________________________,

______________________________, and

______________________________.

42. What safety measures are practiced when a person is receiving strong pain-relieving drugs?

A. ______________________________

B. ______________________________

C. ______________________________

D. ______________________________

E. ______________________________

F. ______________________________

43. Why must you check with the nurse before picking up and holding a child?

____

____

44. During which phase of sleep does mental restoration occur?

____

45. List 7 factors that affect the amount and quality of sleep.

A. ______________________________

B. ______________________________

C. ______________________________

D. ______________________________

E. ______________________________

F. ______________________________

G. ______________________________

46. Alcohol causes drowsiness and sleep. However, it interferes with ______________________________.

47. Describe the 3 forms of insomnia.

A. ______________________________

B. ______________________________

C. ______________________________

48. With sleep deprivation the ______________

and ______________________________

of sleep are decreased.

Multiple Choice

Circle the BEST answer.

49. Comfort, rest, and sleep
   A. Are needed for well-being.
   B. Affect the total person.
   C. Are affected by pain.
   D. All of the above are correct.

50. Which room temperature range is usually comfortable for most healthy people?
   A. 68° F to 74° F
   B. 75° F to 80° F
   C. 65° F to 68° F
   D. 82° F to 90° F

51. Infants and older persons often need higher room temperatures for comfort.
   A. True
   B. False

52. Comfort and discomfort are subjective. This means
   A. You can see, hear, touch, and smell the person's comfort or discomfort.
   B. The person cannot explain his or her discomfort to you.
   C. You must rely on what the person tells you.
   D. You do not report complaints of discomfort to the nurse.

53. Persons with decreased sensation to pain are at increased risk for undetected disease or injury.
   A. True
   B. False

54. Which statement about pain in children is *true?*
   A. Children may not understand pain.
   B. Children know more ways of dealing with pain than do adults.
   C. Children usually have a lot of pain experiences.
   D. It is easy for children to relieve their pain.

55. Which of these measures will *not* promote comfort?
   A. Giving a back massage
   B. Providing soft music
   C. Keeping the room cool and well lighted
   D. Good body alignment

56. Mr. White receives strong pain medication every four hours. You provide for his safety by
   A. Keeping the bed in the highest position.
   B. Checking on him every 3 hours.
   C. Asking family members to leave.
   D. Providing assistance when he is up.

57. You help promote a person's safety and security needs by doing all of the following *except*
   A. Keeping the signal light within reach.
   B. Explaining treatments to the person.
   C. Following the person's routines and rituals.
   D. Checking on the person every 4 hours.

58. Which statement about sleep is *false?*
   A. Tissue healing and repair occur during sleep.
   B. Body functions speed up.
   C. Sleep is a basic need.
   D. Sleep is a part of circadian rhythm.

59. Health care often interferes with a person's circadian rhythm and the sleep-wake cycle.
   A. True
   B. False

60. The amount of sleep needed increases with age.
   A. True
   B. False

61. Which is *not* a symptom of sleep deprivation?
   A. Irritability
   B. Irregular pulse
   C. Increased attention span
   D. Slurred speech

62. Mrs. Adams asks for a bedtime snack. Which will *not* help promote sleep?
   A. Coffee and a brownie
   B. Milk
   C. Toast
   D. Crackers and milk

63. Danny Fisher is walking in his sleep. You should
    A. Allow him to walk about until he wakes up on his own.
    B. Play soft, relaxing music.
    C. Take him back to his room and restrain him in bed.
    D. Protect him from injury and guide him back to bed.

64. Which measure promotes sleep?
    A. Exercising before bedtime
    B. Making sure the person is in bed by 2000
    C. Reducing noise
    D. Providing a bedtime snack of hot chocolate

ADDITIONAL LEARNING ACTIVITIES

1. Make a list of factors that affect your comfort. Answer these questions:
    A. What temperatures are most comfortable for you?
    B. How do you adapt to changes in temperature?
    C. Are there certain odors that cause you discomfort?
    D. How do you control the odors in your environment?
    E. How do noises and sounds affect your comfort?
        (1) What sounds decrease your comfort?
        (2) What sounds help you relax?
    F. How do you control the light in your environment to meet your comfort needs?
    G. How will you use what you know about your comfort needs to help you provide better care?

2. Think of an experience you have had with pain. Answer these questions:
    A. What caused the pain?
    B. What type of pain was it?
    C. What words would you use to describe the pain?
    D. How intense was the pain?
    E. How did it affect your daily activities?
    F. What factors affected your reaction to the pain?
    G. What measures did you use to relieve the pain?
    H. How will your personal experience with pain affect how you care for persons with pain?

3. Think about your needs for rest and sleep. Answer these questions:
   A. How much sleep do you need to feel rested?
   B. Do you have certain rituals that help you sleep? Explain.
   C. What are some physical and psychological factors that prevent you from sleeping well?
   D. How does lack of sleep and rest affect your daily activities?
   E. How will you use what you know about your needs for rest to help you provide better care?

4. Read the vignette. Then answer the questions that follow.
   Miss Ann Green is a patient on the orthopedic unit at Center Hospital. She is 70 years old. She has a diagnosis of a fractured left wrist. The fracture was surgically repaired. Miss Green also has rheumatoid arthritis. She has had two surgeries in the past 6 years related to her arthritis. She was in the hospital for pneumonia 2 years ago.

   Miss Green receives pain-relieving drugs as needed for pain related to the surgical repair of her left wrist. She receives routine pain-relieving drugs related to her rheumatoid arthritis. Frequent position changes are needed. She requires assistance with ADL.

   Miss Green's friend visits her every day and often reads to her before she goes to sleep. This helps Miss Green fall asleep. The friend is taking care of Miss Green's dog until she returns home.
   A. What types of pain is Miss Green likely to have? Explain.
   B. What factors might affect her pain?
   C. What questions will you ask Miss Green about her pain to help the nurse assess the pain?
   D. What safety measures will you practice when caring for Miss Green?
   E. Why are frequent position changes an important part of Miss Green's care?
   F. How will you promote Miss Green's comfort when assisting with position changes?

5. Read the vignette. Then answer the questions that follow.
   John Frank is 8 years old. He had an emergency appendectomy (his appendix was removed surgically). This is his first day after surgery. Sometimes he cries because he is having pain. His mother tells you that he is embarrassed. His care plan involves deep breathing and coughing every 2 hours during the day. John is embarrassed when he needs assistance to and from the bathroom.

   His mother and father take turns staying with him day and night. John has never been in the hospital before. He is missing a trip to the zoo and museum with his scout troop.
   A. What type of pain is John having?
   B. What factors might be affecting his pain?
   C. How can you meet John's comfort needs when helping him with deep breathing and coughing?
   D. How will you meet John's needs for privacy?

19

Urinary Elimination

OBJECTIVES

The questions and student activities in this chapter will help you meet these objectives.

- Define the key terms listed in Chapter 19
- Describe normal urine
- Describe the rules for normal urination
- Describe urinary incontinence and the care required
- Explain why catheters are used
- Explain how to care for persons with catheters
- Describe straight, indwelling, and condom catheters
- Explain the purpose of bladder irrigations
- Describe two methods of bladder training
- Perform the procedures described in Chapter 19

STUDY QUESTIONS

Complete the Crossword

Across

3. Scant amount of urine
7. Blood in the urine
8. The process of emptying urine from the bladder: micturition, or voiding

Down

1. Abnormally large amounts of urine
2. Urination or voiding
4. Used by men for urinating
5. Painful or difficult urination
6. A tube used to drain or inject fluid through a body opening

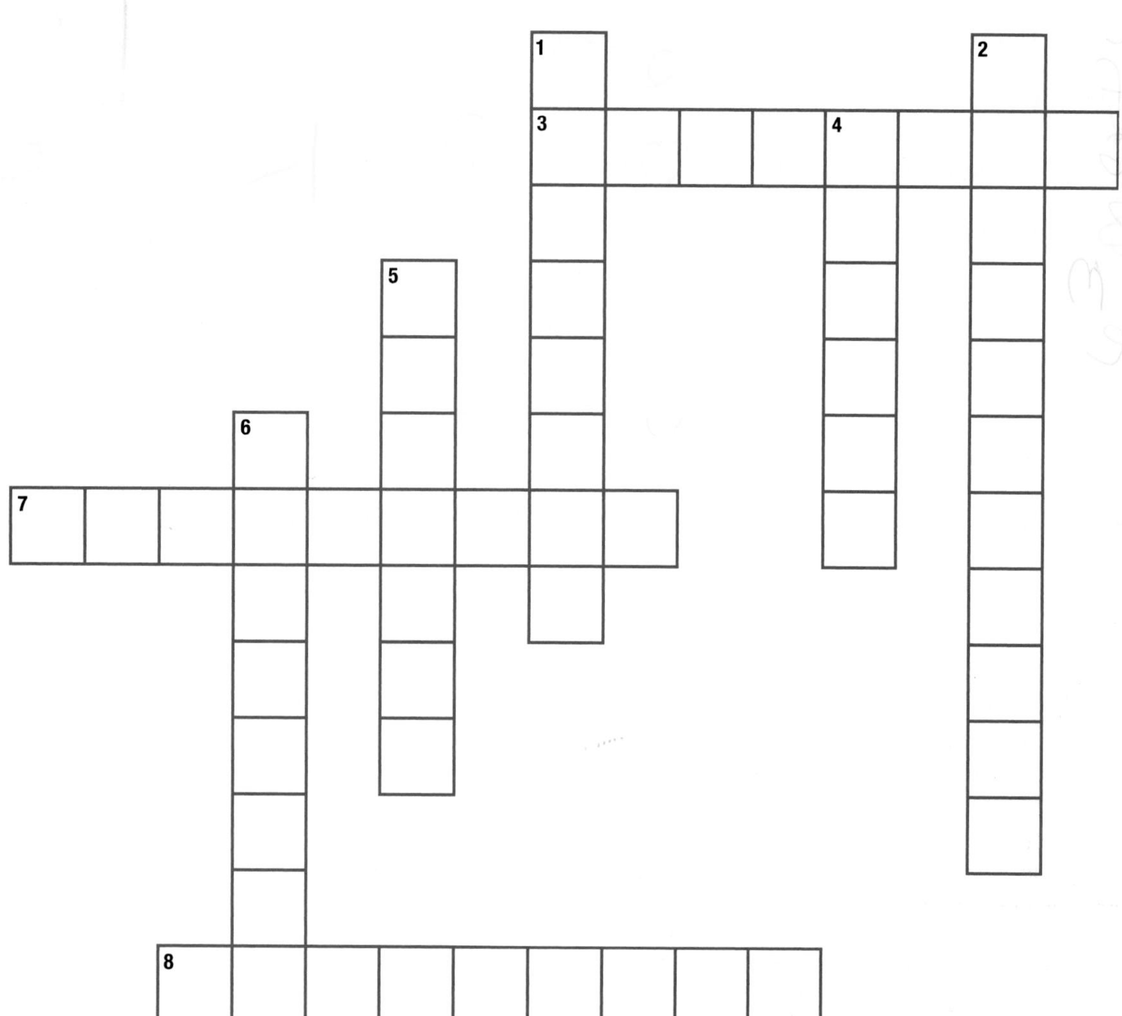

Matching

Match the following terms with the correct definitions.

A. Overflow incontinence
B. Urinary frequency
C. Residual urine
D. Functional incontinence
E. Urinary urgency
F. Stress incontinence
G. Mixed incontinence
H. Reflex incontinence
I. Urge incontinence
J. Irrigation
K. Catheterization
L. Nocturia
M. Urinary incontinence

1. K The process of inserting a catheter
2. D The person has bladder control, but cannot use the toilet in time
3. J The process of washing out, flushing out, clearing, or cleaning a tube or body cavity
4. G When more than one type of incontinence is present
5. L Frequent urination at night
6. a Urine leaks when the bladder is too full
7. H The loss of urine at predictable intervals when the bladder is full

8. C The amount of urine left in the bladder after voiding

9. f When urine leaks during exercise and certain movements

10. G The loss of urine in response to a sudden, urgent need to void

11. B Voiding at frequent intervals

12. M The loss of bladder control

13. e The need to void at once

Fill in the Blanks

14. Which systems remove waste from the body?

    A. __________

    B. __________

    C. __________

    D. __________

15. The __________ removes waste products from the blood and maintains the body's water balance.

16. List 7 factors that affect urine production.

    A. __________

    B. __________

    C. __________

    D. __________

    E. __________

    F. __________

    G. __________

17. Why is it important to tell the nurse if an infant does not have a wet diaper for several hours?

    ____

    ____

18. Urine is observed for __________, __________, __________, __________, and __________.

19. A fracture pan is a bed pan with a thin rim. Fracture pans are used:

    A. __________

    B. __________

    C. __________

    D. __________

    E. __________

20. You assist Mrs. Lind with urinary elimination. What do you need to report and record?

    A. __________

    B. __________

    C. __________

    D. __________

    E. __________

    F. __________

    G. __________

    H. __________

I. ______________________________

J. ______________________________

K. ______________________________

21. Mrs. Lind cannot assist in getting on the bedpan. How will you give her the bedpan?

A. ______________________________

____

B. ______________________________

____

C. ______________________________

____

D. ______________________________

____

E. ______________________________

____

22. Why are urinals *not* placed on overbed tables or bedside stands?

____

____

____

23. What information do you need from the nurse and the care plan before assisting with urinals?

A. ______________________________

B. ______________________________

C. ______________________________

D. ______________________________

E. ______________________________

24. Mr. Lopez stands to use the urinal. How do you give him the urinal?

A. ______________________________

B. ______________________________

C. ______________________________

D. ______________________________

25. Why are urinals emptied promptly?

____

____

____

26. A ______________________________ is a chair or wheelchair with an opening for the bedpan or container.

27. List 4 causes of urge incontinence.

A. ______________________________

B. ______________________________

C. ______________________________

D. ______________________________

28. List 3 measures that help prevent urinary tract infections.

A. ______________________________

B. ______________________________

C. ______________________________

29. Miss Breeze is incontinent of urine. She is at risk for:

A. ______________________________

B. ______________________________

C. ______________________________

D. ______________________________

30. Caring for persons with incontinence is stressful. What should you do if you find yourself becoming impatient?

____

____

31. A(n) _______________ is left in the bladder. Urine drains from the bladder constantly.

32. You are giving catheter care to Mr. Green. What observations do you need to report and record?

A. _______________

B. _______________

C. _______________

D. _______________

E. _______________

33. Why is a closed drainage system used for indwelling catheters?

____

____

____

34. Why must the urinary drainage bag be kept lower than the bladder?

____

____

____

35. What should you do if a urinary drainage system is accidentally disconnected?

A. _______________

B. _______________

C. _______________

D. _______________

E. _______________

F. _______________

G. _______________

36. You empty Mr. Green's urinary drainage bag at the end of your shift. What observations do you need to report and record?

A. _______________

B. _______________

C. _______________

D. _______________

E. _______________

37. A straight catheter is used to:

A. _______________

B. _______________

38. Greg Lewis is 15. He has an erection while you are preparing to insert an indwelling catheter. What should you do?

____

____

39. Before performing a catheterization, you must make sure that:

A. _______________

B. _______________

C. _______________

D. _______________

E. _______________

F. _______________

G. _______________

40. Why should you get an extra catheter and an extra pair of gloves when you collect your equipment and supplies to perform a catheterization?

____

____

41. You are catheterizing Miss Hall. You insert the catheter into the vagina. What should you do?

____

____

____

____

____

____

42. Before removing a catheter, make sure that:

A. _______________

B. _______________

C. _______________

D. _______________

E. _______________

F. _______________

43. If allowed to remove catheters and other needed conditions are met, what information do you need from the nurse before removing a catheter?

A. _______________

B. _______________

C. _______________

D. _______________

44. Why is adhesive tape *never* used to secure a condom catheter?

____

____

____

45. Do *not* apply a condom catheter if

____

_______________.

46. Why are bladder irrigations done?

____

____

47. What is the goal of a bladder training program?

____

Multiple Choice

Circle the BEST answer.

48. How much urine does the healthy adult excrete each day?
   A. About 500 ml
   B. About 1500 ml
   C. About 3000 ml
   D. About 700 ml

49. Normal urine
   A. Is pale yellow, straw colored, or amber.
   B. Does not have an odor.
   C. Is cloudy.
   D. Contains particles.

50. You promote normal elimination by
   A. Setting new voiding routines for the person.
   B. Asking the person to hurry.
   C. Providing only small amounts of fluid.
   D. Providing privacy.

51. Urinary incontinence is always permanent.
   A. True
   B. False

52. Which is *not* a nursing measure for persons with urinary incontinence?
   A. Increase fluid intake at bedtime.
   B. Provide good skin care.
   C. Answer signal lights promptly.
   D. Encourage urination at scheduled intervals.

53. You feel impatient when caring for a person with incontinence. You must
   A. Tell a co-worker to take care of the person for you.
   B. Wait to do the person's care until you feel less stressed.
   C. Discuss the problem with the nurse at once.
   D. Refuse to care for the person.

54. Catheters are used for all of the following reasons *except*
 A. As a first choice to treat incontinence.
 B. To keep the bladder empty before, during, and after surgery.
 C. To protect wounds from urine.
 D. To collect sterile urine specimens.

55. The catheter drainage bag is attached to the bed rail.
 A. True
 B. False

56. Catheterizations decrease the risk of urinary tract infections.
 A. True
 B. False

57. You are going to insert an indwelling catheter in Mr. Clark. He has an erection. You
 A. Continue the procedure.
 B. Get the nurse.
 C. Leave the room immediately.
 D. Cover him and tell him you will give him some time alone.

58. You insert a catheter into a female. No urine flows. This means
 A. There is no urine in the bladder.
 B. The catheter could be in the vagina.
 C. The catheter is plugged.
 D. The person is not relaxed.

59. You are inserting a catheter into a male. You meet resistance. You
 A. Attempt to force the catheter.
 B. Remove the catheter and try again.
 C. Stop the procedure and call for the nurse.
 D. Try a smaller catheter.

60. You are inserting an indwelling catheter. Which is *incorrect?*
 A. Lubricate the catheter.
 B. Clean the meatus.
 C. Insert the catheter until urine appears.
 D. Inflate the balloon as soon as urine appears.

ADDITIONAL LEARNING ACTIVITIES

1. Think of your personal urination patterns.
 A. List the factors that affect your daily patterns.
 B. Do changes in your personal patterns affect your comfort? How?

2. Carefully review and practice the procedure for giving a bedpan. Work with a classmate. Use a regular bedpan and a fracture pan.
 A. Use the procedure checklists provided on page 343 through 344 as a guide.
 B. Take your turn being the patient or resident. Discuss your experience.
  (1) Did you have concerns about dignity and privacy?
  (2) Was the experience physically comfortable? Explain.
  (3) Was it difficult to position the bedpan correctly? Explain.
  (4) Would you like to be left on a bedpan for 15 minutes or 1/2 hour?
  (5) How will your experience affect the care you give?

4. Carefully review all the procedures in Chapter 19. Under the supervision of your instructor, practice the procedures in Chapter 19. Use the procedure checklists provided on pages 345 through 363 as a guide.
   A. If you are embarrassed by any of these procedures, discuss your feelings with your instructor or nurse preceptor. Remember, some states and agencies do not allow assistive personnel to perform some of the procedures in Chapter 19.

5. Read the vignette. Then answer the questions that follow.
   Miss Breeze is an 85-year-old nursing center resident. She has dementia and is incontinent. She wears incontinence briefs. Sometimes she removes her incontinence brief and urinates on the floor. Her care plan includes taking her to the bathroom every 2 hours.
   A. What care needs related to incontinence does Miss Breeze have?
   B. What complications is Miss Breeze at risk for?
   C. How will you promote her safety?
   D. How will you promote her dignity?
   E. What observations do you need to report and record?
   F. What nursing measures might be part of Miss Breeze's care plan?
   G. What must you remember when providing perineal care?

20 Bowel Elimination

OBJECTIVES

The questions and student activities in this chapter will help you meet these objectives.

- Define the key terms listed in Chapter 20
- Describe normal defecation
- List the observations to make about defecation
- Identify the factors that affect bowel elimination
- Describe common bowel elimination problems
- Explain how to promote comfort and safety during defecation
- Describe bowel training
- Explain why enemas are given
- Describe the common enema solutions
- Describe the rules for giving enemas
- Explain the purpose of rectal tubes
- Describe how to care for a person with an ostomy
- Perform the procedures described in Chapter 20

STUDY QUESTIONS

Complete the Crossword

Across

2. The semisolid mass of waste products in the colon
6. The passage of a hard, dry stool
8. Gas or air passed through the anus
9. The frequent passage of liquid stools

Down

1. The alternating contraction and relaxation of intestinal muscles
3. A surgically created opening
4. Excreted feces
5. A surgically created opening between the colon and abdominal wall
7. The introduction of fluid into the rectum and lower colon

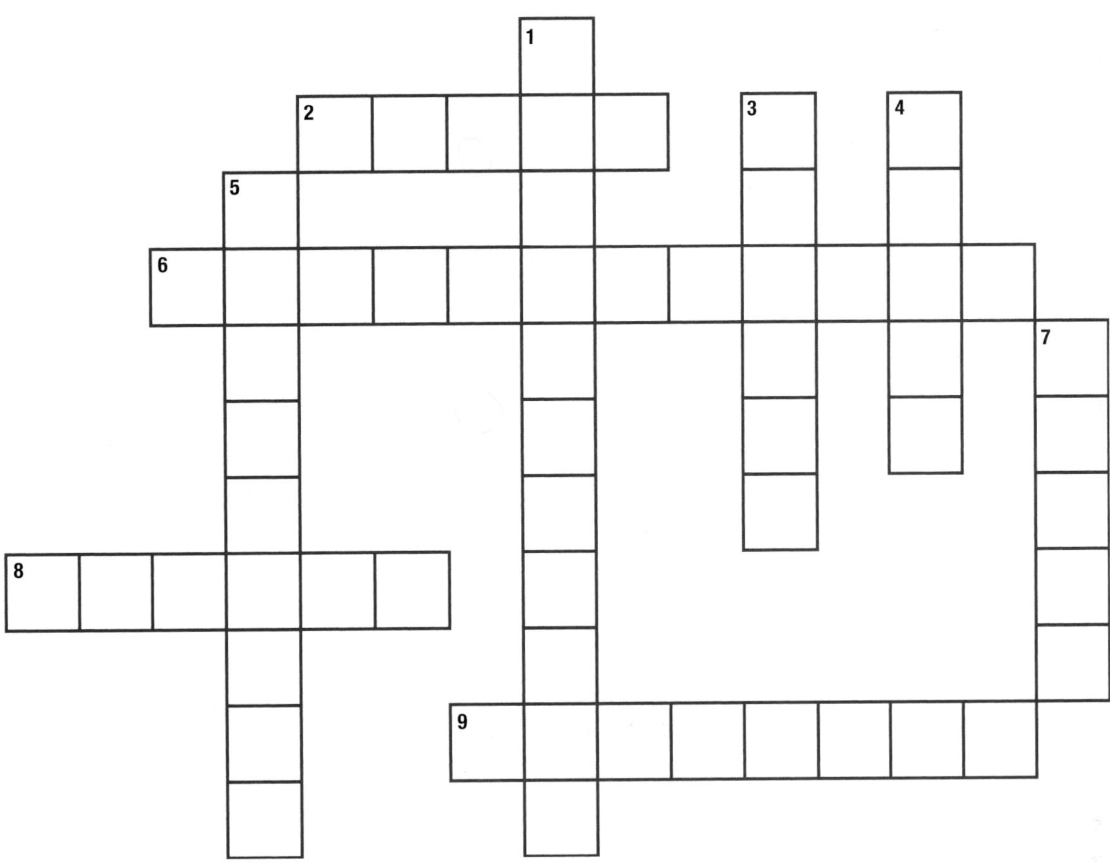

Matching

Match the following terms with the correct definitions.

A. Flatulence
B. Stoma
C. Fecal impaction
D. Ileostomy
E. Suppository
F. Defecation
G. Fecal incontinence
H. Dehydration

1. G The inability to control the passage of feces and gas through the anus
2. f The process of excreting feces from the rectum through the anus; a bowel movement
3. h The excessive loss of water from tissues
4. C The prolonged retention and buildup of feces in the rectum
5. a The excessive formation of gas in the stomach and intestines
6. D A surgically created opening between the ileum (small intestine) and the abdominal wall
7. B An opening
8. e A cone-shaped, solid drug that is inserted into a body opening; it melts at body temperature

Fill in the Blanks

9. Stools are normally ______________________,

______________________,

______________________,

______________________,

and ______________________.

10. When do newborns usually have bowel movements?

____

11. You must carefully observe stools before disposing of them. What should you observe and report to the nurse?

A. ______________________

B. ______________________

C. ______________________

D. ______________________

E. ______________________

F. ______________________

G. ______________________

12. What factors affect stool frequency, consistency, color, and odor?

A. ______________________

B. ______________________

C. ______________________

D. ______________________

E. ______________________

F. ______________________

G. ______________________

H. ______________________

13. Why is constipation a risk for older persons?

____

____

____

14. ______________________ results if constipation is not relieved.

15. Why is checking for and removing a fecal impaction dangerous?

____

____

____

____

16. You are removing a fecal impaction. You check the person's pulse rate and observe that the pulse rate has slowed and is irregular. What must you do?

____

17. Causes of diarrhea include

______________________,

______________________,

______________________,

and ______________________.

18. When caring for persons with diarrhea, you need to:

A. ______________________

B. ______________________

C. ______________________

19. ______________________ and

______________________ are

serious signs of dehydration.

20. List 8 causes of fecal incontinence.

A. ______

B. ______

C. ______

D. ______

E. ______

F. ______

G. ______

H. ______

21. What happens if flatus is not expelled?

______

______

______

22. List 3 measures that help produce flatus.

A. ______

B. ______

C. ______

23. What are the two goals of bowel training?

A. ______

B. ______

24. Doctors order enemas to:

A. ______

B. ______

C. ______

25. The doctor orders enemas until clear. This means ______

______

______.

26. How would you prepare a soapsuds enema?

______

______

27. Why can tap-water enemas be dangerous?

______

______

28. Only ______ are used for cleansing enemas in children.

29. How far is the enema tube inserted in infants?

______

30. How do small-volume enemas cause defecation?

______

______

31. Why is an oil-retention enema retained for 30 to 60 minutes or longer?

______

______

32. What is the purpose of a rectal tube?

______

______

33. What information do you need from the nurse and the care plan before inserting a rectal tube?

A. ______

B. ______

C. ______

D. ______

E. ______

34. Mr. Jordan has a colostomy. The colostomy is near the start of the colon. What kind of stools will he have?

____

35. How are odors prevented in Mr. Jordan's ostomy pouch?

A. ______________________________

B. ______________________________

C. ______________________________

D. ______________________________

36. You are changing Mr. Jordan's colostomy pouch. What observations do you need to report and record?

A. ______________________________

B. ______________________________

C. ______________________________

37. You are changing Mr. Jordan's ostomy pouch. You notice signs of skin breakdown. What should you do?

____

____

Multiple Choice

Circle the BEST answer.

38. Normal stools are
   A. Black in color.
   B. Soft, formed, and moist.
   C. Hard and marble sized.
   D. Liquid and pale in color.

39. Breast-fed infants have
   A. Black stools.
   B. Brown stools.
   C. Red-colored stools.
   D. Yellow stools.

40. Normal bowel movements are promoted by all of the following *except*
   A. Drinking 6 to 8 glasses of water every day.
   B. Eating a well-balanced diet.
   C. Ignoring the urge to defecate.
   D. Regular exercise.

41. Mrs. Smith has had a bowel movement. The stool is black in color and has a tarry consistency. You should
   A. Ask Mrs. Smith if she has had anything unusual to eat.
   B. Ask the nurse to observe the stool.
   C. Dispose of the stool and report the color to the nurse.
   D. Ask a co-worker if this is normal for Mrs. Smith.

42. You assist Mr. Ryan to the commode for a bowel movement. To promote comfort and safety
   A. Encourage his roommate's visitors to stay in the room.
   B. Place the signal light within reach.
   C. Check on him every 5 minutes.
   D. Leave the door open so you can check on him easily.

43. Standard Precautions and the Bloodborne Pathogen Standard are followed when in contact with stools.
   A. True
   B. False

44. David Gomez is 2 years old. He has diarrhea. Which is *false?*
   A. He is at low risk for dehydration.
   B. Death can occur quickly.
   C. Report any liquid stools to the nurse at once.
   D. Ask the nurse to observe his stools.

45. Which statement about fecal incontinence is *false?*
   A. A bowel training program may be effective.
   B. Fecal incontinence affects the person emotionally.
   C. Fecal incontinence is always permanent.
   D. Fecal incontinence can result from unanswered signal lights.

46. You promote comfort and safety during bowel elimination by
    A. Positioning the person in the supine position.
    B. Asking the person to wait until you have time.
    C. Assisting the person onto a cold bedpan.
    D. Leaving the room if the person can be left alone, and placing the signal light and toilet tissue within reach.

47. Which measure does *not* promote comfort and safety when giving an enema to an adult?
    A. A comfortable, right side-lying position.
    B. Raising the enema bag 12 inches above the anus.
    C. Taking 10 to 15 minutes to give the solution.
    D. Making sure the bathroom will not be used by another person.

48. You are giving an enema to a 3-year-old child. Which is *false?*
    A. Only saline enemas are used.
    B. The tube is inserted two inches.
    C. Give 500 ml of solution.
    D. The enema solution is usually given at 100° F.

49. A rectal tube is
    A. Used after rectal surgery.
    B. Inserted 2 inches into the adult rectum.
    C. Left in place for 1 hour.
    D. Used to relieve intestinal distention.

50. Ostomy stomas are painful when touched.
    A. True
    B. False

51. Ostomy pouches are emptied
    A. When full.
    B. Every shift.
    C. When feces is present.
    D. Every 4 hours.

52. Mr. Jordan has a colostomy. Which statement is *false?*
    A. The entire large intestine has been removed.
    B. Good skin care is very important.
    C. Colostomies can be permanent or temporary.
    D. Feces and flatus pass through a stoma located on the abdominal wall.

53. With an ileostomy, the entire colon is removed. Liquid feces drain constantly from an ileostomy.
    A. True
    B. False

ADDITIONAL LEARNING ACTIVITIES

1. Think of your personal elimination routines. Answer the following questions.
    A. How important are these routines to your physical and psychological comfort? Explain.
    B. Are you aware of how your diet, fluid intake, and level of activity affect your bowel elimination routines? Explain.
    C. Have you had personal experience with constipation or diarrhea? How did the experience affect your comfort?

2. Do you know anyone with a colostomy or ileostomy? If the person is willing, discuss how the ostomy has affected his or her life. Answer these questions.
    A. How did the person adjust?
    B. What is the person's daily routine?
    C. How is the skin cared for?

3. If available at your school or place of work, examine several types of colostomy and ileostomy pouches. Read the manufacturer's instructions. Practice handling the pouches and applying them on yourself and a willing classmate.

4. Handle the various types of enema equipment and become familiar with how each is used. This will increase your comfort and confidence.

5. Read the vignette. Then answer the questions that follow.
   Mr. Chan is an 81-year-old resident of Pine Ridge Nursing Center. He has problems with constipation. He has not had a bowel movement for 4 days. He is complaining of abdominal discomfort. The nurse checked Mr. Chan for a fecal impaction. The doctor ordered an oil-retention enema for Mr. Chan. The nurse delegated the procedure to you.
   A. What information do you need from the nurse before you give the enema?
   B. What items do you need to collect for the procedure?
   C. How will you explain the procedure to Mr. Chan?
   D. How will you provide for Mr. Chan's privacy?
   E. How will you provide for Mr. Chan's safety?
   F. How long should Mr. Chan retain the enema?
   G. What observations do you need to report and record?

6. Carefully review the procedures in Chapter 20. Under the supervision of your instructor, practice each procedure. Use the procedure checklists provided on pages 364 through 378 as a guide. Remember, some states and agencies do not allow assistive personnel to perform some of the procedures in Chapter 20.

21

Nutrition

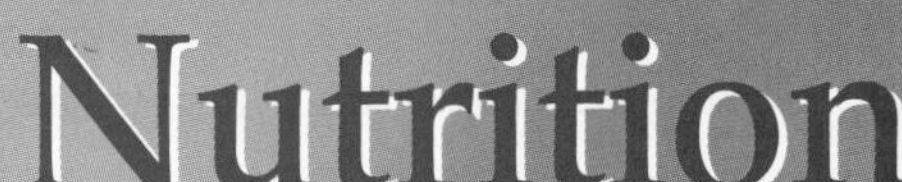

OBJECTIVES

The questions and student activities in this chapter will help you meet these objectives.

- Define the key terms listed in Chapter 21
- Explain the purpose and use of the Food Guide Pyramid
- Explain how to use the Dietary Guidelines for Americans
- Describe the functions and major sources of nutrients
- Explain how to use food labels
- Describe factors that affect eating and nutrition
- Describe the special diets and between-meal nourishments
- Explain how to assist the person with eating
- Explain how to assist with calorie counts
- Explain the purpose of enteral nutrition
- Explain the difference between scheduled and continuous feedings
- Identify the signs, symptoms, and precautions relating to regurgitation and aspiration
- Describe the comfort and safety measures for enteral nutrition
- Identify the reasons for removing a nasogastric tube
- Perform the procedures described in Chapter 21

STUDY QUESTIONS

Matching

Match the following terms with the correct definitions.

A. Percutaneous endoscopic gastrostomy (PEG) tube
B. Calorie
C. Nasogastric (NG) tube
D. Regurgitation
E. Dysphagia
F. Aspiration
G. Nasointestinal tube
H. Jejunostomy tube
I. Daily Reference Values (DRVs)
J. Nutrient
K. Gastrostomy tube
L. Daily Value (DV)
M. Nutrition
N. Enteral nutrition
O. Gavage
P. Anorexia

1. P The loss of appetite
2. F Breathing fluid or an object into the lungs

3. B ____ The amount of energy produced when the body burns food

4. I ____ The maximum daily intake values for total fat, saturated fat, cholesterol, sodium, carbohydrate, and dietary fiber

5. L ____ How a serving fits into the daily diet; expressed in a percent (%) based on a daily diet of 2,000 calories

6. E ____ Difficulty swallowing

7. n ____ Giving nutrients through the gastrointestinal tract

8. K ____ A tube inserted through a surgically created opening in the stomach

9. O ____ Tube feeding

10. h ____ A tube inserted into the intestines through a surgically created opening into the middle part of the small intestine

11. C ____ A tube inserted through the nose into the stomach

12. G ____ A tube inserted through the nose into the small intestine

13. J ____ A substance that is ingested, digested, absorbed, and used by the body

14. m ____ The many processes involved in the ingestion, digestion, absorption, and use of foods and fluids by the body

15. d ____ A tube inserted into the stomach through a stab or puncture wound made through the skin; a lighted instrument allows the doctor to see inside a body cavity or organ

16. D ____ The backward flow of food from the stomach into the mouth

Fill in the Blanks

17. List 5 results of a poor diet and poor eating habits.

A. ____________________

B. ____________________

C. ____________________

D. ____________________

E. ____________________

18. Nutrients are grouped into

____________________,

____________________,

____________________,

____________________,

____________________,

and ____________________.

19. List the 6 food groups in the Food Guide Pyramid, starting at the bottom level.

A. ____________________

B. ____________________

C. ____________________

D. ____________________

E. ____________________

F. ____________________

20. List 7 factors affecting eating and nutrition.

A. ______

B. ______

C. ______

D. ______

E. ______

F. ______

G. ______

21. List the OBRA requirements for food served in long-term care centers.

A. ______

______

B. ______

______

C. ______

______

D. ______

______

E. ______

______

F. ______

______

G. ______

______

H. ______

______

22. Why do doctors order special diets?

A. ______

B. ______

C. ______

23. Regular diet, general diet, and house diet mean

______.

24. What is the average amount of sodium in the daily diet?

______

How much sodium does the body need each day?

______

25. Diabetes is a chromic disease from lack of insulin. What happens when the body does not have enough insulin?

______

______

______

26. Diabetes is usually treated with

______,

______,

and ______.

27. Mr. Lane has dysphagia. How will you promote his safety?

A. ______

______

B. ______

______

C. ______

______

D. ______________________

____

E. ______________________

____

F. ______________________

____

28. Mr. Gomez frequently coughs or chokes after swallowing. This is a sign of

______________________.

29. Miss Andrews eats her meals in bed. She has a hearing aid, wears eyeglasses, and has dentures. She is continent of bowel and bladder. How will you prepare her for her meal?

A. ______________________

B. ______________________

C. ______________________

D. ______________________

E. ______________________

F. ______________________

G. ______________________

H. ______________________

30. Nursing centers have special dining programs. Briefly describe these programs.

A. Social dining

____

____

B. Family dining

____

____

C. Assistive dining

____

____

D. Low-stimulation dining

____

____

31. What information do you need from the nurse and the care plan before serving each person's meal tray?

A. ______________________

B. ______________________

C. ______________________

D. ______________________

32. How do you help a visually impaired person locate foods on the tray?

____

____

33 You are feeding Mr. Gomez his breakfast. What observations do you need to report and record?

A. ______________________

B. ______________________

C. ______________________

34. When are feeding tubes used?

____

____

35. ______________________ is a major risk of enteral nutrition.

36. Why does the RN check tube placement before every scheduled tube feeding and every 4 hours for continuous tube feedings?

____

____

____

37. Mr. Evans receives enteral nutrition through an NG tube. What measures are taken to prevent regurgitation?

A. _______________

____

B. _______________

____

C. _______________

____

38. Mr. Martin receives enteral nutrition through a gastrostomy tube. What do you need to report to the nurse at once?

A. _______________

B. _______________

C. _______________

D. _______________

E. _______________

F. _______________

G. _______________

H. _______________

I. _______________

J. _______________

K. _______________

L. _______________

39. Mr. Martin has an intravenous infusion, a breathing tube, and a gastrostomy tube. Why is it important to always check and inspect his feeding tube with the nurse before giving a tube feeding?

____

____

____

_______________.

40. A nasogastric tube is removed when

____

_______________.

41. Before giving a tube feeding you must make sure that:

A. _______________

B. _______________

C. _______________

D. _______________

E. _______________

F. _______________

G. _______________

Multiple Choice

Circle the BEST answer.

42. The Dietary Guidelines for Americans encourage:
    A. A high fat diet
    B. Eating a variety of foods
    C. A diet high in sodium
    D. Eating only small amounts of fruits and vegetables

43. How many servings from the vegetable group are recommended daily?
    A. 1-2 servings
    B. 5-7 servings
    C. 3-5 servings
    D. 7-9 servings

44. The meat, poultry, fish, dry beans, eggs, and nuts group
    A. Is high in protein, fat, iron, and thiamine.
    B. Is lower in fat than the milk, yogurt, and cheese group.
    C. Contains some sugar.
    D. Is high in fiber, vitamin E, and minerals.

45. Which group is the base of the pyramid? It allows the most servings.
    A. The fruit group
    B. The vegetable group
    C. Breads, cereals, rice and pasta group
    D. Milk, yogurt, and cheese group

46. Protein is an important nutrient because
    A. It provides fiber for bowel elimination.
    B. It is needed for tissue growth and repair.
    C. It helps the body use certain vitamins.
    D. It does not provide calories.

47. What percent of calories in the daily diet should come from fat?
    A. About 10%
    B. 15%
    C. No more than 30%
    D. No more than 50%

48. Which nutrient provides energy and fiber for bowel elimination?
    A. Carbohydrates
    B. Fats
    C. Vitamins
    D. Minerals

49. Which vitamins must be ingested daily because they are not stored by the body?
    A. Vitamins A and K
    B. Vitamins D and E
    C. Vitamin C and the B complex vitamins
    D. Vitamins K and B

50. Which foods are high in vitamin C?
    A. Whole grains
    B. Dairy products
    C. Citrus fruits
    D. Fish liver oils

51. Which mineral allows the red blood cells to carry oxygen?
    A. Iron
    B. Iodine
    C. Calcium
    D. Phosphorus

52. The Food Guide Pyramid does *not* apply to children under 6 years of age.
    A. True
    B. False

53. Which is *not* one of the Dietary Guidelines for Americans?
    A. Choose a diet high in saturated fat and cholesterol.
    B. Choose a variety of fruits and vegetables daily.
    C. Keep food safe to eat.
    D. Choose and prepare foods with less salt.

54. Nutritional needs decrease during illness and recovery from injury.
    A. True
    B. False

55. In what country is the main meal eaten at midday?
    A. United States
    B. England
    C. South Korea
    D. Austria

56. Beef is not eaten in
    A. England.
    B. China.
    C. Poland.
    D. India.

57. A low-sodium diet may be ordered for persons with
    A. Anemia.
    B. Heart disease.
    C. Disease of the colon.
    D. Ulcers.

58. Which foods are *not* allowed on a fiber and residue restricted diet?
    A. Creamed cereal
    B. Plain puddings
    C. Raw fruits
    D. Boiled potatoes

59. Formation of bones and teeth is a major function of
    A. Iron.
    B. Sodium and potassium.
    C. Iodine.
    D. Calcium and phosphorus.

60. Diabetes is a chronic disease from lack of insulin. Insulin allows the body to use
   A. Sugar.
   B. Fat.
   C. Protein.
   D. Minerals.

61. Which is a sign of dysphagia?
   A. Increased appetite
   B. Weight gain
   C. The person eats only solid foods.
   D. Food spills out of the person's mouth while eating.

62. When feeding a person
   A. Always use a fork.
   B. Stand facing the person.
   C. Serve foods in the order the person prefers.
   D. Offer fluids at the end of the meal.

63. Scheduled tube feedings require electronic pumps.
   A. True
   B. False

64. To prevent regurgitation and aspiration in the person receiving a tube feeding, you must
   A. Provide frequent oral hygiene.
   B. Position the person in the left side-lying position for the tube feeding.
   C. Give formula rapidly.
   D. Position the person in the Fowler's or semi-Fowler's position for at least 1 hour after a tube feeding.

65. Lisa Adams is 6 months old. Holding and cuddling her during the tube feeding is preferred.
   A. True
   B. False

66. The water used to flush the tube after a tube feeding is counted as intake.
   A. True
   B. False

67. When removing a nasogastric tube, do all of the following *except*
   A. Use Standard Precautions and the Bloodborne Pathogen Standard.
   B. Explain the procedure to the person.
   C. Position the person in a sitting or semi-Fowler's position.
   D. Withdraw the tube slowly.

ADDITIONAL LEARNING ACTIVITIES

1. Discuss the importance of food in your life. Answer these questions.
   A. Besides meeting physical needs, what role does food play in your life?
   B. Does your cultural background or religious beliefs affect the food you eat and how you prepare your food? Explain.
   C. What role does food play in your social life?

2. Has illness ever affected your appetite or your ability to eat certain foods?
   A. How will your experience affect the care you provide?

3. Review the Food Guide Pyramid (page 399 in the textbook).
   A. Are you making wise food choices? Explain.
   B. Is your diet well balanced? Explain.

4. List the age-related changes in the digestive system. Discuss how these changes affect:
   A. What the person eats
   B. How the person prepares food
   C. The person's enjoyment of food

5. Carefully review the procedures for serving meal trays and feeding a person.
   A. Use the procedure checklists on pages 381 through 383 as a guide.
   B. Practice the procedures with a classmate using various food consistencies.
   C. Take your turn being the patient or resident. Discuss your experience. Answer these questions:
      (1) How does it feel to be fed by another person?
      (2) Did you enjoy your meal? Explain.
      (3) Were you fed too fast or too slow?
      (4) Was the amount given with each bite right for you?
      (5) Were liquids offered during the meal?
      (6) Did your food remain at the right temperature throughout the meal?
      (7) How will your experience affect the care you give?

6. Carefully review the procedures for giving tube feedings and removing a nasogastric tube. You must be supervised by a nurse when practicing these procedures.
   Remember, some states and agencies do not allow assistive personnel to perform these procedures.

22

Fluids and Blood

OBJECTIVES

The questions and student activities in this chapter will help you meet these objectives.

- Define the key terms listed in Chapter 22
- Describe fluid requirements and the causes of dehydration
- Explain what to do when the person has special fluid orders
- Explain the purpose of intake and output records
- Identify the food and fluid that is counted as fluid intake
- Explain how to assist with fluid needs
- Know the types of IV solutions
- Explain the difference between peripheral IV sites and central venous sites
- Describe the equipment used in IV therapy
- Describe how you assist with maintaining the IV flow rate
- Explain the safety measures necessary for IV therapy
- Identify the signs and symptoms of IV therapy complications
- Know the four blood groups in the ABO system
- Know the difference between Rh-positive and Rh-negative blood
- Know the common blood products used for transfusions
- Explain how to obtain blood from the blood bank
- Explain how to assist with the administration of blood
- Identify the signs and symptoms of a transfusion reaction
- Perform the procedures described in Chapter 22

STUDY QUESTIONS

Complete the Crossword

Across

3. A cell necessary for the clotting of blood; thrombocyte
5. The substance in the red blood cells that picks up oxygen in the lungs and carries it to the cells
6. The amount of fluid taken in
7. The liquid portion of the blood
8. The amount of fluid lost
9. The swelling of body tissues with water

Down

1. A substance that the body reacts to
2. Inflammation of a vein
4. White blood cell; protects the body against infection

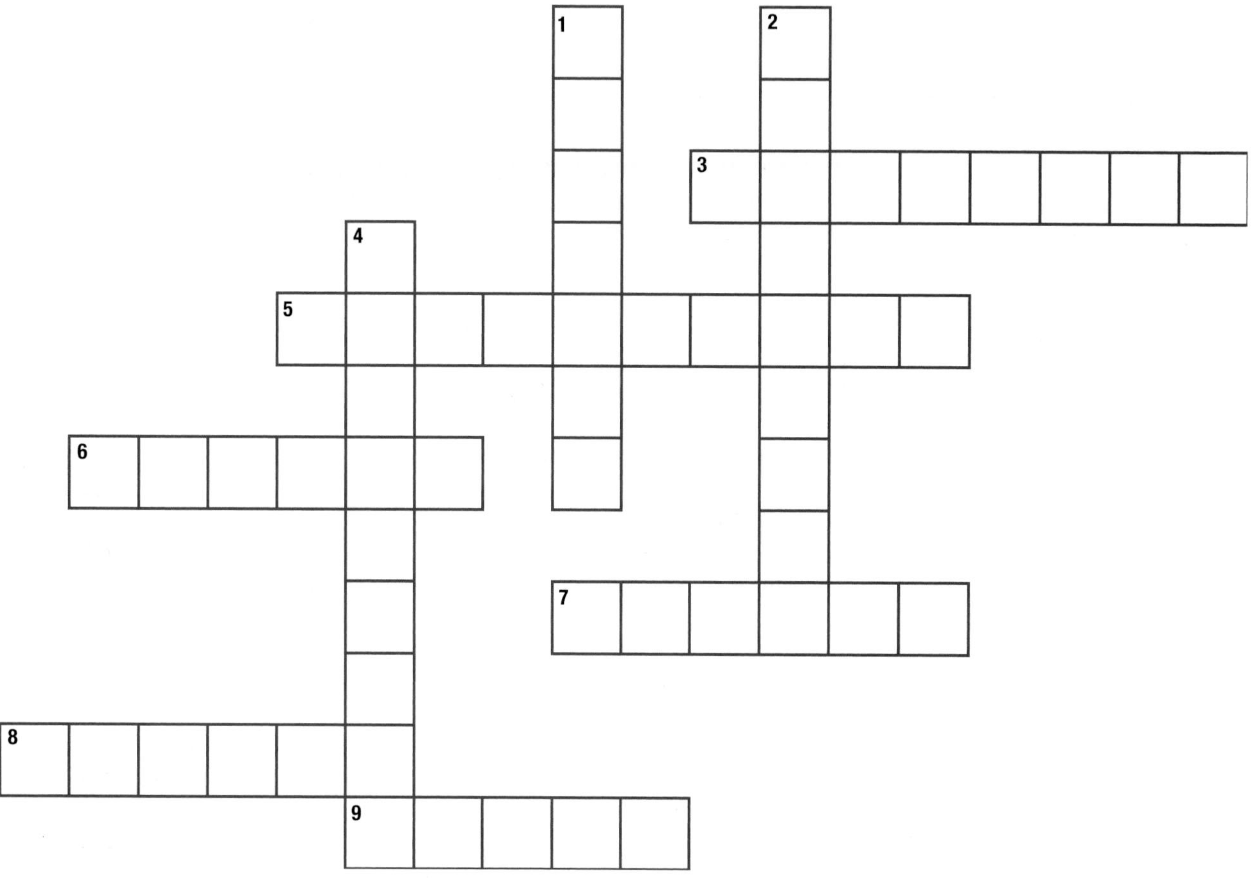

Matching

Match the following terms with the correct definitions.

1. ______ Air that enters the cardiovascular system and travels to the lungs where it obstructs blood flow
2. ______ A substance in the plasma that fights or attacks antigens
3. ______ The intravenous administration of blood or its products
4. ______ A decrease in the amount of water in body tissues
5. ______ Red blood cell; carries oxygen to the cells
6. ______ The number of drops per minute (gtt/min)
7. ______ A measuring container for fluid
8. ______ Blood is destroyed
9. ______ Giving fluids through a needle or catheter inserted into a vein
10. ______ A cell necessary for the clotting of blood

A. Intravenous (IV) therapy
B. Hemolysis
C. Flow rate
D. Blood transfusion
E. Air embolism
F. Graduate
G. Thrombocyte
H. Erythrocyte
I. Dehydration
J. Antibody

Fill in the Blanks

11. After oxygen, ______________________________ is the most important physical need for survival.

12. Fluid balance is needed for health. The amount of fluid ______________________________ and the amount of fluid ______________________ must be equal.

13. List 6 common causes of dehydration.

    A. ______________________________
    B. ______________________________
    C. ______________________________
    D. ______________________________
    E. ______________________________
    F. ______________________________

14. How much fluid intake is needed per day for normal fluid balance?

    ____

15. Why do infants and young children need more fluids than adults do?

    ____
    ____

16. Mrs. Sanchez has an NPO order. This means ______________________________.

17. List 3 reasons that intake and output records are kept.

    A. ______________________________
    B. ______________________________
    C. ______________________________

18. The nurse tells you to measure Mr. Smith's output. Output includes ______________________________.

19. What information do you need from the nurse and the care plan when measuring intake and output?

 A. ______________________________

 B. ______________________________

 C. ______________________________

 D. ______________________________

20. When do patients and residents need fresh drinking water?

 A. ______________________________

 B. ______________________________

21. List 4 reasons why doctors order IV therapy?

 A. ______________________________

 B. ______________________________

 C. ______________________________

 D. ______________________________

22. Nutrient IV solutions are given for ______________________________.

23. Where are the peripheral IV sites for adults located?

 ____

 ____

24. ______________________________ are peripheral IV sites in infants.

25. The ______________________________ and the ______________________________ are central venous sites. The ______________________________ are also used.

26. What parts of the IV infusion set are sterile?

 A. ______________________________

 B. ______________________________

27. The RN tells you to check the flow rate on an IV infusion. What observations do you report to the RN at once?

 A. ______________________________

 B. ______________________________

 C. ______________________________

28. Before priming IV tubing, changing an IV dressing, or discontinuing an IV, you must make sure that:

 A. ______________________________

 B. ______________________________

 C. ______________________________

 D. ______________________________

 E. ______________________________

 F. ______________________________

 If the above conditions are met, what information do you need from the nurse?

 G. ______________________________

 H. ______________________________

 I. ______________________________

 J. ______________________________

 K. ______________________________

 L. ______________________________

 M. ______________________________

29. When checking an IV bag, you must make sure that:

    A. ______________________________

    B. ______________________________

    C. ______________________________

    D. ______________________________

30. Who is responsible for blood transfusions?

    ____

31. List five blood products often ordered by the doctor.

    A. ______________________________

    B. ______________________________

    C. ______________________________

    D. ______________________________

    E. ______________________________

32. Why are blood groups and types important?

    ____

    ____

    ____

33. You are obtaining blood from the blood bank. What information must you check with the laboratory technician and read aloud?

    A. ______________________________

    B. ______________________________

    C. ______________________________

    D. ______________________________

    E. ______________________________

    F. ______________________________

34. Transfusion reactions occur when

    ____

    ______________________________.

35. Why are the person's vital signs taken before a blood transfusion?

    ____

    ____

    ____

    ____

36. The RN tells you to check the flow rate on a blood transfusion. What observations do you report to the RN at once?

    A. ______________________________

    B. ______________________________

    C. ______________________________

    D. ______________________________

37. A person receiving a blood transfusion is anxious and complains of itching. What should you do?

    ____

Labeling

38. Label equipment used for IV therapy.

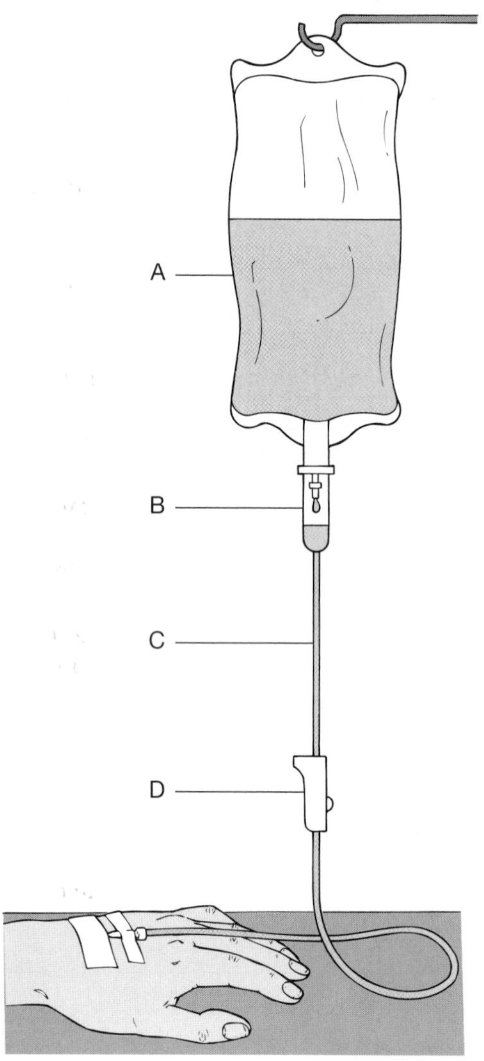

A. ______________________

B. ______________________

C. ______________________

D. ______________________

39. Label the parts of the infusion set.

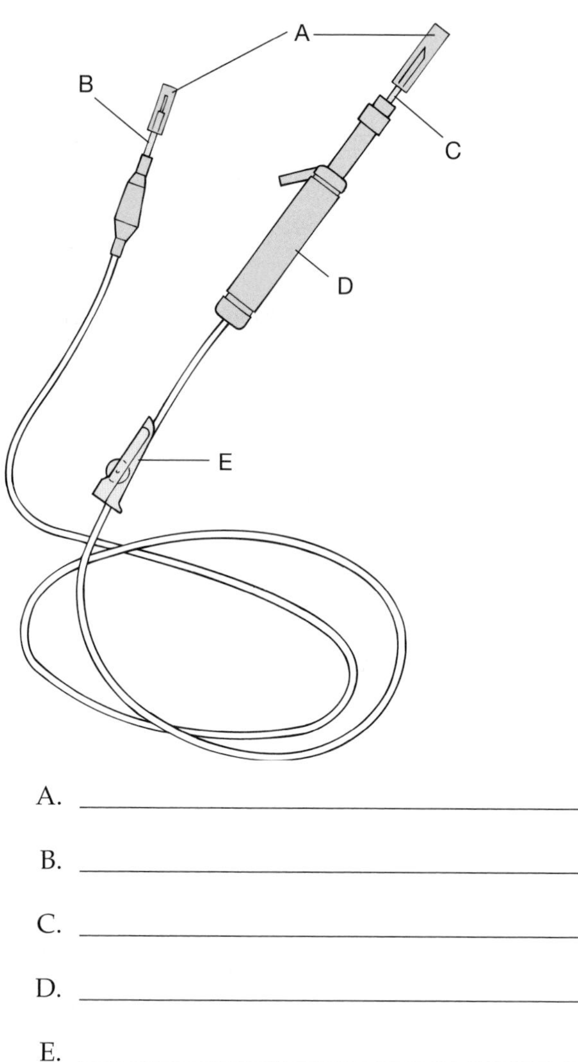

A. ______________________

B. ______________________

C. ______________________

D. ______________________

E. ______________________

Multiple Choice

Circle the BEST answer.

40. Mr. White has a "restrict fluids order." Which is *false?*
    A. Offer fluids frequently.
    B. Fluids are limited to a certain amount.
    C. Accurate intake and output records are kept.
    D. Oral hygiene is important.

41. To measure fluid intake, only fluid ingested by the person through the mouth is measured.
    A. True
    B. False

42. One ounce equals 30 milliliters (ml).
    A. True
    B. False

43. One ounce equals
    A. 10 ml
    B. 20 ml
    C. 30 ml
    D. 50 ml

44. You are providing drinking water to patients. Which action will *not* prevent the spread of microbes?
    A. Labeling the water pitcher with the person's name and room and bed number
    B. Not touching the inside of the water glass or pitcher
    C. Preventing the scoop from touching the rim and inside of the water glass and pitcher
    D. Storing the scoop in the ice container

45. You will care for persons receiving IV therapy. Which is *false?*
    A. Fluid enters the person's vein through a needle or catheter.
    B. IV therapy is given in hospital, outpatient, long-term care, and home settings.
    C. The doctor orders the types of IV solutions to use.
    D. Assistive personnel are responsible for IV therapy.

46. The RN tells you to collect the IV solution for Mrs. Marsh. You must do all of the following *except*
    A. Make sure you understand what the RN asks you to collect.
    B. Repeat the information back to the RN.
    C. Check the bag for cracks or leaks.
    D. Add medication to the IV solution as directed by the RN.

47. A bag of IV solution is *not* used if the expiration date has passed.
    A. True
    B. False

48. Mrs. Lund is receiving IV therapy. An electronic infusion pump is used. An alarm sounds. You must
    A. Turn off the pump.
    B. Reset the flow rate.
    C. Tell the nurse at once.
    D. Turn off the alarm.

49. IV tubing is primed
    A. To remove air from the tubing before administering IV fluid.
    B. Only before administering blood.
    C. When adding medication to the IV solution.
    D. Before discontinuing IV therapy.

50. When changing IV dressings, which is *incorrect?*
    A. Make sure you have good lighting.
    B. Be careful not to move the needle or catheter.
    C. Report any redness, swelling, or drainage to the RN at once.
    D. Cover the needle adapter with the dressing.

51. You have removed a peripheral IV needle from a patient. How long is pressure applied to the IV site?
    A. 30 seconds
    B. 1 minute
    C. 2 to 3 minutes
    D. 10 minutes

52. What type blood is called the universal donor?
    A. Type B
    B. Type O
    C. Type AB
    D. Type A

ADDITIONAL LEARNING ACTIVITIES

1. Obtain samples of I&O flow sheets. Practice filling out these forms.

2. Practice measuring and recording a variety of liquids as intake. Use food containers available in the classroom and in the home (for example, cups, glasses, bowls).

3. Practice measuring and recording liquids as output. Use containers available in the classroom (for example, graduates, urinals, emesis basins).

4. If you have had a personal experience receiving IV therapy, discuss your experience with your classmates. Answer these questions:
   A. Were you afraid? Explain.
   B. Were you physically comfortable?
   C. How did the health care team meet your needs?
   D. How will your experience affect the care you give?

   Remember, some states and agencies do not allow assistive personnel to perform some of the procedures in Chapter 22.

23

Oxygen Needs

OBJECTIVES

The questions and student activities in this chapter will help you meet these objectives.

- Define the key terms listed in Chapter 23
- Describe the factors affecting oxygen needs
- Identify the signs and symptoms of hypoxia and altered respiratory function
- Describe the tests used to diagnose respiratory problems
- Explain the measures that promote oxygenation
- Describe the oxygen devices
- Explain how to safely assist with oxygen therapy
- Explain how to assist in the care of persons with artificial airways
- Describe the safety measures for suctioning
- Explain how to assist in the care of persons on mechanical ventilation
- Explain how to assist in the care of persons with chest tubes
- Perform the procedures described in Chapter 23

STUDY QUESTIONS

Matching

Match the following terms with the correct definitions.

A. Mechanical ventilation
B. Pneumothorax
C. Tachypnea
D. Cheyne-Stokes
E. Hemothorax
F. Intubation
G. Orthopnea
H. Pollutant
I. Allergy
J. Dyspnea
K. Oxygen concentration
L. Respiratory arrest
M. Suction
N. Hypoventilation
O. Hyperventilation
P. Bradypnea
Q. Kussmaul respirations
R. Pleural effusion
S. Orthopneic position
T. Respiratory depression
U. Hypoxia
V. Hemoptysis
W. Hypoxemia
X. Apnea
Y. Biot's respirations

1. ___I___ A sensitivity to a substance that causes the body to react with signs and symptoms

2. ___X___ The lack or absence of breathing

3. ______ Rapid or deep respirations followed by 10 to 30 seconds of apnea
4. ______ Slow breathing; respirations are fewer than 12 per minute
5. ______ Respirations gradually increase in rate and depth and then become shallow and slow; breathing may stop for 10 to 20 seconds
6. ______ Difficult, labored, or painful breathing
7. ______ Bloody sputum
8. ______ Blood in the pleural space
9. ______ Respirations are rapid and deeper than normal
10. ______ Respirations are slow, shallow, and sometimes irregular
11. ______ A reduced amount of oxygen in the blood
12. ______ Cells do not have enough oxygen
13. ______ Inserting an artificial airway
14. ______ Very deep and rapid respirations
15. ______ Using a machine to move air into and out of the lungs
16. ______ Breathing deeply and comfortably only while sitting
17. ______ Sitting up and leaning over a table to breathe
18. ______ The amount of hemoglobin containing oxygen
19. ______ The escape and collection of fluid in the pleural space
20. ______ Air in the pleural space
21. ______ A harmful chemical or substance in the air or water
22. ______ When breathing stops
23. ______ Slow, weak respirations at a rate of less than 12 per minute
24. ______ The process of withdrawing or sucking up fluid (secretions)
25. ______ Rapid breathing; respirations are 24 or more per minute

Fill in the Blanks

26. Oxygen is a ______________________________.

    It has no ______________________________,

    ______________________________,

    or ______________________________.

27. How are oxygen needs affected by respiratory status?

    ____

    ____

28. How are oxygen needs affected by fever?

    ____

    ____

29. Substance abusers are at risk for

    ____

    and ______________________________.

30. How are oxygen needs affected by alcohol?

    ____

    ____

    ____

    ____

31. Describe the 3 processes involved in respiratory function.

    A. ______________________________

    B. ______________________________

    C. ______________________________

32. Early signs of hypoxia are

    ______________________________,

    ______________________________,

    and ______________________________.

33. An SpO_2 measurement between __________%

    and __________% is within normal range.

34. Cyanosis is ______________________________

    ______________________________.

35. Normal respirations are

    ______________________________,

    ______________________________,

    and ______________________________.

36. Common causes of orthopnea include

    ______________________________,

    ______________________________,

    ______________________________,

    ______________________________,

    and ______________________________.

37. What is the purpose of a lung scan?

    ____

    ____

38. Miss Darby had a thoracentesis. Afterward she

    is observed for ______________________________,

    ______________________________,

    ______________________________,

    ______________________________,

    ______________________________,

    ______________________________,

    ______________________________,

    and ______________________________.

39. Miss Darby has a pulse oximeter sensor attached to her finger. The oximeter alarm will sound if:

    A. ______________________

    B. ______________________

    C. ______________________

40. Mucus from the respiratory system is called

    ______________________ when

    expectorated through the mouth.

41. Mr. Jenson has difficulty breathing. He prefers the orthopneic position. What can you do to increase his comfort?

    ____

42. How do coughing and deep breathing exercises help persons with respiratory problems?

    A. ______________________

    B. ______________________

43. The nurse delegates coughing and deep breathing exercises to you. What information do you need from the nurse and the care plan?

    A. ______________________

    B. ______________________

    C. ______________________

44. What is the goal of incentive spirometry?

    ____

45. Oxygen is treated as a ______________________.

46. List 4 ways that oxygen is supplied.

    A. ______________________

    B. ______________________

    C. ______________________

    D. ______________________

47. The amount of oxygen given is called

    ______________________.

48. Why is oxygen humidified?

    ____

    ____

49. When are artificial airways needed?

    A. ______________________

    ____

    B. ______________________

    ____

    C. ______________________

    ____

    D. ______________________

    ____

50. Which airway is inserted through the mouth and into the pharynx?

    ____

51. What should you do if an airway comes out or is dislodged?

    ____

52. A person has a tracheostomy. List 8 safety measures needed to prevent aspiration.

    A. ______________________

    ____

    B. ______________________

    ____

    C. ______________________

    ____

    D. ______________________

    ____

E. ______________________

____

F. ______________________

____

G. ______________________

____

H. ______________________

____

53. What does tracheostomy care involve?

A. ______________________

____

B. ______________________

____

C. ______________________

____

54. How many staff members are needed for tracheostomy care?

____

55. When giving tracheostomy care, you must call for the nurse at once if:

A. ______________________

B. ______________________

56. One complete suctioning cycle involves:

A. ______________________

B. ______________________

C. ______________________

57. The length of a suction cycle for adults is ______________________. The length of a suction cycle for infants and children is ______________________.

58. How many times is a suction catheter passed?

____

Labeling

59. Label the parts of a tracheostomy tube.

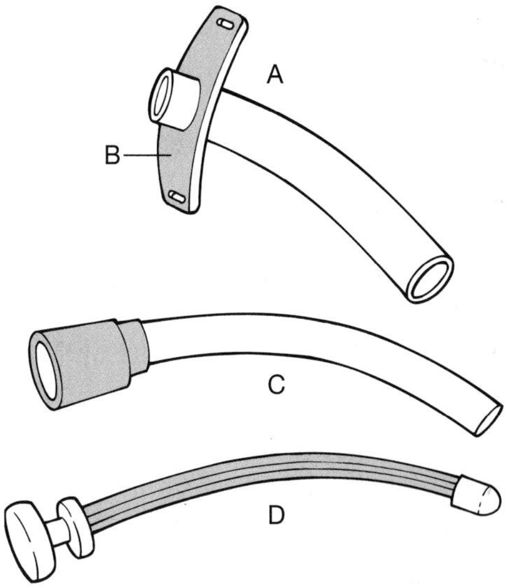

A ______________________

B ______________________

C ______________________

D ______________________

A. ______________________

B. ______________________

C. ______________________

D. ______________________

Multiple Choice

Circle the BEST answer.

60. Altered function of any system affects oxygen needs.
   A. True
   B. False

61. Aging affects oxygen needs because
   A. Older people have heart disease.
   B. Older people do not exercise.
   C. Respiratory muscles weaken and lung tissue becomes less elastic.
   D. Most older people have diets poor in iron and vitamins.

62. How often do normal respirations occur in a healthy adult?
    A. 12 to 20 times per minute
    B. 20 to 30 times per minute
    C. 5 to 10 times per minute
    D. 35 times per minute

63. During a pulmonary function test
    A. The person removes all jewelry.
    B. The amount of air moving in and out of the lungs is measured.
    C. A sputum specimen is collected.
    D. The pleura is punctured and fluid is aspirated.

64. A person has a pulse oximeter. This means
    A. You do not need to observe the person as often.
    B. The person's blood pressure is being measured.
    C. Oxygen concentration in arterial blood is being measured.
    D. Blood is taken from the radial artery to be tested.

65. A pulse oximeter is used on Ann Blake. She is 2 years old and moves around a lot. What is the better site for the sensor?
    A. The foot
    B. The palm of the hand
    C. A finger
    D. The earlobe

66. Collapse of a portion of the lung is
    A. Atelectasis.
    B. Pneumothorax.
    C. Pneumonia.
    D. Cyanosis.

67. You are assisting Mrs. Lopez with coughing and deep breathing exercises. Which is *incorrect?*
    A. Have her place her hands over her rib cage.
    B. Have her take a deep breath in through her nose.
    C. Ask her to hold the breath for 3 seconds.
    D. Ask her to exhale slowly through her nose.

68. Mr. Jones is receiving continuous oxygen therapy. This means
    A. The oxygen is stopped only for meals.
    B. Oxygen is given only for symptom relief.
    C. Oxygen is given only when the person is in bed.
    D. Oxygen is not interrupted for any reason.

69. Which does *not* promote safety when using oxygen?
    A. "No Smoking" signs in the room and on the room door.
    B. Keeping oxygen tanks away from heaters.
    C. Using electrical equipment with two-pronged plugs.
    D. Turning off electrical items before unplugging them.

70. An airway comes out. You should
    A. Call the nurse at once.
    B. Take the person's vital signs.
    C. Try to put the airway back in.
    D. Turn up the oxygen flow rate.

71. A person has a tracheostomy. The purpose of the obturator is
    A. To insert the inner cannula.
    B. To insert the outer cannula.
    C. To hold the tracheostomy cannula in place.
    D. To suction the tracheostomy.

72. You are suctioning Mr. Brown's tracheostomy. Suction is applied while inserting the catheter.
    A. True
    B. False

73. You are caring for a person on a mechanical ventilator. The alarm sounds. What should you do first?
    A. Call the nurse.
    B. Turn off the alarm.
    C. Get the Ambu bag.
    D. Check to see if the person's endotracheal tube or tracheostomy tube is attached to the ventilator.

74. Mrs. Jones has chest tubes. Which is *incorrect?*
    A. Make sure the tubing is not kinked.
    B. Keep the drainage system below the level of her chest.
    C. If a chest tube comes out, reinsert it at once.
    D. Report any change in chest drainage to the nurse at once.

ADDITIONAL LEARNING ACTIVITIES

1. Read each vignette. Then answer the questions that follow.

   Mr. Brown is a 50-year-old patient at Northeast Medical Center. His doctor has ordered a bronchoscopy.

   A. What is the purpose of a bronchoscopy?
   B. How is Mr. Brown prepared for the procedure?
   C. How is the procedure done?
   D. Who performs the procedure?
   E. What observations are made after the procedure?

   Mrs. Green is a 70-year-old resident of Valley View Nursing Center. Her doctor has ordered pulse oximetry. You have been assigned to assist with her pulse oximetry.

   A. What is the purpose of pulse oximetry?
   B. What information do you need from the nurse and the care plan?
   C. What observations do you need to report and record?
   D. How would you record an oxygen concentration value of 98?

   Miss Reed is a patient on the medical unit at Northridge Hospital. She is recovering from pneumonia. Her treatment plan includes the use of incentive spirometry. You have been assigned to assist her.

   A. What is the purpose of incentive spirometry?
   B. What is another name for incentive spirometry?
   C. How is the spirometer used?
   D. What information do you need from the nurse and the care plan?

   Mr. Blanc is a 20-year-old college student. He was in a car accident. As a result of his injuries, he needs mechanical ventilation to breathe. Mr. Blanc's parents visit every day. The nurse asks you to assist with Mr. Blanc's care.

   A. What is mechanical ventilation?
   B. What psychosocial needs might Mr. Blanc have?
   C. What care measures will you practice?

2. Define each of the following devices used to give oxygen.
   A. Nasal cannula

   B. Simple facemask

   C. Partial-rebreather mask

   D. Non-rebreather facemask

   E. Venturi mask

3. An RN delegates tracheostomy care to you. What information must you have before you proceed?

4. Discuss why it is important to know and follow the correct procedure when suctioning an airway.
   A. What safety measures must be practiced?
   Remember, some states and agencies do not allow assistive personnel to perform the procedures in Chapter 23.

24

Exercise and Activity

OBJECTIVES

The questions and student activities in this chapter will help you meet these objectives.

- Define the key terms listed in Chapter 24
- Describe bedrest
- Describe how to prevent the complications of bedrest
- Describe the devices used to support and maintain body alignment
- Explain the purpose of a trapeze
- Describe range-of-motion exercises
- Explain how to help a falling person
- Describe four walking aids
- Perform the procedures described in Chapter 24

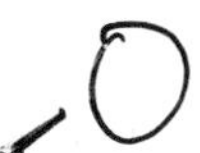

STUDY QUESTIONS

Matching

Match the following terms with the correct definitions.

A. Adduction
B. Dorsiflexion
C. Hyperextension
D. Orthostatic hypotension
E. Pronation
F. Internal rotation
G. Abduction
H. Syncope
I. External rotation
J. Contracture
K. Flexion
L. Plantar flexion
M. Supination
N. Atrophy
O. Extension
P. Range of motion
Q. Rotation
R. Footdrop

1. ______ Moving a body part away from the midline of the body
2. ______ Moving a body part toward the midline of the body
3. ______ A decrease in size or a wasting away of tissue
4. ______ The lack of joint mobility caused by abnormal shortening of a muscle
5. ______ Bending the toes and foot up at the ankle
6. ______ Straightening a body part

7. I ____ Turning the joint outward

8. K ____ Bending a body part

9. C ____ Excessive straightening of a body part

10. f ____ Turning the joint inward

11. D ____ Abnormally low blood pressure when the person suddenly stands up; postural hypotension

12. L ____ The foot is bent; bending down at the ankle

13. e ____ Turning the joint downward

14. P ____ The movement of a joint to the extent possible without causing pain

15. m ____ Turning the joint upward

16. H ____ A brief loss of consciousness; fainting

17. R ____ The foot falls down at the ankle; permanent plantar flexion

18. Q ____ Turning the joint

Fill in the Blanks

19. Being active is important for

____________________ and

____________________ well-being.

20. List 5 reasons why bedrest is ordered.

A. ____________________

B. ____________________

C. ____________________

D. ____________________

E. ____________________

21. Define these types of bedrest.

A. Bedrest

____

____

B. Strict bedrest

____

____

C. Bedrest with commode privileges

____

____

D. Bedrest with bathroom privileges

____

____

22. List 3 nursing measures that help prevent complications of bedrest.

A. ____________________

B. ____________________

C. ____________________

23. What are 2 complications of bedrest involving the musculoskeletal system?

____

____

24. What are 2 complications of bedrest involving the cardiovascular system?

____

____

25. ______________________________ is key to preventing orthostatic hypotension.

26. Trochanter rolls keep the hips and legs from ______________________________.

27. Foot boards prevent ______________________________

____

______________________________.

28. Exercise helps prevent ______________________________, ______________________________, and other complications of ______________________________.

29. List 3 ways a trapeze is used.

A. ______________________________

B. ______________________________

C. ______________________________

30. Mary Adams performs range-of-motion exercises to her knees and hips with some help from you. This is called ______________________________.

31. OBRA requires activity programs for nursing center residents. Activities must meet each person's ______________________________ and ______________________________, ______________________________, and ______________________________ needs.

32. You have been delegated range-of-motion exercises for Miss Mary Adams. What information do you need from the nurse and the care plan?

A. ______________________________

B. ______________________________

C. ______________________________

D. ______________________________

E. ______________________________

33. When can you perform range-of-motion exercises to a person's neck?

____

____

34. List and describe the range-of-motion exercises performed to the hips.

A. ______________________________

B. ______________________________

C. ______________________________

D. ______________________________

E. ______________________________

F. ______________________________

35. The act of walking is called ______________________________.

36. Why should you ease a person to the floor if the person starts to fall?

A. ______________________________

B. ______________________________

37. Mr. Reese lost his balance while you were assisting him with ambulation. You eased him to the floor. What must you report to the nurse?

A. ______________________________

B. ______________________________

C. ______________________________

D. ______________________

E. ______________________

38. List 8 safety measures for a person using crutches.

A. ______________________

____

B. ______________________

____

C. ______________________

____

D. ______________________

____

E. ______________________

____

F. ______________________

____

G. ______________________

____

H. ______________________

____

39. Braces are used to:

A. ______________________

B. ______________________

C. ______________________

40. You are applying a knee brace to Mr. Reese's left knee. What observations do you need to report to the nurse at once?

A. ______________________

B. ______________________

Multiple Choice

Circle the BEST answer.

41. Complications of bedrest include all of the following *except*
    A. Pneumonia
    B. Muscle atrophy
    C. Pressure ulcers
    D. Dorsiflexion

42. Footboards are used to
    A. Prevent the mattress from sagging.
    B. Prevent plantar flexion.
    C. Prevent orthostatic hypotension.
    D. Strengthen the feet.

43. Active range-of-motion exercises are performed
    A. By the person.
    B. With some help from a health team member.
    C. By a health team member.
    D. Only while a person is on bedrest.

44. Most any play activity promotes active range-of-motion exercises in children.
    A. True
    B. False

45. You are assisting Miss Mary Adams with range-of-motion exercises. Which is *incorrect?*
    A. Exercise only the joints the nurse tells you to exercise.
    B. Expose only the body part being exercised.
    C. Move the joint slowly, smoothly, and gently.
    D. Move the joint slightly beyond the point of pain.

46. Mrs. Smith is weak and unsteady from bedrest. You assist her to ambulate. Which is *false?*
    A. A gait belt is used.
    B. You check her for orthostatic hypotension.
    C. Handrails along the wall are used for additional support.
    D. Encourage her to walk bent forward and to slide her feet.

47. The patient or resident decides which crutch gait to use.
    A. True
    B. False

48. When using a cane to walk
    A. The cane tip is about 16 inches to the side of the foot.
    B. The grip is level with the waist.
    C. The cane is held on the strong side.
    D. The strong leg is moved forward first.

ADDITIONAL LEARNING ACTIVITIES

1. Make a list of activities in your daily life which provide ROM for your joints.
   A. How do these activities promote your physical, social, and emotional well-being?
   B. How can you use daily activities to promote ROM for patients and residents?

2. Practice active range-of-motion exercises. Use the procedure checklist on pages 412 through 415 as a guide. This will help you better understand the ROM of each joint.

3. Under the supervision of your instructor, practice the procedures in Chapter 24. Use the procedure checklists on pages 412 through 418 as a guide.
   A. Take your turn being the patient or resident.
   B. Discuss your experience.

4. Read the vignettes. Then answer the questions that follow.
   Mrs. Gomez is an 80-year-old resident of Northridge Nursing Center. She has been on bedrest for 3 days. She has been performing active-assistive ROM to her arms and legs while on bedrest. Her doctor wants her to begin walking. The nurse assigned you to care for Mrs. Gomez. The nurse reminds you that Mrs. Gomez is weak and unsteady from bedrest.
   A. What complications is Mrs. Gomez at risk for?
   B. How should Mrs. Gomez's activity be increased?
   C. Will you need to use a gait belt? Explain.
   D. What information will you need from the nurse and the care plan before helping Mrs. Gomez with ambulation?
   E. What supplies do you need to collect?
   F. How will you provide for privacy?
   G. What safety measures will you practice?
   H. What observations do you need to report and record after assisting Mrs. Gomez with ambulation?

   Mr. Reese needs passive ROM exercises to his left knee. The nurse delegates the ROM exercises to you.
   A. What information do you need from the nurse and the care plan before you begin?
   B. How will you provide for privacy?
   C. How will you position Mr. Reese?
   D. How will you support his leg?
   E. What exercises will you perform?
   F. How many times will you repeat each exercise?
   G. What safety measures will you practice?
   H. How will you provide for Mr. Reese's comfort when you complete the exercises?
   I. What do you need to report and record?

25

Measuring Vital Signs

OBJECTIVES

The questions and student activities in this chapter will help you meet these objectives.

- Define the key terms listed in Chapter 25
- Explain why vital signs are measured
- List the factors affecting vital signs
- Identify the normal ranges for each temperature site
- Know when to use each temperature site
- Identify the pulse sites
- Describe normal respirations
- Describe the factors affecting blood pressure
- Describe the practices followed when measuring blood pressure
- Know the normal vital signs for different age-groups
- Perform the procedures described in Chapter 25

STUDY QUESTIONS

Matching

Match the following terms with the correct definitions.

A. Hypertension
B. Blood pressure
C. Respiration
D. Systole
E. Pulse
F. Diastole
G. Apical-radial pulse
H. Pulse deficit
I. Stethoscope
J. Tachycardia
K. Hypotension
L. Diastolic pressure
M. Bradycardia
N. Pulse rate
O. Sphygmomanometer
P. Vital signs
Q. Body temperature
R. Systolic pressure

1. ___G___ Taking the apical and radial pulses at the same time
2. ___B___ The amount of force exerted against the walls of an artery by the blood
3. ___Q___ The amount of heat in the body that is a balance between the amount of heat produced and the amount lost by the body

4. M A slow heart rate; the rate is less than 60 beats per minute
5. f The period of heart muscle relaxation
6. L The pressure in the arteries when the heart is at rest
7. A Blood pressure that remains above the normal systolic (140 mm Hg) or diastolic (90 mm Hg) pressures
8. K When the systolic blood pressure is below 90 mm Hg and the diastolic pressure is below 60 mm Hg
9. e The beat of the heart felt at an artery as a wave of blood passes through the artery
10. H The difference between the apical and radial pulse rates
11. N The number of heartbeats or pulses felt in 1 minute
12. C Breathing air into (inhalation) and out of (exhalation) the lungs
13. O A cuff and measuring device used to measure blood pressure
14. i An instrument used to listen to the sounds produced by the heart, lungs, and other body organs
15. D The period of heart muscle contraction
16. R The amount of force needed to pump blood out of the heart into the arterial circulation
17. J A rapid heart rate; the heart rate is over 100 beats per minute
18. P Temperature, pulse, respirations, and blood pressure

Fill in the Blanks

19. Accuracy is essential when you

_______________,

_______________, and

_______________ vital signs.

20. Vital signs show even minor changes in a person's condition. Therefore you must report the following at once:

A. _______________

B. _______________

C. _______________

21. List the sites for measuring body temperature.

A. _______________

B. _______________

C. _______________

D. _______________

22. What is the normal range for body temperature for the rectal site?

____

____

23. Oral temperatures are not taken if the person:

A. ____________________

B. ____________________

C. ____________________

D. ____________________

E. ____________________

F. ____________________

G. ____________________

H. ____________________

I. ____________________

J. ____________________

24. Mr. Lewis has heart disease. Which temperature sites can you use?

____

____

25. Which temperature site is *not* used for infants and children under 6 years of age?

____

26. Why are rectal temperatures dangerous for persons with heart disease?

____

____

____

____

27. Which temperature site is the least reliable?

____

28. If a mercury-glass thermometer breaks, you must ____________________. Do not ____________________ and do not ____________________.

29. What do the short lines on a Fahrenheit thermometer mean?

____

30. What does each long line on a centigrade thermometer mean?

____

31. List 4 special measures needed when taking a rectal temperature with a glass thermometer.

A. ____________________

____

B. ____________________

____

C. ____________________

____

D. ____________________

____

32. Tympanic membrane thermometers are gently inserted into the ____________________.

33. Which site is used most often for taking a pulse?

____

34. Which pulse site is used during CPR and other emergencies?

____

35. List the rules to follow when using a stethoscope.

A. ____________________

____

B. ____________________

____

C. ____________________

____

D. ________________________________

____

E. ________________________________

____

36. The normal adult pulse rate is between

________________________________ and

________________________ beats per minute.

37. You are taking a radial pulse on Mr. Adams. What observations do you need to report and record?

A. ________________________________

____

B. ________________________________

____

C. ________________________________

____

38. You do not use your thumb to take a pulse because ________________________________

________________________________.

39. The healthy adult has ____________________ respirations per minute.

40. Respirations are normally

________________________________,

________________________________,

and ________________________________.

41. When are respirations usually counted?

____

42. You have counted Mr. Wilson's respirations. What observations do you need to report and record?

A. ________________________________

B. ________________________________

C. ________________________________

D. ________________________________

E. ________________________________

F. ________________________________

43. Blood pressure is controlled by:

A. ________________________________

B. ________________________________

C. ________________________________

44. Report any systolic pressure above

________________________________ and any diastolic pressure above ____________________.

45. List and briefly describe 3 types of sphygmomanometers.

A. ________________________________

____

B. ________________________________

____

C. ________________________________

____

Labeling

46. Label the pulse sites.

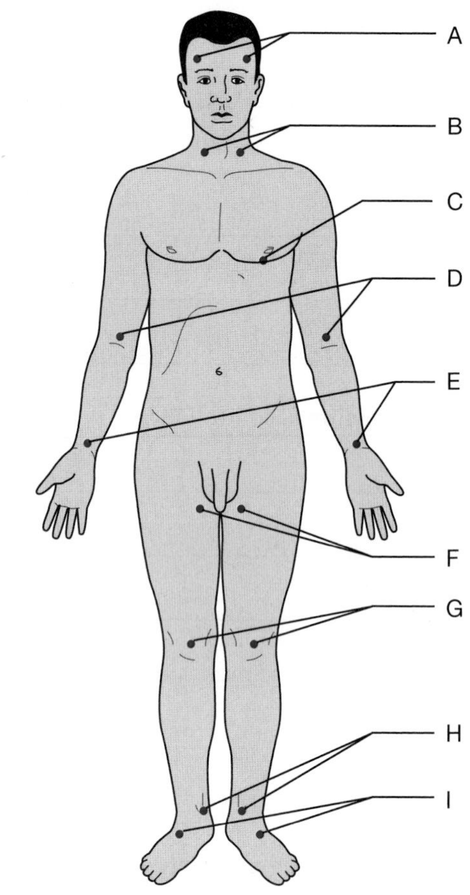

A. ____________________

B. ____________________

C. ____________________

D. ____________________

E. ____________________

F. ____________________

G. ____________________

H. ____________________

I. ____________________

47. Label the parts of a stethoscope.

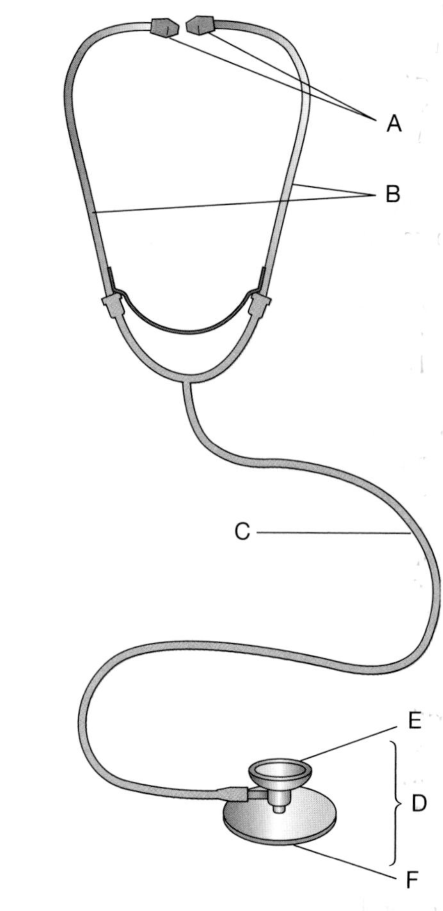

A. ____________________

B. ____________________

C. ____________________

D. ____________________

E. ____________________

F. ____________________

48. Place an X at the apical pulse site.

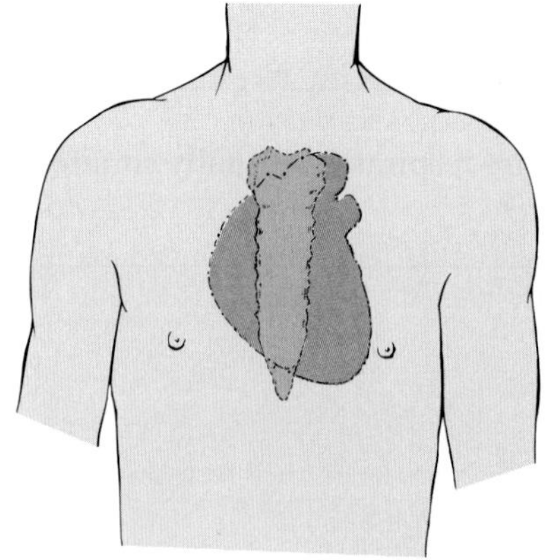

Multiple Choice

Circle the BEST answer.

49. Unless otherwise ordered, vital signs are taken
    A. After the person's bath.
    B. With the person lying or sitting.
    C. After breakfast.
    D. After performing ROM exercise.

50. Do *not* take an oral temperature if
    A. The person is unconscious.
    B. The person has diarrhea.
    C. The person has just had a bath.
    D. The person has heart disease.

51. You are taking a rectal temperature with a glass thermometer. Which is *incorrect?*
    A. Privacy is important.
    B. The thermometer is lubricated before insertion.
    C. The thermometer is held in place.
    D. The thermometer remains in the rectum for 1 minute.

52. Axillary temperatures
    A. Are more reliable than oral temperatures.
    B. Are taken right after bathing the person.
    C. Are taken for three minutes.
    D. Are used when other routes cannot be used.

53. Pacifier thermometers can be used for children under 5 years of age.
    A. True
    B. False

54. Which pulse site is used for children under 2 years of age?
    A. The radial site
    B. The brachial site
    C. The apical site
    D. The carotid site

55. Gregg Smith is 6 years old. What is the normal range for his pulse rate?
    A. 60 to 100 beats per minute
    B. 75 to 120 beats per minute
    C. 80 to 130 beats per minute
    D. 100 to 120 beats per minute

56. The force of a pulse relates to
    A. How regular the pulse is.
    B. The strength of the pulse.
    C. The number of beats per minute.
    D. The number of skipped beats.

57. An apical pulse is counted for
    A. 30 seconds
    B. 1 minute
    C. 2 minutes
    D. 5 minutes

58. You and a co-worker take an apical-radial pulse. Which is *false?*
    A. The apical and radial pulses are taken at the same time.
    B. There may be a difference between the apical and radial pulse rates.
    C. The apical rate may be less than the radial rate.
    D. The radial rate may be less than the apical rate.

59. The normal respiratory rate for a 2-year-old is
    A. 17 per minute.
    B. 20 per minute.
    C. 25 per minute.
    D. 35 per minute.

60. Which adult blood pressure is reported to the nurse at once?
    A. 142/90
    B. 118/80
    C. 120/80
    D. 116/78

61. Infants and children have higher blood pressures than adults.
    A. True
    B. False

62. Older persons are at risk for orthostatic hypotension.
    A. True
    B. False

63. Blood pressure is usually measured
    A. In the radial artery.
    B. At the apical site.
    C. In the popliteal artery.
    D. In the brachial artery.

64. Women usually have higher blood pressure than men do.
    A. True
    B. False

65. Blood pressure decreases with
    A. Age.
    B. Severe blood loss.
    C. Exercise.
    D. Smoking.

66. Which action is correct when measuring blood pressure?
    A. Taking the blood pressure on an arm with an IV infusion
    B. Applying the cuff over clothing
    C. Using a regular size cuff for a person with a very large arm
    D. Making sure the room is quiet

ADDITIONAL LEARNING ACTIVITIES

1. Practice the procedures in Chapter 25 with a classmate. Use the procedure checklist as a guide. Practice with various partners. Take your turn being the patient or resident. *Use a simulator for practicing rectal temperature.*
   A. Temperature
      (1) Practice reading a glass thermometer.
      (2) If available, practice taking temperatures with different types of thermometers. Discuss the advantages and disadvantages of each.
   B. Pulse
      (1) Practice with various classmates. Locate the following pulse sites: carotid, radial, brachial, popliteal, posterior tibial, and dorsalis pedis.
      (2) Take radial pulses on various persons. Do you notice differences in rate, rhythm, and force?
      (3) Take a person's pulse before and after exercise. Notice and record the differences in rate, rhythm, and force.
   C. Respirations
      (1) Practice with various people. Note differences in respiratory rates. Does the respiratory rate and depth of respirations change with exercise?
   D. Blood pressure
      (1) Practice with various people.
      (2) Take and record blood pressure before and after exercise.
      (3) Take and record blood pressure with the person lying, sitting, and standing.
      (4) If available, practice using different types of blood pressure equipment. Discuss advantages and disadvantages of each.

2. Read the vignette. Then answer the questions that follow.
   Mrs. Herman is a 65-year-old patient on the medical unit at Westlake Hospital. She has heart disease. She is also confused and restless. She has an IV infusion in her left arm. You have been assigned to measure Mrs. Herman's vital signs before she has her breakfast.
   A. What temperature sites can you use? Explain.
   B. Which arm will you take the blood pressure in? Explain.
   C. What information do you need from the nurse and the care plan before measuring:
      (1) Temperature?
      (2) Pulse?
      (3) Respirations?
      (4) Blood pressure?
   D. How will you protect Mrs. Herman's privacy when measuring her vital signs?
   E. What observations do you need to report and record when measuring:
      (1) Temperature?
      (2) Pulse?
      (3) Respirations?
      (4) Blood pressure?
   F. What are the normal ranges for Mrs. Herman's:
      (1) Temperature?
      (2) Pulse?
      (3) Respirations?
      (4) Blood pressure?

26

Obtaining an Electrocardiogram

OBJECTIVES

The questions and student activities in this chapter will help you meet these objectives.

- Define the key terms listed in Chapter 26
- Explain the purpose of electrocardiograms and telemetry
- Describe the structures and functions of the heart
- Explain the conduction system of the heart
- Identify the normal waves of an electrocardiogram
- Locate the sites for limb leads and chest leads
- Identify the functions of the electrocardiograph
- Describe electrocardiograph paper
- Calculate the heart rate using a 6-second strip
- Explain how to prepare the person for an electrocardiogram
- Know the dysrhythmias that are life-threatening
- Perform the procedure described in Chapter 26

STUDY QUESTIONS

Matching

Match the following terms with the correct definitions.

1. _____ Without a rhythm
2. _____ Interference on the electrocardiogram
3. _____ An abnormal rhythm
4. _____ A recording of the electrical activity of the heart; ECG or EKG
5. _____ An instrument that records the electrical activity of the heart
6. _____ A pair of electrodes; electrical activity is recorded between the electrodes
7. _____ Means to measure a person's heart rhythm and rate from a distant point

A. Lead
B. Arrhythmia
C. Electrocardiogram
D. Artifact
E. Telemetry
F. Electrocardiograph
G. Dysrhythmia

Fill in the Blanks

8. Doctors order electrocardiograms (ECGs) for persons with the following symptoms of heart disease:

   A. ______________________

   B. ______________________

   C. ______________________

   D. ______________________

9. Why are ECGs done before surgery?

   ____

   ____

10. The heart is hollow and has three layers. List the 3 layers of the heart.

    A. The ______________________ is the outer layer. It is a thin sac covering the heart.

    B. The ______________________ is the second layer. It is the thick muscular portion of the heart.

    C. The ______________________ is the inner layer. It is the membrane lining the inner surface of the heart.

11. List and briefly describe the functions of the 4 chambers of the heart.

    A. ______________________

    ____

    B. ______________________

    ____

    C. ______________________

    ____

    D. ______________________

    ____

12. Systole and diastole make up the

    ______________________.

13. The ______________________

    controls the cardiac cycle.

14. List the 4 structures that make up the heart's conduction system. Briefly describe the function of each structure.

    A. ______________________

    ____

    ____

    B. ______________________

    ____

    ____

    C. ______________________

    ____

    ____

    D. ______________________

    ____

    ____

15. What happens when an area outside the SA node starts an impulse?

    ____

    ____

16. Blocks can occur in the conduction system. What does a block do?

    ____

    ____

17. The ______________, ______________,

    and ______________________ are the major

    parts of the cardiac cycle.

18. The doctor studies the ECG to:

    A. ______________________

    B. ______________________

19. A standard ECG has 6 ____________________ leads and 6 ____________________ leads.

20. Chest leads are also called ____________________ ____________________.

21. Electrocardiograph paper is divided into squares. Moving vertically, the squares represent ____________________. Voltage is a measure of ____________________.

22. Using an electrocardiograph strip, how would you estimate the heart rate?
____
____

23. Interference occurring on an ECG is called artifact. List 5 causes of artifact.
A. ____________________
B. ____________________
C. ____________________
D. ____________________
E. ____________________

24. The doctor orders a *stat* ECG. What does this mean?
____
____

25. What is the preferred position for an ECG?
____

26. You are obtaining an ECG. You call the nurse immediately if the person has any of the following:
A. ____________________
B. ____________________
C. ____________________
D. ____________________
E. ____________________
F. ____________________
G. ____________________
H. ____________________

27. If you see anything abnormal on an ECG tracing, you must ____________________ ____________________.

28. The following dysrhythmias are life threatening:
A. ____________________
B. ____________________
C. ____________________
D. ____________________
E. ____________________

29. Initiate your agency's emergency response system if the person:
A. ____________________
B. ____________________
C. ____________________

30. Telemetry involves:
A. ____________________
____
B. ____________________
____
C. ____________________
____
D. ____________________
____

Labeling

31. Label the major parts of the cardiac cycle.

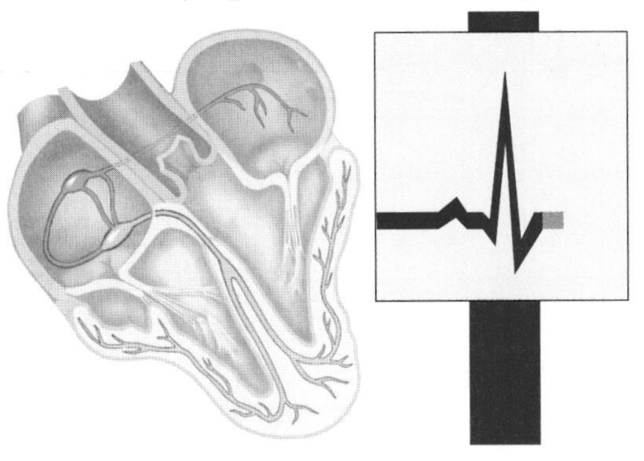

A. ______________________________

B. ______________________________

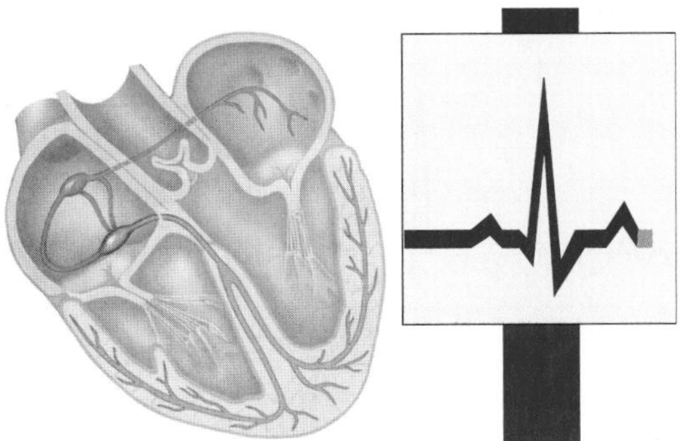

C. ______________________________

32. Place an X where each chest lead is placed for an ECG.

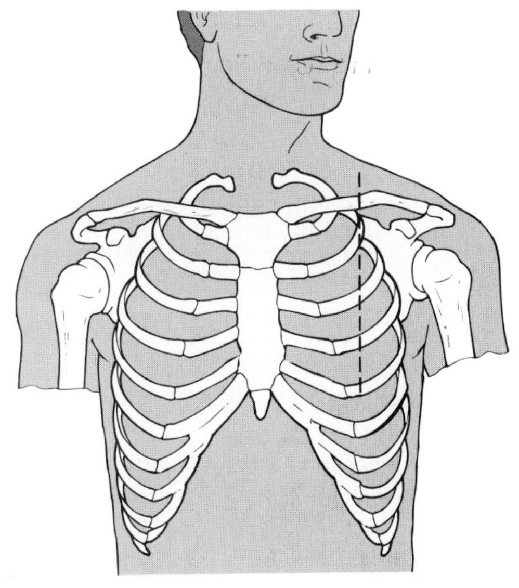

33. Calculate the heart rates using these 6-second charts.

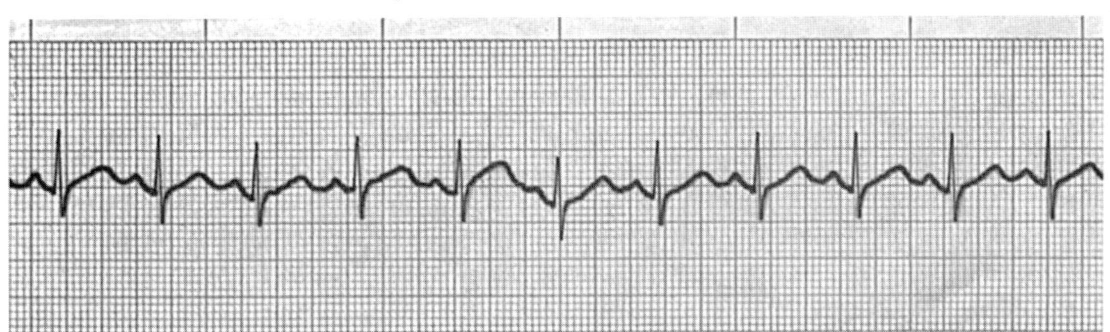

A. ______________________________

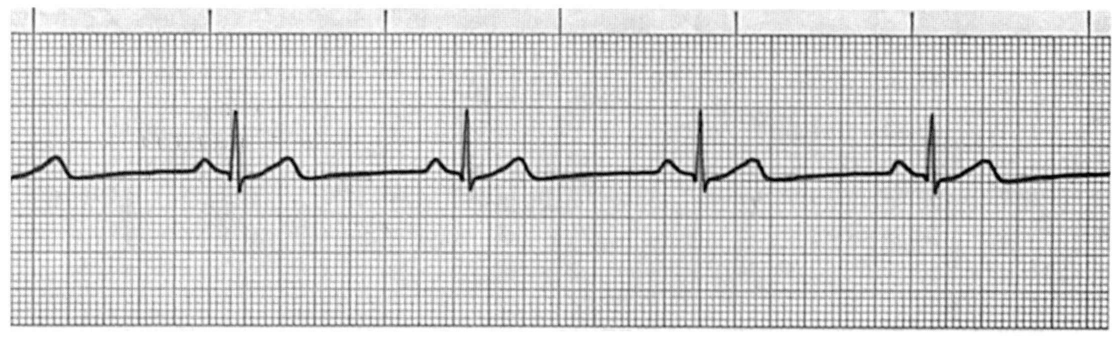

B. ______________________________

34. Identify the type of rhythm on each strip.

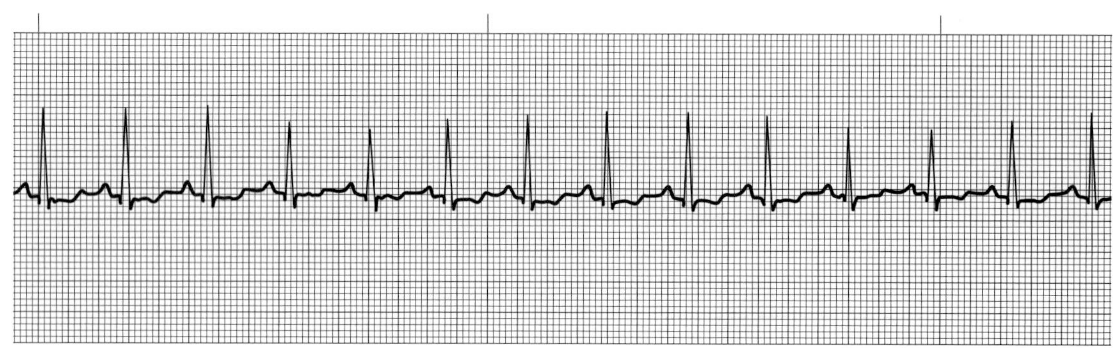

A.______________________________

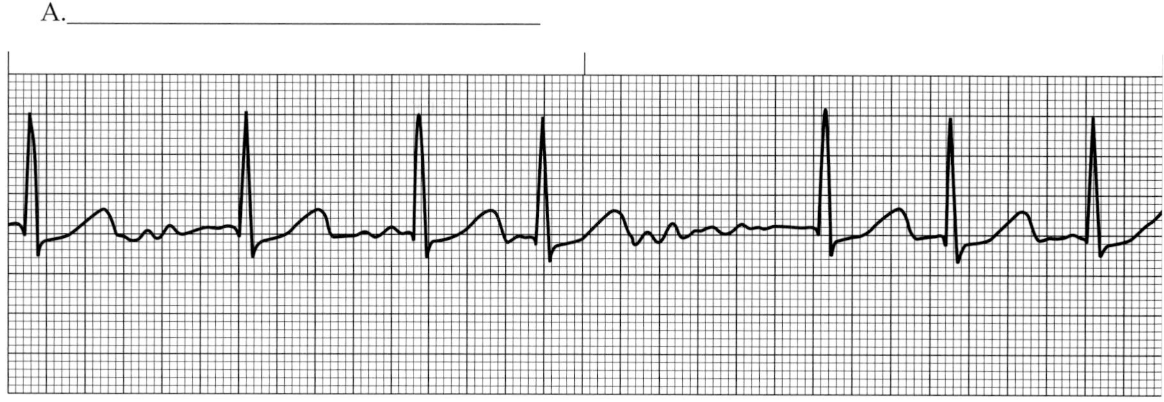

B.______________________________

Multiple Choice

Circle the BEST answer.

35. The heart chambers fill with blood during
    A. Systole.
    B. Diastole.
    C. Arrhythmia.
    D. Contraction.

36. The pace of the heart is set by
    A. The SA node.
    B. The AV node.
    C. The AV bundle.
    D. The Purkinje fibers.

37. Which causes artifact on an ECG?
    A. Increased heart rate
    B. Heart block
    C. Poorly connected or loose electrodes
    D. Abnormal heart rhythm

38. How many leads does a standard ECG involve?
    A. 10
    B. 12
    C. 14
    D. 16

39. You prepare the person's skin for an ECG by
    A. Shaving excess body hair and wiping electrode sites with alcohol.
    B. Wiping the electrode sites with a warm damp cloth.
    C. Applying lotion to prevent irritation.
    D. No skin preparation is needed.

40. You are obtaining an ECG from Mr. Eckhart. He complains of chest pain and shortness of breath. You should
    A. Discontinue the procedure, tell him you will be right back, and get the nurse.
    B. Put on his signal light and continue the procedure until the nurse arrives.
    C. Call for the nurse at once and stay with Mr. Eckhart until the nurse arrives.
    D. Report Mr. Eckhart's complaints to the nurse when you finish the procedure.

41. You are obtaining an ECG. The tracing appears to show asystole. Start your agency's life support procedures
    A. Immediately.
    B. After you call the nurse to check the tracing.
    C. After you disconnect the electrodes.
    D. If the person is unresponsive, not breathing, or has no pulse.

ADDITIONAL LEARNING ACTIVITIES

1. Work with a classmate. Use the procedure checklist on page 431 through 432 as a guide. Practice applying electrodes to the chest, arms, and legs. The more you practice the more skilled and confident you will become.
   A. Take your turn being the patient or resident.

2. Ask your instructor to obtain a variety of ECG strips for you to look at and interpret. This will help you become familiar with normal rhythm and the different dysrhythmias.

3. Read the vignette. Then answer the questions that follow.
   Miss Abbot was admitted to Evergreen Hospital by way of the emergency room. She has complaints of chest pain and dizziness. She is anxious. The doctor ordered a stat ECG. The nurse tells you to obtain the ECG.
   A. What information do you need from the nurse?
   B. How can you help Miss Abbot relax?
   C. What equipment and supplies do you need to collect?
   D. How will you prepare the electrode sites?
   E. What length tracing of each lead do you need to obtain?
   F. What observations do you need to report to the nurse at once?
   G. Why must you look at Miss Abbot if you notice ECG patterns similar to ventricular tachycardia, ventricular fibrillation, and asystole?
   H. How will you label Miss Abbot's ECG tracing?
   Remember, some states and agencies do not allow assistive personnel to perform the procedure in Chapter 26.

100%

27

Collecting and Testing Specimens

OBJECTIVES

The questions and student activities in this chapter will help you meet these objectives.

- Define the key terms listed in Chapter 27
- Explain why specimens are collected
- Describe the different types of urine specimens
- Explain why urine, stools, sputum, and blood are tested
- Explain the rules for collecting specimens
- Identify the sources of blood specimens
- Identify the sites for skin punctures and venipunctures
- Explain how to select tubes for blood specimens
- Perform the procedures described in Chapter 27

STUDY QUESTIONS

Complete the Crossword

Across

2. A swelling that contains blood
5. A short, pointed blade
6. A technique in which a vein is punctured

Down

1. The study of blood
3. A constricting device applied to a limb to control bleeding
4. A thick, hardened area on the skin

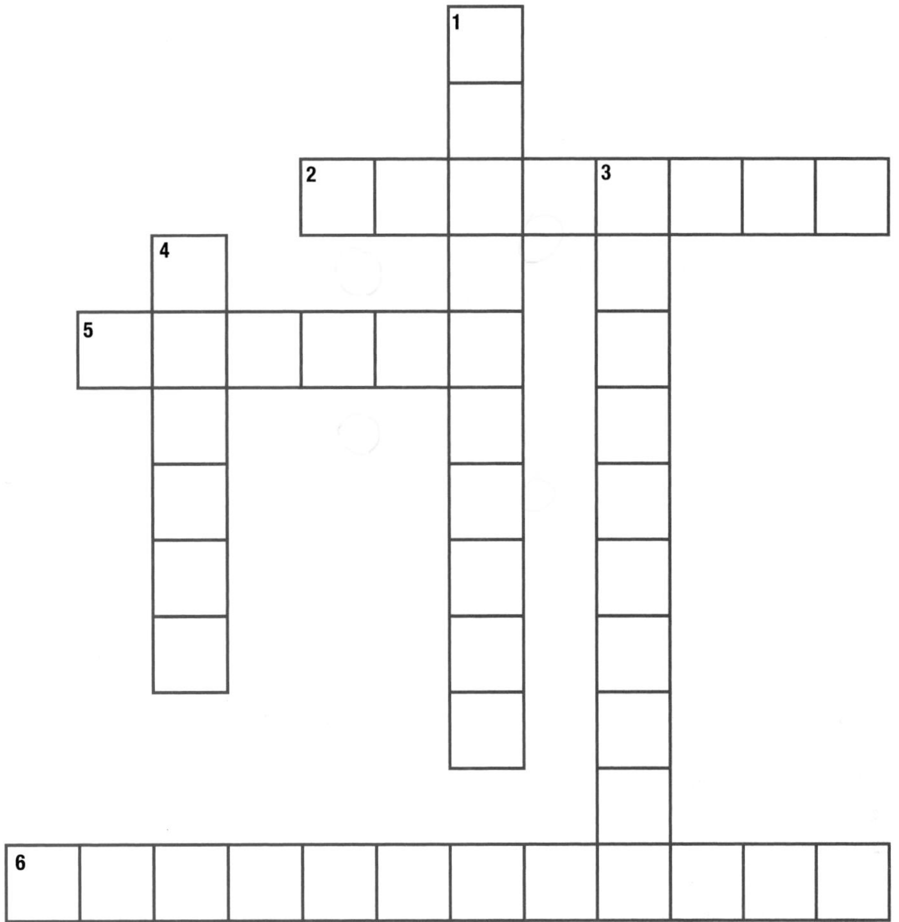

Matching

Match the following terms with the correct definitions.

A. Hematuria
B. Ketone body
C. Sputum
D. Melena
E. Glucosuria
F. Palpate
G. Hemoptysis

1. E Sugar in the urine; glycosuria
2. A Blood in the urine
3. G Bloody sputum
4. B Acetone; ketone
5. D A black, tarry stool
6. F To feel or touch using your hands or fingers
7. C Mucus from the respiratory system that is expectorated through the mouth

Fill in the Blanks

8. Specimens are collected and tested to ______________________________ ______________________________.

9. What information do you need from the nurse before collecting a urine specimen?

   A. ______________________________
   B. ______________________________
   C. ______________________________
   D. ______________________________
   E. ______________________________

10. The midstream specimen is also called ______________________________ ______________________________.

11. The nurse tells you to collect a midstream specimen from Mrs. Peterson. What equipment and supplies do you need to collect?

   A. ______________________________
   B. ______________________________
   C. ______________________________
   D. ______________________________
   E. ______________________________
   F. ______________________________
   G. ______________________________

12. How do you prevent the growth of microbes when collecting a 24-hour urine specimen?

____
____

13. Fresh-fractional specimens are used to test urine for ______________________________.

14. How would you collect a sterile urine specimen from a person with a catheter?

____
____

15. What parts of a syringe are sterile?

____
____

16. List and briefly describe the parts of a needle.

   A. ______________________________
   ____
   B. ______________________________
   ____
   C. ______________________________
   ____

17. Urine pH tests if urine is ______________________________ ______________________________.

18. Ketone bodies appear in the urine from ______________________________.

19. How can you make sure that you use reagent strips correctly?

____
____

20. A urinometer measures ______________________________ ______________________________.

21. What information do you need from the nurse before collecting a stool specimen?

   A. ______________________________
   B. ______________________________
   C. ______________________________
   D. ______________________________

22. When collecting stool specimens, you must follow ______________________ and the ______________________.

23. Sputum specimens are studied for ______________________, ______________________, and ______________________.

24. What is the purpose of postural drainage?

____

____

____

25. The nurse asks you to collect a sputum specimen from Mr. Juarez. What observations do you need to report and record?

A. ______________________

B. ______________________

C. ______________________

D. ______________________

E. ______________________

F. ______________________

G. ______________________

H. ______________________

26. When collecting a sputum specimen from a person who has or may have TB, you need to follow Standard Precautions, the Bloodborne Pathogen Standard, and ______________________ ______________________.

27. Blood tests are ordered and used to ______________________, ______________________, and ______________________ disease.

28. The nurse asks you to do a skin puncture on Mr. Duval. He has poor circulation in his hands. What can you do to increase blood flow to his fingers?

____

____

29. What are the most common venipuncture sites?

____

____

30. You are selecting an arm for a venipuncture. You should *not* choose the arm on the side:

A. ______________________

B. ______________________

C. ______________________

D. ______________________

31. You apply a tourniquet to Miss Mann's left arm. You do not feel a radial pulse in the arm. What should you do?

____

____

32. When selecting a vein for venipuncture, you should avoid veins that are:

A. ______________________

B. ______________________

C. ______________________

D. ______________________

33. How do you hold the needle and syringe for a venipuncture?

____

____

34. Blood glucose testing is used for persons with

_______________________________________.

The doctor uses the results to _______________

_______________________________________.

Labeling

35. Place an X on the sites for skin puncture.

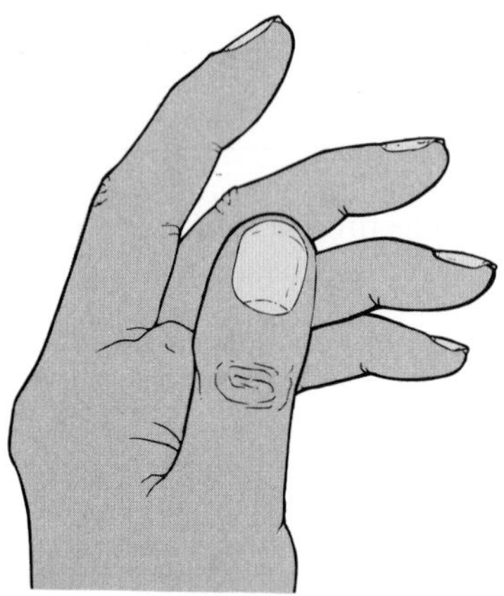

36. Label the parts of the vacutainer.

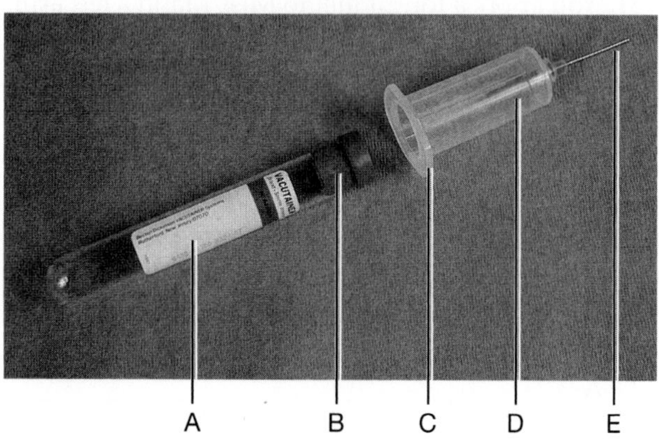

A. _______________________________________

B. _______________________________________

C. _______________________________________

D. _______________________________________

E. _______________________________________

Multiple Choice

Circle the BEST answer.

37. What type of specimen is collected for a urinalysis?
    A. A midstream specimen
    B. A 24-hour specimen
    C. A double-voided specimen
    D. A random specimen

38. You are assisting Mr. Clark to collect a 24-hour urine specimen. He voids to begin the test. Discard this voiding.
    A. True
    B. False

39. Which action is correct when using needles and syringes?
    A. Remove the needle from the syringe after use.
    B. Discard the needle and syringe into a sharps disposal container.
    C. Recap the needle after use.
    D. Bend or break the needle before discarding it.

40. To collect a urine specimen from an infant, a collection bag is applied over the urethra.
    A. True
    B. False

41. The body needs insulin to
    A. Maintain fluid balance.
    B. Use protein for tissue repair.
    C. Produce urine.
    D. Use sugar for energy.

42. What kind of urine specimen is needed to test for blood?
    A. A routine specimen
    B. A clean-catch specimen
    C. A double-voided specimen
    D. An early morning specimen

43. The normal specific gravity of urine is between
    A. 1.000 and 1.0100.
    B. 1.003 and 1.030.
    C. 1.035 and 1.0400.
    D. 1.0400 and 1.045.

44. Urine is strained to check for
    A. Occult blood.
    B. Ketones.
    C. Stones.
    D. Sugar.

45. Which statement about collecting sputum specimens is *false?*
    A. It is easier to collect a specimen in the morning.
    B. The person coughs up sputum from the bronchi and trachea.
    C. The person uses mouthwash to rinse before coughing up sputum.
    D. Privacy is important.

46. Use the center, fleshy part of the fingertip for skin punctures.
    A. True
    B. False

47. The heel is used for skin punctures in infants who are not walking.
    A. True
    B. False

48. You apply a tourniquet to perform a venipuncture on a vein in the antecubital space. Which is *incorrect?*
    A. The tourniquet is applied 1 inch above the elbow.
    B. You should feel the radial pulse.
    C. The veins below the tourniquet should distend.
    D. The tourniquet is applied no longer than 1 minute.

ADDITIONAL LEARNING ACTIVITIES

1. Have you had a skin puncture or venipuncture performed on you? Discuss your experience. Answer these questions.
   A. Was the person performing the procedure skilled?
   B. Was the procedure explained to you?
   C. Did you feel afraid or anxious? Explain.
   D. Did you experience pain or discomfort?
   E. How will your experience affect the care you provide?

2. What special measures are needed when collecting sputum specimens from infants and small children?

3. Read each of the following situations. Then answer the questions that follow.
   The nurse asks you to collect a 24-hour urine specimen from Mrs. Smith.
   A. What additional information do you need from the nurse before you collect the specimen?
   B. What equipment and supplies do you need to collect?
   C. How will you explain the procedure to Mrs. Smith?
   D. What are the steps involved in collecting a 24-hour urine specimen?
   E. What observations do you need to report and record?

Miss Norris has an indwelling catheter. The nurse asks you to collect a sterile urine specimen.

A. What conditions must be met before you collect a sterile urine specimen?
B. What information do you need from the nurse before you collect the specimen?
C. What equipment and supplies do you need to collect?
D. What steps are involved in collecting the specimen?
E. What safety measures will you practice when handling the needle and syringe?
F. How will you provide for Miss Norris's comfort and privacy?

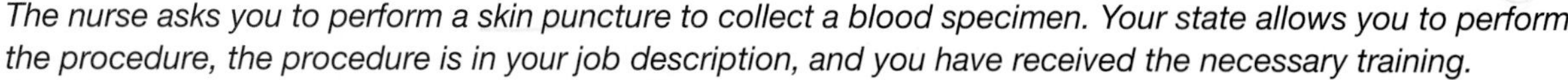

The nurse asks you to perform a skin puncture to collect a blood specimen. Your state allows you to perform the procedure, the procedure is in your job description, and you have received the necessary training.

A. What other conditions must be met before you perform the procedure?
B. What information do you need from the nurse before you perform the procedure?
C. What safety measures do you need to practice?
D. How will you prepare the puncture site?
E. What do you need to report and record after you perform the procedure?

Remember, some states and agencies do not allow assistive personnel to perform some of the procedures in this chapter.

28

Assisting With the Physical Examination

OBJECTIVES

The questions and student activities in this chapter will help you meet these objectives.

- Define the key terms listed in Chapter 28
- Explain what to do before, during, and after an examination
- Identify the equipment used for an examination
- Describe how to prepare and drape a person for an examination
- Explain the rules for assisting with an examination
- Perform the procedures described in Chapter 28

STUDY QUESTIONS

Matching

Match the following terms with the correct definitions.

A. Ophthalmoscope
B. Lithotomy position
C. Knee-chest position
D. Dorsal recumbent position
E. Percussion hammer
F. Otoscope
G. Nasal speculum
H. Laryngeal mirror
I. Vaginal speculum
J. Tuning fork

1. ______ The supine position with the legs together; horizontal recumbent position
2. ______ The person kneels and rests the body on the knees and chest; the head is turned to one side, arms are above the head or flexed at the elbows, the back is straight, and the body is flexed about 90 degrees at the hips
3. ______ An instrument used to examine the mouth, teeth, and throat
4. ______ The person lies on the back with the hips at the edge of the examination table, knees are flexed, hips are externally rotated, and feet are in stirrups
5. ______ An instrument used to examine the inside of the nose
6. ______ A lighted instrument used to examine the internal structures of the eye

7. ______ A lighted instrument used to examine the external ear and the eardrum

8. ______ An instrument used to tap body parts to test reflexes

9. ______ An instrument vibrated to test hearing

10. ______ An instrument used to open the vagina so it and the cervix can be examined

Fill in the Blanks

11. Examinations are done to:

    A. ______________________________

    B. ______________________________

    C. ______________________________

12. What you do to assist with examinations depends on:

    A. ______________________________

    B. ______________________________

13. Why does the person void before the examination?

    A. ______________________________

    ____

    B. ______________________________

    ____

14. Describe how you would measure length in a child under 2 years of age.

    ____

    ____

    ____

    ____

    ____

15. The nurse tells you to position Mrs. Sanchez in the lithotomy position. What do you need to explain to Mrs. Sanchez before you help her assume the position?

    A. ______________________________

    B. ______________________________

    C. ______________________________

    D. ______________________________

16. The dorsal recumbent position is used to examine the ______________________________,

    ______________________________,

    and ______________________________.

17. Which position is used to examine the vagina?

    ____

18. The ______________________________ position is used to examine the rectum in older persons.

19. A ______________________________ draws blood for laboratory study.

Labeling

20. Label these instruments used for a physical examination.

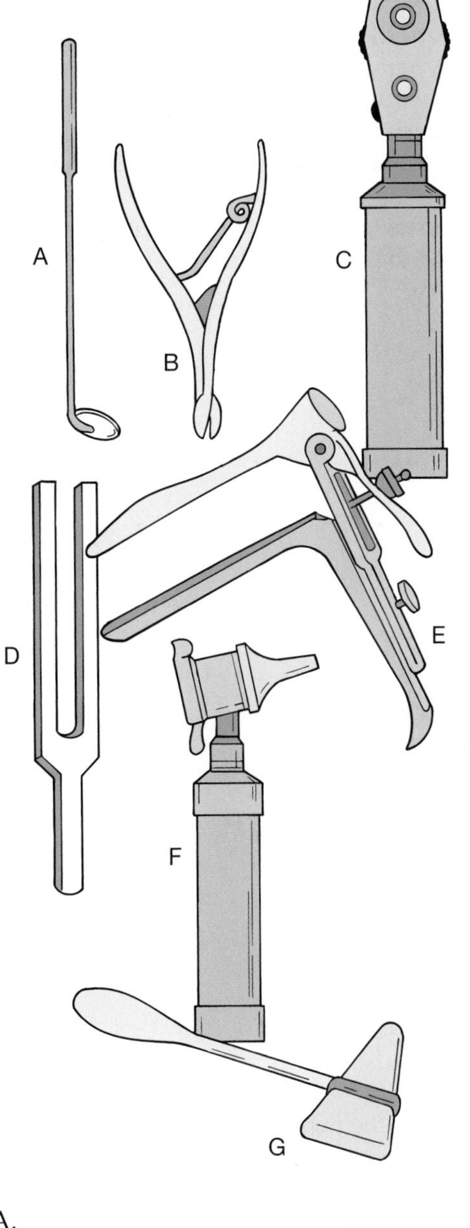

A. ____________________

B. ____________________

C. ____________________

D. ____________________

E. ____________________

F. ____________________

G. ____________________

21. Label these examination positions.

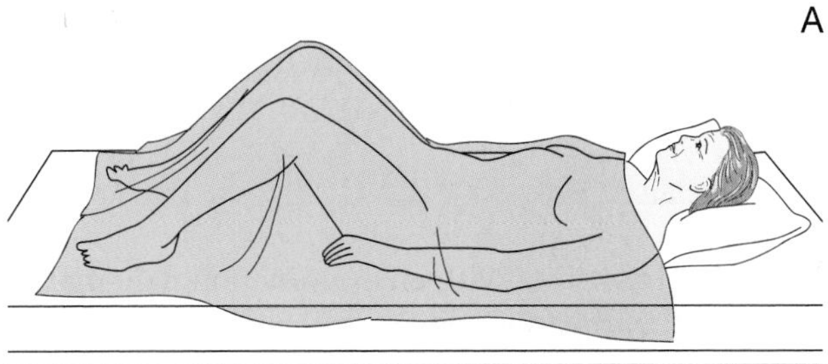

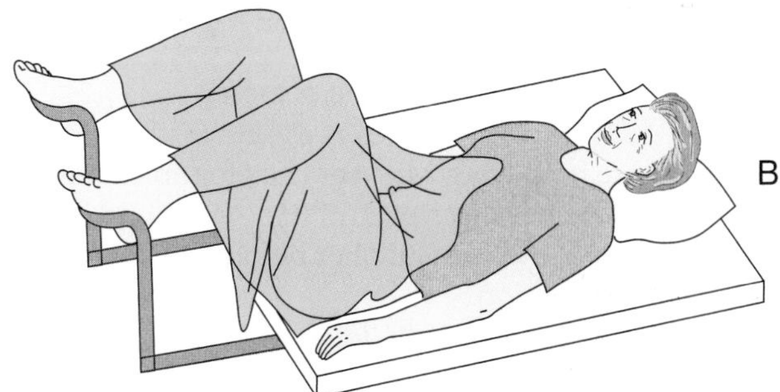

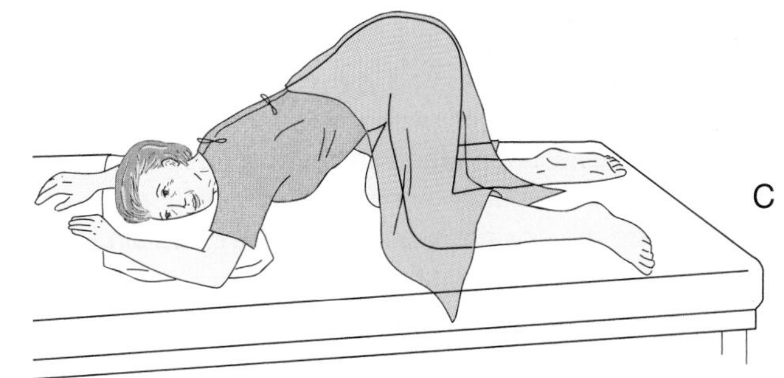

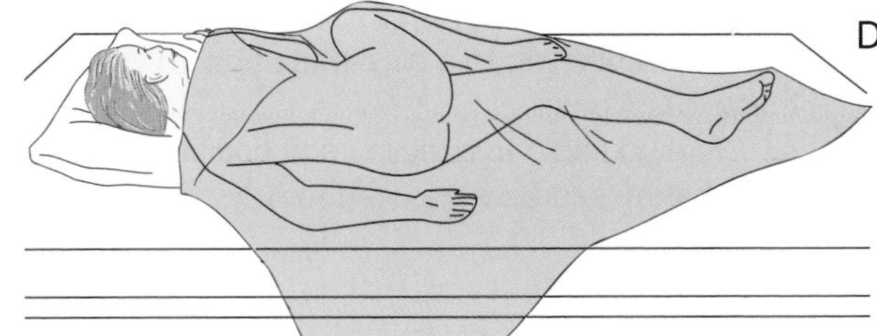

A. ____________________

B. ____________________

C. ____________________

D. ____________________

Multiple Choice

Circle the BEST answer.

22. An examination is done only if the person gives consent.
    A. True
    B. False

23. When assisting with an examination, you may do all of the following *except*
    A. Prepare the room.
    B. Explain the purpose of the examination to the person.
    C. Transport the person to and from the exam room.
    D. Position and drape the person.

24. You are preparing Mrs. Sanchez for an examination. Which is *incorrect?*
    A. Weigh and measure her before the examination.
    B. Clothes are usually left on.
    C. Only the body part being examined is exposed.
    D. She is protected from chilling.

25. To obtain an accurate weight, the person wears only a gown or pajamas.
    A. True
    B. False

26. You are assisting with the examination of a 2-year-old girl. Which is *false?*
    A. A parent is present during the exam.
    B. Toys are used to assess development.
    C. A small vaginal speculum is used.
    D. A calm manner helps the child and parent.

27. A person who resists an exam is restrained and forced to have the exam.
    A. True
    B. False

ADDITIONAL LEARNING ACTIVITIES

1. Practice assuming the various positions which are commonly assumed for examinations. Stay in each position for 10 minutes. Answer these questions:
   A. Are the positions uncomfortable? Explain.
   B. Did you feel dignified?
   C. How would you want your right to privacy protected?
   D. How will your experience affect the care you provide?

2. Practice explaining to a classmate how to assume each position and the purpose of each position. Answer these questions:
   A. Were you able to explain each position so the other person understood?
   B. What measures were used to help the person relax and decrease anxiety?

3. Handle and practice setting up the equipment used for an examination.

4. Read the vignette. Then answer the questions that follow.
Miss Mary Martin is an 80-year-old resident of Pine Ridge Nursing Center. She has joint stiffness due to arthritis. She also has poor circulation in her lower legs and feet. She is able to ambulate with a walker. Dr. Robert Moore has scheduled Miss Martin for her annual physical exam. Miss Martin does not like to undress in front of others. She says that she likes Dr. Moore, but he is so young. The nurse asks you to prepare the exam room, prepare Miss Martin, and assist with the physical exam. She tells you that the doctor wants Miss Martin's height and weight and vital signs. He also ordered a urinalysis.
   A. What additional information do you need from the nurse before you begin?
   B. How will you prepare the exam room?
   C. What fears might Miss Martin have?
   D. How is Miss Martin's right to personal choice protected?
   E. How will you prepare Miss Martin for her exam?
   F. How will you protect Miss Martin's right to privacy?
   G. How will you promote Miss Martin's comfort and safety?
   H. When will you obtain her vital signs and height and weight?
   I. When will you obtain the urine specimen?
   J. How will you position and drape Miss Martin? Explain.
   K. What positions might be uncomfortable for Miss Martin? Why?
   L. What observations and information do you need to report and record?
   M. What do you need to do after the exam to promote Miss Martin's comfort and safety?
   N. How will you clean the exam room after the exam?

100%

29 The Surgical Patient

OBJECTIVES

The questions and student activities in this chapter will help you meet these objectives.

- Define the key terms listed in Chapter 29
- Describe the common fears and concerns of surgical patients
- Explain how people are prepared for surgery
- Describe how to prepare a room for the postoperative patient
- List the signs and symptoms to report postoperatively
- Explain how to meet the person's needs after surgery
- Perform the procedures described in Chapter 29

STUDY QUESTIONS

Matching

Match the following terms with the correct definitions.

A. Thrombus
B. Postoperative
C. Embolus
D. Anesthesia
E. Preoperative
F. Urgent surgery
G. Emergency surgery
H. Elective surgery
I. Local anesthesia
J. Regional anesthesia
K. General anesthesia

1. D The loss of feeling or sensation produced by a drug
2. h Scheduled surgery done by choice to improve the person's life or well-being
3. C A blood clot that travels through the vascular system until it lodges in a distant blood vessel
4. G Surgery done immediately to save life or function
5. K The loss of consciousness and all feeling or sensation
6. I The loss of sensation or feeling in a small area

7. B After surgery

8. e Before surgery

9. J The loss of sensation or feeling in a larger area of the body

10. a A blood clot

11. f Surgery needed for the person's health; it is done soon to prevent further damage or disease

Fill in the Blanks

12. List 8 reasons that surgery is done.

A. ______

B. ______

C. ______

D. ______

E. ______

F. ______

G. ______

H. ______

13. Mrs. Wind is having same-day surgery. This means ______

______

______.

14. List 4 tests done before surgery.

A. ______

B. ______

C. ______

D. ______

15. Why is a person NPO 6-8 hours before surgery?

______

______

16. Personal care before surgery usually involves the following measures. Describe what is involved and the purpose of each.

A. A complete bed bath, shower, or tub bath:

______

______

______

B. Removing makeup, nail polish, and artificial nails:

______

______

______

C. Hair care:

______

______

______

D. Oral hygiene:

______

______

______

E. Removing dentures:

______

______

______

F. Checking for loose teeth in children:

____

____

____

G. Removing other prostheses:

____

____

____

17. You are preparing Mrs. Young for surgery. She is wearing a watch, earrings, and her wedding ring. What is done with this jewelry?

____

____

____

____

18. The skin is prepped before surgery to

____

______________________.

19. Why is the surgical site marked before the person goes to surgery?

____

____

20. Pre-operative medications are given to the person about 45 minutes to 1 hour before surgery. What is the purpose of these medications?

A. ______________________

B. ______________________

C. ______________________

21. What measures prevent falls and accidents after pre-operative medications are given?

A. ______________________

B. ______________________

C. ______________________

22. You have helped transfer Mr. Vincent to the stretcher for transport to the operating room. How will you provide for his comfort and safety?

____

____

____

____

23. The recovery room (RR) may also be called

______________________ or

______________________.

24. After surgery, the person is taken to the recovery room. The person returns to his or her room when:

A. ______________________

B. ______________________

C. ______________________

25. Post-operatively, proper positioning promotes

______________________ and prevents

______________________.

26. You promote the person's comfort during position changes by:

A. ______________________

B. ______________________

C. ______________________

27. What major respiratory complications do coughing and deep breathing exercises and incentive spirometry help prevent?

____

____

28. Leg exercises increase ______________________________ ______________________________ and help prevent ______________________________.

29. The doctor orders leg exercises every 2 hours while awake for Mr. Vincent. The following exercises are done 5 times:

A. ______________________________

B. ______________________________

C. ______________________________

D. ______________________________

30. What is the purpose of elastic stockings?

____

____

31. When applying elastic bandages you must do the following:

A. ______________________________

B. ______________________________

C. ______________________________

D. ______________________________

E. ______________________________

F. ______________________________

G. ______________________________

H. ______________________________

32. What information do you need from the nurse and the care plan before you apply elastic bandages?

A. ______________________________

B. ______________________________

C. ______________________________

D. ______________________________

E. ______________________________

33. You have applied and secured an elastic bandage to Miss Henry's right leg. What do you need to do next?

____

____

____

____

34. Early ambulation after surgery prevents

______________________________,

______________________________,

______________________________,

______________________________,

and ______________________________.

35. Pain is common after surgery. What factors affect the degree of pain?

A. ______________________________

B. ______________________________

C. ______________________________

Multiple Choice

Circle the BEST answer.

36. Mr. Randy Bland was in a car accident. He arrives at the hospital by ambulance. He has a torn artery in his right leg. He is taken to surgery at once to repair the torn artery. This is:
    A. Same-day surgery.
    B. Elective surgery.
    C. Urgent surgery.
    D. Emergency surgery.

37. You assist in providing psychological care to person's having surgery by:
    A. Telling the person not to worry.
    B. Answering questions about the surgery.
    C. Spending as little time with the person as possible.
    D. Reporting verbal and nonverbal signs of patient fear or anxiety to the nurse.

38. A person is NPO 6-8 hours before surgery. Which is *false?*
    A. An NPO sign is placed in the person's room.
    B. The person is allowed only sips of water.
    C. The water pitcher and glass are removed from the person's room.
    D. The person is allowed nothing to eat or drink.

39. You can obtain the person's consent for surgery if an RN delegates the task to you.
    A. True
    B. False

40. What type of bed is made for the person returning from the recovery room?
    A. A closed bed
    B. An open bed
    C. A surgical bed
    D. An occupied bed

41. Elastic stockings prevent
    A. Pain.
    B. Pulmonary complications.
    C. Thrombi.
    D. Aspiration.

42. Elastic stockings are applied
    A. With the person in a sitting position.
    B. Every 4 hours.
    C. Before the person gets out of bed.
    D. When you have time.

43. Early ambulation after surgery is discouraged because it is uncomfortable for the patient.
    A. True
    B. False

44. Notify the nurse if a person has not voided within 8 hours after surgery.
    A. True
    B. False

45. Anesthesia can cause nausea and vomiting.
    A. True
    B. False

ADDITIONAL LEARNING ACTIVITIES

1. Have you or a family member ever had surgery? If so, answer the following questions.
    A. What fears were there before and after surgery?
    B. How did members of the health care team help meet the person's physical and psychological needs?

2. Read the vignette. Then answer the questions that follow.
    Mr. Vincent is a 54-year-old man admitted to the hospital for surgery to remove an abdominal tumor. He is an accountant at a local bank. He has 2 children in high school. Mr. Vincent is scheduled for surgery in the morning. He tells you that he is afraid because his uncle died from colon cancer. Mr. Vincent's wife is with him.
    A. What fears might Mr. Vincent and his wife have?
    B. What do you need to report to the nurse?
    C. What information does the doctor explain to Mr. Vincent and his wife?
    D. What preoperative teaching does the nurse do?
    E. What tests and procedures might the doctor order and why?
    F. How can you assist in Mr. Vincent's psychological care?

The morning of surgery the nurse assigns you to assist Mr. Vincent to get ready for surgery.

A. What personal care will Mr. Vincent need?
B. What information do you need from the nurse before you do the skin prep?
C. What observations about the skin prep do you need to report and record?
D. What safety measures are practiced after Mr. Vincent receives his preoperative medication?
E. How will you prepare Mr. Vincent's room for transfer to the OR?
F. How is Mr. Vincent's safety promoted after he is transferred to the stretcher?

Mr. Vincent is a 54-year-old hospital patient. He had abdominal surgery. After surgery he was taken to the recovery room. His condition is stable and the nurse tells you that he is returning to his room. Mr. Vincent has a catheter. He also has an IV in his left arm and elastic stockings on both legs.

A. How is Mr. Vincent's room prepared for his return from the recovery room?
B. What can you do to help transfer Mr. Vincent to his bed and to position him?
C. How often are vital signs usually measured postoperatively?
D. How often is Mr. Vincent repositioned?
E. What observations related to Mr. Vincent's elastic stockings do you need to report and record?
F. How will you promote Mr. Vincent's comfort and safety during:
   (1) Repositioning?
   (2) Coughing and deep breathing exercises?
   (3) Leg exercises?
G. What measures will help meet Mr. Vincent's needs for:
   (1) Nutrition and fluids?
   (2) Elimination?
   (3) Comfort and rest?
H. What personal hygiene measures are needed to promote Mr. Vincent's physical and mental well-being?

3. Review and practice the procedures in Chapter 29. Use the procedure checklists on pages 468 through 472 as a guide. Take your turn being the patient.
   A. Discuss your experience.
   B. How will your experience affect the care you provide?

4. Review and practice the leg exercises in Chapter 29. Take your turn being the patient.
   A. Discuss your experience.
   B. How will your experience affect the care you provide?

100%

30 Wound Care

OBJECTIVES

The questions and student activities in this chapter will help you meet these objectives.

- Define the key terms listed in Chapter 30
- Describe the different types of wounds
- Describe skin tears, pressure ulcers, and circulatory ulcers and how to prevent them
- Identify the pressure points in each body position
- Describe the process, types, and complications of wound healing
- Describe what to observe about wounds and wound drainage
- Explain how to secure dressings
- Explain the rules for applying dressings
- Explain the rules for cleaning wounds and drain sites
- Explain the purpose of binders and how to apply them
- Describe how to meet the basic needs of persons with wounds
- Perform the procedure described in Chapter 30

STUDY QUESTIONS

Complete the Crossword

Across

1. The separation of the wound along with the protrusion of abdominal organs
4. An open wound with torn tissues and jagged edges
5. A closed wound caused by a blow to the body; bruise
7. A break in the skin or mucous membrane

Down

2. A partial-thickness wound caused by the scraping away or rubbing of the skin
3. The condition that results when there is not enough blood supply to organs and tissues
6. An accident or violent act that injures the skin, mucous membranes, bones, and internal organs

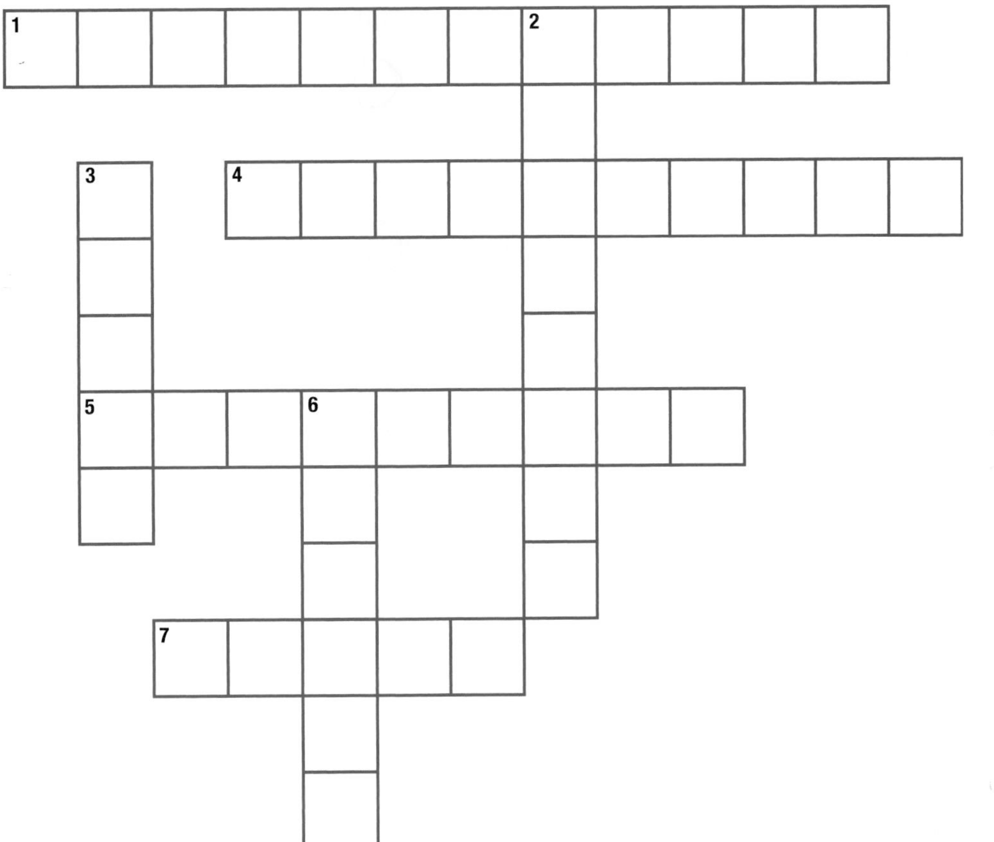

Matching

Match the following terms with the correct definitions.

A. Infected wound
B. Open wound
C. Puncture wound
D. Full-thickness wound
E. Sanguineous drainage
F. Partial-thickness wound
G. Penetrating wound
H. Contaminated wound
I. Clean wound
J. Chronic wound
K. Purulent drainage
L. Closed wound
M. Clean-contaminated wound
N. Intentional wound
O. Serous drainage
P. Unintentional wound
Q. Dehiscence
R. Hematoma
S. Epidermal stripping
T. Serosanguineous drainage

1. ______ A wound that does not heal easily
2. ______ Occurs from the surgical entry of the reproductive, urinary, respiratory, or gastrointestinal system
3. ______ A wound that is not infected; microbes have not entered the wound
4. ______ Tissues are injured but the skin is not broken
5. ______ A wound with a high risk of infection
6. ______ The separation of wound layers
7. ______ The dermis, epidermis, and subcutaneous tissue are penetrated; muscle and bone may be involved
8. ______ A collection of blood under the skin and tissues

9. __a__ A wound containing large amounts of microbes and that shows signs of infection; a dirty wound

10. __n__ A wound created for therapy

11. __B__ The skin or mucous membrane is broken

12. __f__ The dermis and epidermis of the skin are broken

13. __G__ An open wound in which the skin and underlying tissues are pierced

14. __C__ An open wound made by a sharp object; entry of the skin and underlying tissues may be intentional or unintentional

15. __K__ Thick green, yellow, or brown drainage

16. __R__ Bloody drainage

17. __t__ Thin, watery drainage that is blood-tinged

18. __O__ Clear, watery fluid

19. __P__ A wound resulting from trauma

20. __S__ Removing the epidermis as tape is removed from the skin

Fill in the Blanks

21. A ______________________ is a break or rip in the skin. The epidermis separates from the underlying tissues.

22. A stasis ulcer is ______________________

____

______________________.

23. Your role in wound care depends on

______________________,

______________________,

and ______________________.

24. List 8 measures to help prevent skin tears.

A. ______________________

____

B. ______________________

____

C. ______________________

____

D. ______________________

____

E. ______________________

____

F. ______________________

____

G. ______________________

____

H. ______________________

____

25. ______________________________,

______________________________,

and ______________________________

are common causes of skin breakdown and pressure ulcers. Other factors include

______________________________,

______________________________,

______________________________,

______________________________,

and ______________________________.

26. Shearing is when ______________________________

____

____

______________________________.

27. Persons at risk for pressure ulcers are those who:

A. ______________________________

B. ______________________________

C. ______________________________

D. ______________________________

E. ______________________________

F. ______________________________

G. ______________________________

H. ______________________________

I. ______________________________

J. ______________________________

28. The first sign of a pressure ulcer is

______________________________.

29. ______________________________ is a condition in which there is death of tissue.

30. ______________________________ are open wounds on the lower legs and feet caused by decreased blood flow through arteries or veins.

31. List 8 risk factors for stasis ulcers.

A. ______________________________

B. ______________________________

C. ______________________________

D. ______________________________

E. ______________________________

F. ______________________________

G. ______________________________

H. ______________________________

32. What are common sites for arterial ulcers?

____

____

____

33. Briefly describe the three phases of wound healing.

A. Inflammation phase:

____

____

B. Proliferative phase:

____

____

C. Maturation phase:

____

____

34. ______________________ is the excessive loss of blood in a short time.

35. ______________________ is bleeding inside the body into tissues and body cavities.

36. Describe three ways to measure wound drainage.

A. ______________________

____

B. ______________________

____

C. ______________________

____

37. List 7 functions of wound dressings.

A. ______________________

B. ______________________

C. ______________________

D. ______________________

E. ______________________

F. ______________________

G. ______________________

38. ______________________ are used for large dressings and frequent dressing changes.

39. You are changing Mr. Burt's abdominal dressing. What observations do you need to report and record?

A. ______________________

____

B. ______________________

____

C. ______________________

____

D. ______________________

____

E. ______________________

____

F. ______________________

____

G. ______________________

____

H. ______________________

____

I. ______________________

____

40. List 5 ways that binders promote wound healing.

A. ______________________

B. ______________________

C. ______________________

D. ______________________

E. ______________________

41. Incorrect application of binders can cause:

A. ______________________

B. ______________________

C. ______________________

42. Whatever the wound site and size, it affects

______________________.

Labeling

43. Place an X on the pressure points for each position.

A

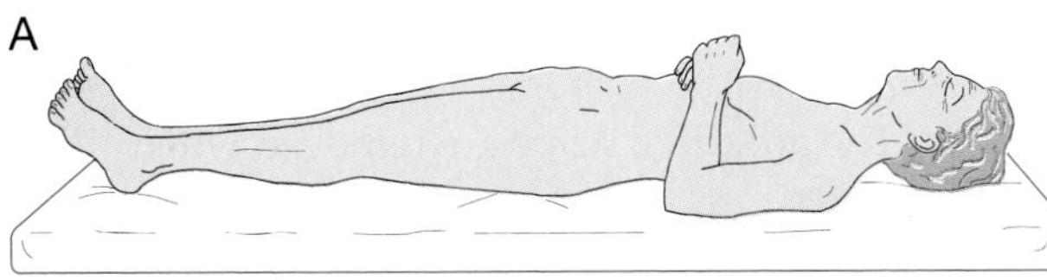

B

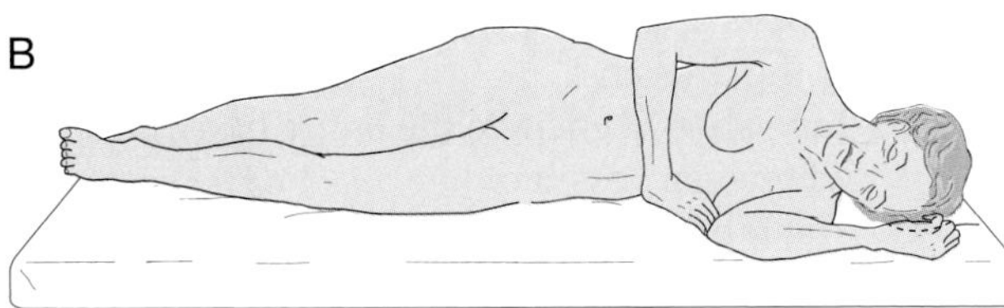

C

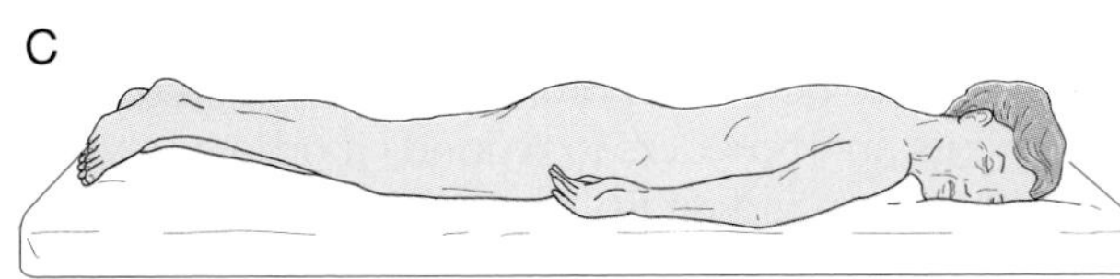

D

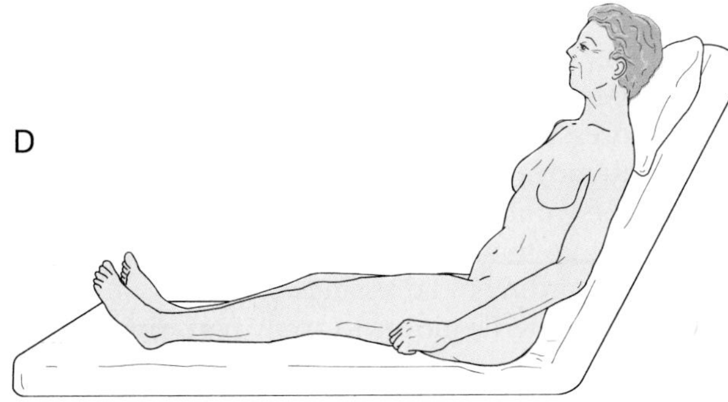

E

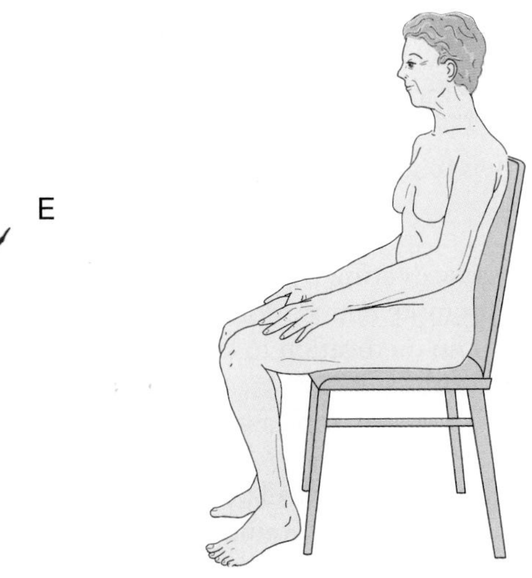

Multiple Choice

Circle the BEST answer.

44. Any injury caused by unrelieved pressure is
    A. A skin tear.
    B. An intentional wound.
    C. A pressure ulcer.
    D. A chronic wound.

45. Miss Paul has a stage 2 decubitus ulcer. This means
    A. The skin is red but intact.
    B. The skin is cracked and there is a shallow crater.
    C. The skin is gone. The underlying tissue is gone. There is drainage.
    D. Muscle and bone are exposed and damaged.

46. Which measure helps prevent pressure ulcers?
    A. Repositioning the person every 4 hours
    B. Raising the head of the bed 45 to 60 degrees when the person is in bed
    C. Vigorously rubbing the skin dry after bathing
    D. Positioning the person in the 30-degree lateral position

47. A metal frame placed on the bed and over the person to keep top linens off the feet is called
    A. A bed cradle.
    B. A heel elevator.
    C. A flotation pad.
    D. An eggcrate-like mattress.

48. Open wounds on the lower legs and feet caused by poor blood return through the veins are called
    A. Arterial ulcers.
    B. Pressure ulcers.
    C. Epidermal ulcers.
    D. Stasis ulcers.

49. Arterial ulcers are often painful at rest and are usually worse at night.
    A. True
    B. False

50. A venipuncture is
    A. An intentional wound.
    B. A contaminated wound.
    C. An unintentional wound.
    D. A closed wound.

51. A wound is healing by secondary intention. Which is *false?*
    A. The wound edges are brought together.
    B. The wound gaps.
    C. Healing occurs naturally.
    D. Healing takes longer.

52. Which is *not* a sign or symptom of shock?
    A. Falling blood pressure
    B. A strong, regular pulse
    C. Cold, moist, and pale skin
    D. Restlessness

53. Mrs. Adams has a surgical incision. The incision is reddened and has drainage. Mrs. Adams has a fever and complains of pain at her incision site. These are signs and symptoms of
    A. A healing wound.
    B. An infected wound.
    C. Hemorrhage.
    D. Shock.

54. Dehiscence and evisceration are surgical emergencies.
    A. True
    B. False

55. A signed consent is *not* needed before taking a photograph of a person's wound.
    A. True
    B. False

56. Serous drainage is
    A. Blood-tinged.
    B. Thick and green.
    C. Clear and watery.
    D. Dark red.

57. A transparent adhesive film dressing
    A. Absorbs drainage.
    B. Keeps the wound moist.
    C. Helps control bleeding.
    D. Prevents pain.

58. A gauze dressing saturated with a solution is applied over the wound. More dressings are applied as needed. They are also saturated with solution. The dead tissue is absorbed by the dressing and removed with the dressing. The dressings are removed when dry. This is a
    A. Nonadherent dressing.
    B. Wet-to-dry dressing.
    C. Dry-to-dry dressing.
    D. Wet-to-wet dressing.

59. Montgomery ties are used to secure a dressing. Which is *incorrect?*
    A. The adhesive strips are removed with each dressing change.
    B. Cloth ties are secured over the dressing.
    C. The cloth ties are undone for dressing changes.
    D. The adhesive strips are removed when soiled.

60. Which is correct when applying tape to secure a dressing?
    A. Tape is applied to secure the top and bottom of the dressing.
    B. Tape should encircle the entire body part whenever possible.
    C. The tape extends 1 inch on each side of the dressing.
    D. Tape is applied to secure the top, middle, and bottom of the dressing.

61. Assistive personnel can apply medicated ointments and powders to wounds if ordered by the doctor and an RN is available to supervise.
    A. True
    B. False

62. Which is correct when applying sterile dressings?
    A. Wear sterile gloves for removing old dressings.
    B. Remove tape by gently pulling it away from the wound.
    C. Set up your sterile field before removing and discarding old dressings.
    D. Wear sterile gloves to apply new dressings.

63. You are cleaning a drain site. Which is *incorrect?*
    A. Use a circular motion.
    B. Clean from the surrounding skin toward the drain site.
    C. Use a sterile forceps to hold the sterile gauze.
    D. Use a different gauze dressing for each stroke.

64. Mrs. Gomez is recovering from a traumatic wound. You promote her comfort by
    A. Allowing pain medication to take effect before giving care.
    B. Telling her to ignore unpleasant odors caused by drainage.
    C. Telling her that she will feel better if she does not talk about her wound.
    D. Encouraging her to look at her wound.

ADDITIONAL LEARNING ACTIVITIES

1. If available, handle the various types of dressings commonly used for wound care. Practice opening packages and applying various types of dressings. Also practice applying and removing various types of tape. The greater your skill, the better care you can provide.

2. Mr. Norris has a sterile abdominal dressing. The nurse tells you to change the dressing.
   A. What conditions must be in place before you can change a sterile dressing?

3. You are allowed to change sterile dressings in your state and agency, and you have the necessary training and supervision.
   A. What information do you need from the nurse before you change a dressing?

4. List the rules for applying binders.

5. Read the vignette. Then answer the questions that follow.
   Miss Bonnie Lee is a 62-year-old hospital patient. Miss Lee has high blood pressure and smokes a pack of cigarettes a day. She is diabetic and is being treated for a large stasis ulcer on her right leg. She has been trying to heal the wound at home for the past 6 months, but it keeps getting worse. The ulcer is painful and drains a clear, yellow fluid. Miss Lee tells you that she cannot afford to be away from work. She is also worried that she will lose her leg if the ulcer will not heal.
   A. What type of wound does Miss Lee have?
   B. What risk factors for developing circulatory ulcers does Miss Lee have?
   C. What fears are Miss Lee expressing?
   D. What type of drainage is there?
   E. How can you promote Miss Lee's safety and comfort?
   Remember, some states and agencies do not allow assistive personnel to perform the procedure in Chapter 30.

31

Heat and Cold Applications

OBJECTIVES

The questions and student activities in this chapter will help you meet these objectives.

- Define the key terms listed in Chapter 31
- Identify the purposes, effects, and complications of heat and cold applications
- Identify the persons at risk for complications from heat and cold applications
- Explain the differences between moist and dry heat and cold applications
- Describe the rules for applying heat and cold
- Explain how cooling and warming blankets are used
- Perform the procedures described in Chapter 31

STUDY QUESTIONS

Matching

Match the following terms with the correct definitions.

A. Cyanosis
B. Hypothermia
C. Constrict
D. Compress
E. Hyperthermia
F. Dilate
G. Pack

1. ______ A soft pad applied over a body area
2. ______ To narrow
3. ______ Bluish skin color
4. ______ To expand or open wider
5. ______ A body temperature that is much higher than the person's normal range
6. ______ A very low body temperature
7. ______ A treatment that involves wrapping a body part with a wet or dry application

Fill in the Blanks

8. Heat applications are used to:

   A. ______________________________

   B. ______________________________

   C. ______________________________

   D. ______________________________

   E. ______________________________

9. What happens when heat is applied too long?

   ____

   ____

   ____

10. Persons at great risk for complications from heat applications are:

    A. ______________________________

    B. ______________________________

    C. ______________________________

    D. ______________________________

    E. ______________________________

11. How do infants and young children communicate pain?

    ____

12. What are the advantages of dry heat?

    A. ______________________________

    B. ______________________________

13. Heat and cold are applied for no longer than

    ______________________________.

14. When cold is applied to the skin, blood vessels

    ______________________________.

15. You applied a hot compress to Miss White's right forearm. When you check her, she complains of pain and numbness in her right forearm. What should you do?

    ____

    ____

16. A hot soak involves

    ____

    ______________________________.

17. Provide the temperature range in Fahrenheit and Centigrade for each of the following.

    A. Hot ______________________________

    ____

    B. Tepid ______________________________

    ____

    C. Cold ______________________________

    ____

18. Sitz baths are used to:

    A. ______________________________

    B. ______________________________

    C. ______________________________

    D. ______________________________

    E. ______________________________

19. You are assisting Mrs. Lopez with a sitz bath.

    You must observe her for signs of

    ______________________________,

    ______________________________,

    and ______________________________.

20. What should you do if the edge of the sitz bath causes pressure under the person's knees?

____

21. _______________________________________ and

_______________________________________ to

safely use a commercial hot pack.

22. List 4 effects of cold applications.

A. _______________________________________

B. _______________________________________

C. _______________________________________

D. _______________________________________

23. Complications of cold applications are

_______________________________________,

_______________________________________,

and _______________________________________.

24. Why are vital signs measured frequently when hypothermia and hyperthermia blankets are used?

____

____

Multiple Choice

Circle the BEST answer.

25. Heat is *not* applied to a pregnant woman's abdomen because heat can affect fetal growth.
   A. True
   B. False

26. Moist heat has greater and faster effects than dry heat.
   A. True
   B. False

27. Which is a moist cold application?
   A. Ice bag
   B. Ice collar
   C. Ice glove
   D. Cold compress

28. The prolonged application of cold has the same effects as heat applications.
   A. True
   B. False

29. You have applied an ice pack to Mr. Wilson's left knee. How often do you need to check the skin at the application site?
   A. Every 5 minutes
   B. Every 10 minutes
   C. Every 15 minutes
   D. Frequently

30. To safely apply an aquathermia pad
   A. Keep the heating unit below the pad and connecting hoses.
   B. Hoses are free of kinks and bubbles.
   C. The temperature is set at 108° F.
   D. The pad is secured with pins.

31. Cold applications are used for all of the following *except*
   A. To reduce pain.
   B. To cool the body when fever is present.
   C. To increase circulation to an area.
   D. To prevent swelling.

32. Intense cold causes burns and blisters.
   A. True
   B. False

33. You give Mr. Adams a hot foot soak. Which is *incorrect?*
   A. Position him in good body alignment.
   B. Measure the water temperature every 5 minutes. Change water as necessary.
   C. Check his feet every 5 minutes for complications.
   D. Remove his feet from the water in 30 minutes.

ADDITIONAL LEARNING ACTIVITIES

1. Under the supervision of your instructor, practice the procedures in Chapter 31. Use the procedure checklists on pages 476 through 487 as a guide. Take your turn being the patient or resident.
   A. Answer these questions:
      (1) Were you comfortable?
      (2) Did you feel safe?
   B. Discuss ways to promote the person's safety, comfort, and dignity when performing each procedure.
   C. How will your experience affect the care you provide?

2. List the conditions that must be in place before you can apply a heat or cold application.

3. If your state and agency allow you to apply heat and cold applications, what information do you need from the nurse and the care plan?

4. What observations do you need to report and record for heat and cold applications?
   Remember, some states and agencies do not allow assistive personnel to perform the procedures in Chapter 31.

32

Hearing and Vision Problems

OBJECTIVES

The questions and student activities in this chapter will help you meet these objectives.

- Define the key terms listed in Chapter 32
- Explain otitis media and Meniere's disease
- Describe the effects of hearing loss and vision loss
- Describe how to communicate with the hearing-impaired person
- Explain how to communicate with the speech-impaired person
- Explain the purpose of a hearing aid
- Describe how to care for a hearing aid
- Explain the differences between glaucoma and cataracts
- Describe how to protect an artificial eye from loss or damage
- Explain how to assist a blind person
- Perform the procedure described in Chapter 32

STUDY QUESTIONS

Matching

Match the following terms with the correct definitions.

A. Deafness
B. Tinnitus
C. Braille
D. Vertigo
E. Cerumen
F. Hearing loss

1. _______ A writing system that uses raised dots for each letter of the alphabet; the first 10 letters also represent 0 through 9
2. _______ Ear wax
3. _______ Hearing loss in which it is impossible for the person to understand speech through hearing alone
4. _______ Difficulty hearing normal conversations
5. _______ Ringing in the ears
6. _______ Dizziness

Fill in the Blanks

7. Common causes of vision or hearing loss include

_______________,

_______________,

_______________,

_______________,

and _______________.

8. The ear functions in _______________ and

_______________.

9. _______________ is

infection of the middle ear.

10. _______________ is a

chronic disease of the inner ear in which

tinnitus, hearing loss, and vertigo occur.

11. List 10 common causes of hearing loss.

A. _______________

B. _______________

C. _______________

D. _______________

E. _______________

F. _______________

G. _______________

H. _______________

I. _______________

J. _______________

12. What is the most common cause of hearing loss in children?

____

13. List 5 signs of hearing loss in children and adults.

A. _______________

B. _______________

C. _______________

D. _______________

E. _______________

14. List 4 simple measures to try when a hearing aid does not seem to be working properly.

A. _______________

B. _______________

C. _______________

D. _______________

15. List 5 risk factors for glaucoma.

A. _______________

B. _______________

C. _______________

D. _______________

E. _______________

16. Treatment for glaucoma involves

_______________ and

_______________.

17. With _______________ the

lens of the eye becomes cloudy. Light cannot

enter the eye.

18. The most common cause of cataract is

_______________.

19. _______________ is the

only treatment for cataract.

20. Postoperative care for cataract surgery includes:

A. ______________________________

____

B. ______________________________

____

C. ______________________________

____

D. ______________________________

____

E. ______________________________

____

21. How do you protect a person's eyeglasses from breakage or other damage?

____

____

____

22. Mrs. Jane Paul wears contact lenses. What observations do you need to report to the nurse at once?

A. ______________________________

B. ______________________________

23. The legally blind person sees at 20 feet what a person with normal vision sees at ______________________________.

24. What 2 aids are used worldwide by persons who are blind?

A. ______________________________

B. ______________________________

Multiple Choice

Circle the BEST answer.

25. Otitis media is most common
   A. Between 6 months and 3 years of age.
   B. After the child reaches puberty.
   C. In middle aged women.
   D. In older persons.

26. A child has chronic otitis media. Which is *false?*
   A. Fluid build-up occurs in the middle ear.
   B. Symptoms include fever and ringing in the ear.
   C. Permanent hearing loss can occur.
   D. There is no treatment.

27. When caring for a person with Meniere's disease, do all of the following *except*
   A. Keep the person's head still.
   B. Assist with ambulation.
   C. Avoid bright, glaring lights.
   D. Encourage the person to be up as much as possible.

28. Treatment of Meniere's disease includes
   A. Antibiotics and encourage fluids.
   B. Drugs, fluid restriction, and a low-salt diet.
   C. ROM exercises to the neck and drugs.
   D. A hearing aid and fluid restrictions.

29. Women are at higher risk for hearing loss than men.
   A. True
   B. False

30. Hearing loss may cause speech problems such as slurred speech, improper pronunciation, and monotone voice.
   A. True
   B. False

31. To remove cerumen from the ear, gently insert a cotton swab about 1/2 inch into the ear canal.
   A. True
   B. False

32. To communicate with a hearing-impaired person
   A. Shout loudly.
   B. Approach the person from behind.
   C. Speak clearly, distinctly, and slowly.
   D. Stand or sit in dim light.

33. A person who uses a hearing aid hears better because
   A. The hearing problem is cured.
   B. Background noise is decreased.
   C. The person's ability to hear improves.
   D. The hearing aid makes sounds louder.

34. To care for a hearing aid correctly, do all of the following *except*
   A. Wash the mold in soapy water every day.
   B. Remove the battery at night.
   C. When not in use, turn the hearing aid off.
   D. Handle the hearing aid carefully.

35. Mrs. Adams has glaucoma. Which is *true?*
   A. There is no treatment.
   B. Glaucoma is corrected with eyeglasses.
   C. The onset is always sudden.
   D. Glaucoma is a major cause of blindness.

36. Mr. Norris has an artificial eye. You are assisting with care of the eye socket after he has removed the artificial eye. Which is *incorrect?*
   A. Wash the eye socket with warm water or saline.
   B. Remove excess moisture with a gauze square.
   C. Wash the eyelid with mild soap and warm water.
   D. Clean from the outer to the inner aspect of the eye.

37. When caring for a blind person, you must avoid using the words *see, look,* or *read.*
   A. True
   B. False

38. Which action will *not* promote safety when caring for a blind person?
   A. Provide lighting as the person prefers.
   B. Orient the person to the room.
   C. Keep doors partly open.
   D. Tell the person when you are leaving the room.

ADDITIONAL LEARNING ACTIVITIES

1. Read the vignettes. Then answer the questions that follow.
   Miss Rita Reed is an 80-year-old resident of Green Valley Nursing Center. She is hearing impaired in both ears. She wears hearing aids and lip reads. She needs assistance putting her hearing aids in and taking them out. Miss Reed also has glaucoma, which is controlled with drugs. She wears eyeglasses. She can see well enough to read large print. She also listens to talking books.
   A. How might Miss Reed's hearing and vision impairment affect her ability to care for herself?
   B. How might Miss Reed's social life be affected by her hearing and vision impairment?
   C. How can you promote Miss Reed's safety?
   D. What measures will you practice when caring for Miss Reed's eyeglasses and hearing aids?
   E. What measures will you practice when communicating with Miss Reed?

   You are assisting Mr. Ted Tanner with ADL in his home. Mr. Tanner has Meniere's disease. He lives alone in his apartment. He is having an attack involving tinnitus vertigo, nausea, and vomiting.
   A. How long does an attack last?
   B. What does treatment of Meniere's disease involve?
   C. What safety measures are practiced during an attack?
   D. How will you communicate with Mr. Tanner during the attack?

2. Simulate hearing loss by using earplugs in both ears. Then participate in these activities:
   A. Watch a movie on TV.
   B. Call a friend on the telephone.
   C. Go to the grocery store and shop for food items. (Do not drive a car with earplugs in place.)
   D. Discuss your experience. Answer the following questions.
      (1) How did you feel when performing these routine activities with a hearing impairment?
      (2) Were you ever frustrated?
      (3) Did you feel others were frustrated or impatient with you?
      (4) Did you feel left out?
      (5) How will your experience affect the care you provide?

3. Simulate vision impairment by wearing a pair of eyeglasses with crushed cellophane or petroleum jelly over the lenses. Then try to do the following:
   A. Write a letter.
   B. Do a load of laundry.
   C. Watch a movie on TV.
   D. Prepare a simple snack.
   E. Discuss your experience. Answer the following questions.
      (1) How did your vision impairment affect your ability to perform these simple activities?
      (2) Did you feel uncertain or unsafe when performing any of the activities?
      (3) How will your experience affect the care you provide?

33

Common Health Problems

OBJECTIVES

The questions and student activities in this chapter will help you meet these objectives.

- Define the key terms listed in Chapter 33
- Describe how cancer is treated
- Describe arthritis and the care required
- Explain how to care for persons in casts, in traction, and with hip pinnings
- Describe the care required for osteoporosis
- Describe the effects of amputation
- Describe signs and symptoms of stroke and the care required
- Describe the care needs of person's with Parkinson's disease and multiple sclerosis
- Identify the causes of head and spinal cord injuries and the care required
- Describe common respiratory disorders and the care required
- Identify the signs, symptoms, and treatment of hypertension
- List the risk factors for coronary artery disease
- Describe the care required by persons with heart disease
- Describe the care required by persons with urinary system disorders
- Identify the signs, symptoms, and complications of diabetes
- Explain the care required by persons with digestive problems
- Describe the signs and symptoms of communicable diseases and the care required

STUDY QUESTIONS

Complete the Crossword

Across

1. Type of tumor that grows slowly and within a local area
7. A broken bone
9. Joint inflammation
10. Hair loss

Down

2. A condition in which there is death of tissue
3. A new growth of abnormal cells
4. The spread of cancer to other body parts
5. The removal of all or part of an extremity
6. Type of tumor that grows fast and invades other tissues
8. The inability to speak

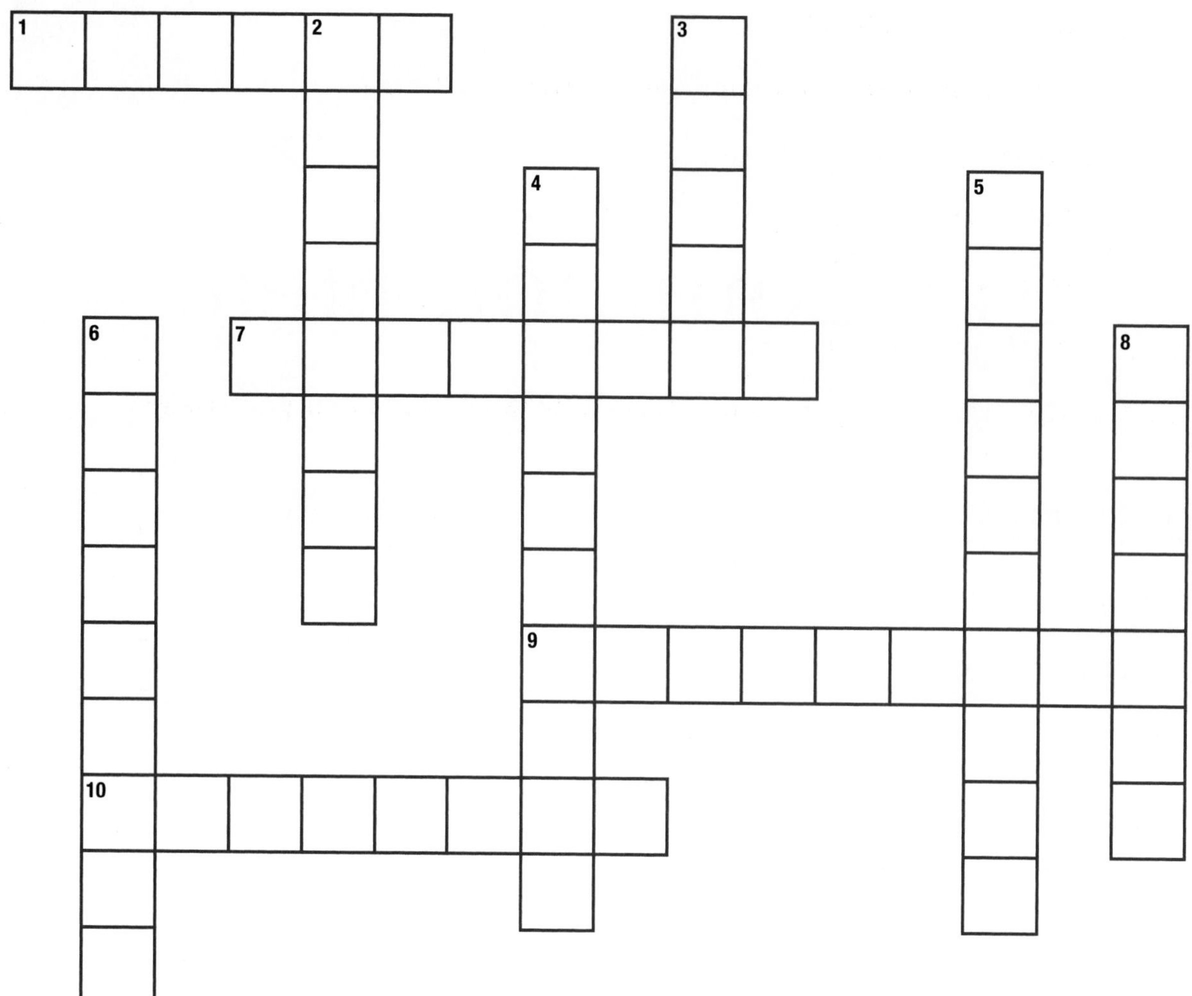

Matching

Match the following terms with the correct definitions.

A. Expressive-receptive aphasia
B. Receptive aphasia
C. Quadriplegia
D. Paraplegia
E. Hemiplegia
F. Open fracture
G. Closed fracture
H. Hypoglycemia
I. Hyperglycemia
J. Stomatitis
K. Cancer
L. Ureterostomy
M. Expressive aphasia
N. Arthroplasty

1. _______ The surgical replacement of a joint
2. _______ Malignant tumor
3. _______ The bone is broken but the skin is intact; simple fracture
4. _______ Difficulty expressing or sending out thoughts
5. _______ Difficulty expressing or sending out thoughts and difficulty receiving information
6. _______ Paralysis on one side of the body
7. _______ High sugar in the blood

8. _______ Low sugar in the blood

9. _______ The broken bone has come through the skin; compound fracture

10. _______ Paralysis from the waist down

11. _______ Paralysis from the neck down

12. _______ Difficulty receiving information

13. _______ Inflammation of the mouth

14. _______ The surgical creation of an artificial opening between the ureter and the abdomen

Fill in the Blanks

15. List the 7 cancer risk factors cited by the National Cancer Institute.

A. ______________________

B. ______________________

C. ______________________

D. ______________________

E. ______________________

F. ______________________

G. ______________________

16. Cancer treatment depends on

______________________,

______________________,

and ______________________.

17. List and briefly describe 5 cancer treatments.

A. ______________________

____

B. ______________________

____

C. ______________________

____

D. ______________________

____

E. ______________________

____

18. ______________________ is the most common type of cancer in children.

19. List 9 warning signs of cancer in children.

A. ______________________

B. ______________________

C. ______________________

D. ______________________

E. ______________________

F. ______________________

G. ______________________

H. ______________________

I. ______________________

20. List and briefly describe the 2 types of arthritis.

A. ______________________________

____

____

B. ______________________________

____

____

21. Treatment for osteoarthritis involves:

A. ______________________________

B. ______________________________

C. ______________________________

D. ______________________________

E. ______________________________

22. Treatment goals for rheumatoid arthritis are to

______________________________,

______________________________,

and ______________________________.

23. When rheumatoid arthritis occurs in children, it is called ______________________________.

24. ______________________________ is a bone disorder in which the bone becomes porous and brittle. Bones are fragile and break easily.

25. List 5 risk factors for osteoporosis.

A. ______________________________

B. ______________________________

C. ______________________________

D. ______________________________

E. ______________________________

26. List 7 signs and symptoms of a fracture.

A. ______________________________

B. ______________________________

C. ______________________________

D. ______________________________

E. ______________________________

F. ______________________________

G. ______________________________

27. A person has a cast. What signs and symptoms are reported to the nurse at once?

A. ______________________________

B. ______________________________

C. ______________________________

D. ______________________________

E. ______________________________

F. ______________________________

G. ______________________________

H. ______________________________

I. ______________________________

J. ______________________________

28. Traction is used to ______________________________ and ______________________________ fractures. It also is used ______________________________,

______________________________,

and ______________________________.

29. A hip fracture is fixed in position with a ____________________, ____________________, ____________________, ____________________, or ____________________.

30. After hip surgery ____________________, ____________________, and ____________________ are avoided.

31. A prosthesis is ____________________.

32. Mr. Bryant's left leg was amputated below the knee. He complains of pain and tingling in his left foot and toes. This is ____________________.

33. ____________________ is a disease affecting the blood vessels that supply blood to the brain.

34. What are the 2 main causes of cerebrovascular accident (CVA)?

A. ____________________

B. ____________________

35. List 5 warning signs of stroke.

A. ____________________

B. ____________________

C. ____________________

D. ____________________

E. ____________________

36. Mrs. Jones had a stroke affecting her left side. She frequently forgets about and ignores her left side. This is called ____________________.

37. After a stroke, rehabilitation starts at once. The health team helps the person ____________________.

38. Mrs. Jones does not know how to use her fork and knife for eating. This is ____________________.

39. Signs and symptoms of Parkinson's disease include:

A. ____________________

B. ____________________

C. ____________________

D. ____________________

E. ____________________

40. ____________________ is a chronic disease in which the myelin in the brain and spinal cord are destroyed.

41. Miss Ann Clark has the primary progressive type of MS. This means ____________________.

42. Mr. Paul Higgins has a head injury as the result of a fall. Nursing care depends on ____________________.

43. Common causes of spinal cord injuries are ____________________, ____________________, ____________________, and ____________________.

44. Three disorders are grouped under chronic obstructive pulmonary disease (COPD). They are ____________________, ____________________, and ____________________.

45. ____________________ is the major cause of chronic bronchitis.

46. In emphysema, the ____________________ enlarge and become less elastic.

47. Asthma is triggered by ____________________, ____________________, ____________________, ____________________, ____________________, and ____________________.

48. Pneumonia is ____________________ ____________________. It is caused by ____________________ ____________________.

49. Tuberculosis (TB) is spread by ____________________ ____________________ with coughing, sneezing, speaking, and singing.

50. List 7 signs and symptoms of TB.

A. ____________________

B. ____________________

C. ____________________

D. ____________________

E. ____________________

F. ____________________

G. ____________________

51. With hypertension the ____________________ ____________________ is too high.

52. Hypertension can damage other organs. It can lead to ____________________, ____________________, ____________________, ____________________, and ____________________.

53. The ____________________ supply the heart with blood.

54. The most common cause of coronary artery disease is ____________________.

55. The major complications of coronary artery disease (CAD) are ____________________ and ____________________.

56. Angina pectoris is chest pain from ____________________ ____________________.

57. Angina pectoris often leads to ______________

____.

58. What occurs when a person has a myocardial infarction (MI)?

____

____

59. ________________________________ occurs when the heart cannot pump blood normally. Blood backs up and tissue congestion occurs.

60. With left-sided heart failure, blood backs up into the ________________________________.

61. ________________________________ can cause heart failure in children.

62. ________________________________ is inflammation of the kidney pelvis.

63. List 4 risk factors for renal calculi.

A. ________________________________

B. ________________________________

C. ________________________________

D. ________________________________

64. Renal failure may be ________________ or ________________________________.

65. Causes of acute renal failure include:

A. ________________________________

B. ________________________________

C. ________________________________

D. ________________________________

E. ________________________________

F. ________________________________

66. ________________________________ and ________________________________ are common causes of chronic renal failure.

________________________________,

________________________________, and

________________________ are other causes.

67. Treatment of chronic renal failure includes

________________________________,

________________________________,

________________________________, and

________________________________.

68. Dialysis is ________________________________

____

________________________________.

69. ________________________________ is the most common endocrine disorder.

70. List and briefly describe the 3 types of diabetes.

A. ________________________________

____

____

B. ________________________________

____

____

C. ________________________________

____

____

71. Which ethnic groups are at risk for type 2 diabetes?

A. ______________________

B. ______________________

C. ______________________

D. ______________________

72. Type 1 diabetes is treated with

______________________,

______________________,

and ______________________.

73. Diverticular disease involves ______________________

____

____

______________________.

74. Mr. Drew is vomiting. You turn his head well to one side to prevent ______________________.

75. Vomitus that looks like coffee grounds contains

______________________.

76. How are communicable diseases transmitted from one person to another?

A. ______________________

B. ______________________

C. ______________________

D. ______________________

E. ______________________

77. ______________________ is an inflammation of the liver.

78. Hepatitis A is spread by ______________________

______________________.

79. The hepatitis B virus is present in

____

____

______________________.

80. The AIDS virus (HIV) is transmitted mainly by:

A. ______________________

B. ______________________

C. ______________________

D. ______________________

81. Sexually transmitted diseases are spread by

______________________.

______________________.

82. Using ______________________ helps prevent the spread of sexually transmitted diseases, especially HIV and AIDS.

Multiple Choice

Circle the BEST answer.

83. Radiation therapy is used to treat cancer. Which is *false?*
   A. X-rays are directed at the tumor.
   B. Only cancer cells are destroyed.
   C. Side effects include nausea, vomiting, and fatigue.
   D. Skin breakdown can occur at the treatment site.

84. Mrs. Andrews has rheumatoid arthritis. Which is *true?*
   A. Joint injury and obesity are causes.
   B. Severe inflammation causes very painful and swollen joints.
   C. Bony growths called Heberden's nodes are common in fingers.
   D. The hips, knees, and spine are affected first.

85. Fractures in infants may be a sign of child abuse.
   A. True
   B. False

86. Traction applied directly to the bone is called
    A. Skeletal traction.
    B. Closed reduction.
    C. Skin traction.
    D. A prosthesis.

87. When caring for a person with a stroke, do all of the following *except*
    A. Perform range-of-motion exercises to prevent contractures.
    B. Give good skin care to prevent pressure sores.
    C. Keep the bed in the flat position.
    D. Encourage coughing and deep breathing.

88. A person has Parkinson's disease. It is important to do everything for the person.
    A. True
    B. False

89. A person has multiple sclerosis. Which is *false?*
    A. There is no known cure.
    B. Muscle weakness and difficulty with balance occur.
    C. Activities should be limited, and the person should stay in bed as much as possible.
    D. The person's condition worsens over time.

90. The major cause of emphysema is
    A. Smoking.
    B. Air pollution.
    C. Industrial dust.
    D. Allergies.

91. Changes from aging, diseases, and decreased mobility increase the risk of pneumonia in older persons.
    A. True
    B. False

92. The leading causes of death in the United States are
    A. Infections.
    B. Pulmonary diseases.
    C. Cardiovascular disorders.
    D. Cancers.

93. Which is *not* a risk factor for hypertension?
    A. Cigarette smoking
    B. A high sodium diet
    C. Regular exercise
    D. Obesity

94. Angina pectoris is relieved by
    A. Exercise.
    B. Rest and nitroglycerin.
    C. Food.
    D. Oxygen.

95. Mr. Smith has had a myocardial infarction. His cardiac rehabilitation will involve all of the following *except*
    A. An exercise program.
    B. Teaching about drugs.
    C. Teaching about dietary changes.
    D. An end to sexual activity.

96. Heart failure cannot be treated.
    A. True
    B. False

97. Women are at high risk for urinary tract infections.
    A. True
    B. False

98. A bladder infection caused by bacteria is
    A. Pyelonephritis.
    B. Renal calculi.
    C. Renal failure.
    D. Cystitis.

99. The diet for a person with chronic renal failure is low in all of the following *except*
    A. Sodium.
    B. Vitamins.
    C. Potassium.
    D. Protein.

100. Mrs. Smith has diabetes. Which is *true?*
    A. Her body cannot produce or use insulin properly.
    B. She is obese.
    C. She cannot eat a balanced diet.
    D. Her diet should be low in protein.

101. Which is a cause of hypoglycemia?
    A. Omitting a meal
    B. Not enough insulin
    C. Eating too much food
    D. Too little exercise

102. The AIDS virus is spread through
    A. Sneezing and coughing.
    B. Holding hands and hugging.
    C. Blood, semen, vaginal secretions, and breast milk.
    D. Insects.

103. All persons infected with the HIV virus have symptoms.
    A. True
    B. False

104. Persons over age 50 are not at risk for AIDS.
    A. True
    B. False

ADDITIONAL LEARNING ACTIVITIES

1. Review with classmates these common health problems discussed in Chapter 33.
   - Cancer
   - Arthritis (osteoarthritis and rheumatoid arthritis)
   - Osteoporosis
   - Fractures
   - Loss of a limb
   - Stroke
   - Parkinson's disease
   - Multiple sclerosis
   - Head and spinal cord injuries
   - COPD
   - Pneumonia
   - Tuberculosis
   - Heart disease
   - Urinary system disorders
   - Diverticular disease
   - Hepatitis
   - AIDS
   - Sexually transmitted diseases

   A. Discuss how each problem affects the individual's physical, psychological, social, and spiritual needs.
   B. Discuss the financial aspects of each health problem.
   C. Discuss measures to promote comfort, safety, and dignity for persons with acute and chronic health problems.
   D. Discuss measures to promote personal choice when caring for persons with common health problems.

2. List and discuss the risk factors for each of the health problems discussed in Chapter 33.
   A. Which risk factors can be controlled and which cannot?
   B. Are there life-style changes you can make to decrease your risks for any common health problems?

3. Read the vignettes. Then answer the questions that follow.
   Mr. Adam Lane is 55 years old. He is married and has 2 teenage children. He is a teacher at the high school. He enjoys hiking and camping with his family. He attends church every Sunday with his family. His wife works part time as a checkout clerk at the local grocery store. Mr. Lane is being treated for colon cancer. He had surgery to remove a tumor and is now receiving radiation therapy.
   A. What fears might Mr. Lane have?
   B. What fears might his family have?
   C. How might Mr. Lane's health problems affect the family financially?
   D. What physical needs does Mr. Lane have?
   E. What are the side effects of radiation therapy?
   F. How can you and other members of the health team help meet Mr. Lane's psychological, social, and spiritual needs?
   G. How can you and other members of the health team provide support for the family?

Mrs. Ann Lopez is a 75-year-old retired nurse. She lives alone in her home. She does volunteer work at the hospital 2 days a week. She is teaching her granddaughter how to quilt. She has a small flower garden and enjoys working in it every day. Mrs. Lopez fell in her driveway and fractured her right hip. She had a hip pinning and is receiving rehabilitation at a skilled nursing center.

A. What are the signs and symptoms of a fracture?
B. What fears might Mrs. Lopez have?
C. How might the hip fracture affect Mrs. Lopez's life-style?
D. What care measures are practiced after an open reduction and pinning of a fractured hip?
E. What complications is Mrs. Lopez at risk for?
   (1) What nursing measures can help prevent these complications?
F. What activities does Mrs. Lopez need to avoid for 6 to 8 weeks after surgery?
G. What assistive devices might Mrs. Lopez need?
H. What are the roles of the occupational therapist and the physical therapist in Mrs. Lopez's care?

34

Mental Health Problems

OBJECTIVES

The questions and student activities in this chapter will help you meet these objectives.

- Define the key terms listed in Chapter 34
- Explain the difference between mental health and mental illness
- List the causes of mental illness
- Explain how personality develops
- Describe three anxiety disorders
- Explain the defense mechanisms used to relieve anxiety
- Describe common phobias
- Explain schizophrenia
- Describe bipolar disorder and depression
- Describe three personality disorders
- Describe substance abuse
- Explain two types of eating disorders
- Describe the care required by persons with mental health disorders

STUDY QUESTIONS

Matching

Match the following terms with the correct definitions.

A. Mental
B. Delusion
C. Phobia
D. Psychosis
E. Stress
F. Ego
G. Id
H. Superego
I. Mental health
J. Defense mechanism
K. Delusion of persecution
L. Obsession
M. Paranoia
N. Stressor
O. Affect
P. Conscious
Q. Panic
R. Unconscious
S. Subconscious
T. Anxiety
U. Mental illness
V. Personality
W. Hallucination
X. Compulsion
Y. Delusion of grandeur

1. _______ Feelings and emotions
2. _______ A vague, uneasy feeling in response to stress
3. _______ The repeating of an act over and over again
4. _______ Awareness of the environment and experiences; the person knows what is happening and can control thoughts and behaviors
5. _______ An unconscious reaction that blocks unpleasant or threatening feelings
6. _______ A false belief
7. _______ An exaggerated belief about one's own importance, wealth, power, or talents
8. _______ A false belief that one is being mistreated, abused, or harassed
9. _______ The part of the personality dealing with reality; deals with thoughts, feelings, good sense, and problem solving
10. _______ Seeing, hearing, or feeling something that is not real
11. _______ The part of the personality at the unconscious level; concerned with pleasure
12. _______ Relating to the mind
13. _______ The person copes with and adjusts to everyday stresses in ways accepted by society
14. _______ A disturbance in the ability to cope or adjust to stress; behavior and functioning are impaired; mental disorder, emotional illness, psychiatric disorder
15. _______ A recurrent, unwanted thought or idea
16. _______ An intense and sudden feeling of fear, anxiety, terror, or dread
17. _______ A disorder of the mind; false beliefs and suspicion about a person or situation
18. _______ The set of attitudes, values, behaviors, and traits of a person
19. _______ Fear, panic, or dread
20. _______ A state of severe mental impairment
21. _______ The response or change in the body caused by any emotional, physical, social, or economic factors
22. _______ Any factor that causes stress
23. _______ Memory, past experiences, and thoughts of which the person is not aware; they are easily recalled
24. _______ The part of the personality concerned with right and wrong
25. _______ Experiences and feelings that cannot be recalled

Fill in the Blanks

26. Causes of mental health disorders include:

    A. ______________________

    B. ______________________

    C. ______________________

    D. ______________________

    E. ______________________

27. When does personality start to develop?

    ____

28. According to Maslow's theory of basic needs, ______________________ must be met before ______________________.

29. Unmet needs at any age affect ______________________.

30. There is a ______________________, ______________________, and ______________________ to growth and development.

31. Freud's theory of personality development involves the ______________________, ______________________, and ______________________.

32. Coping and defense mechanisms are used to ______________________.

33. ______________________ is the highest level of anxiety.

34. ______________________ means split mind. It is a severe, chronic, disabling brain disease.

35. Some persons with schizophrenia regress. To regress means ______________________ ______________________.

36. Affective disorders involve ______________________, ______________________, and ______________________.

37. The person with bipolar disorder has ______________________ ______________________.

38. Why is depression in older persons often untreated?

    ____

    ____

39. ______________________ involve rigid and maladaptive behaviors.

40. Define these personality disorders.

    A. Abusive personality

    ____

    ____

    B. Paranoid personality

    ____

    ____

    C. Antisocial personality

    ____

    ____

41. ______________________ occurs when a person overuses or depends on drugs or alcohol.

42. Two common eating disorders are ____________

____

and _______________________________________.

43. _______________________________________ occurs when a person has an intense fear of weight gain and obesity.

44. Which defense mechanisms are being used in the following situations?

   A. A man has emphysema. He continues to smoke even though the doctor told him he would die if he did not stop smoking.

   ____

   B. Mary's favorite aunt is a professional dancer. Mary dresses up and practices dancing every night in her room.

   ____

   C. A 14-year-old girl starts sucking her thumb when her parents divorce.

   ____

Multiple Choice

Circle the BEST answer.

45. According to Freud, the part of the personality involved with reasoning and good sense is the
   A. Unconscious.
   B. Superego.
   C. Id.
   D. Ego.

46. Which statement about anxiety is *false?*
   A. Anxiety is an abnormal response to stress.
   B. Anxiety occurs when a person's needs are not met.
   C. Anxiety level depends on the stressor.
   D. Defense mechanisms are used to relieve anxiety.

47. All defense mechanisms are unhealthy.
   A. True
   B. False

48. Fear of pain or seeing others in pain is called
   A. Agoraphobia.
   B. Algophobia.
   C. Mysophobia.
   D. Pyrophobia.

49. A person with major depression
   A. Has extreme mood swings.
   B. Sees things that are not real.
   C. Is very sad and loses interest in daily activities.
   D. Regresses back to childhood.

50. Only illegal drugs can be abused.
   A. True
   B. False

51. Anorexia nervosa occurs mostly in teenage boys.
   A. True
   B. False

52. Binge eating and purging the body of food eaten occurs with
   A. Anorexia nervosa.
   B. Depression.
   C. Bulimia nervosa.
   D. Delusions of grandeur.

ADDITIONAL LEARNING ACTIVITIES

1. Review Maslow's theory of basic needs.
   A. How do unmet needs affect personality development?

2. Think of the stressors in your personal life that cause anxiety.
   A. How do you feel when you are anxious?
   B. What defense mechanisms do you use to cope with anxiety?

3. What fears do you have about caring for persons with mental health problems? Discuss your feelings and fears with your instructor.

35 Confusion and Dementia

OBJECTIVES

The questions and student activities in this chapter will help you meet these objectives.

- Define the key terms listed in Chapter 35
- Describe confusion and its causes
- List the measures that help confused persons
- Explain the differences between delirium, depression, and dementia
- Describe Alzheimer's disease (AD)
- Describe the signs, symptoms, and behaviors of AD
- Explain the care required by persons with AD and other dementias
- Describe the effects of AD on the family

STUDY QUESTIONS

Matching

Match the following terms with the correct definitions.

A. Pseudodementia
B. Dementia
C. Delirium
D. Sundowning
E. Hallucination
F. Delusion

1. _______ A state of temporary but acute mental confusion
2. _______ A false belief
3. _______ The loss of cognitive and social function caused by changes in the brain
4. _______ Seeing, hearing, or feeling something that is not real
5. _______ False dementia
6. _______ Signs, symptoms, and behaviors of AD increase during hours of darkness

Fill in the Blanks

7. Cognitive functioning involves:

   A. ______

   B. ______

   C. ______

   D. ______

   E. ______

   F. ______

8. The treatment of acute confusion (delirium) is aimed at ______.

9. ______ is the most common type of dementia.

10. List 8 early warning signs of dementia.

    A. ______

    B. ______

    C. ______

    D. ______

    E. ______

    F. ______

    G. ______

    H. ______

11. List 9 treatable causes of dementia.

    A. ______

    B. ______

    C. ______

    D. ______

    E. ______

    F. ______

    G. ______

    H. ______

    I. ______

12. Multi-infarct dementia is caused by ______.

13. Miss Jean Parma is having problems concentrating. She is agitated and withdrawn. Why is it important to diagnose her problem correctly?

    ______

    ______

14. ______ is the most common mental health problem in older persons.

15. AD is a brain disease. List the functions affected by AD.

    A. ______

    B. ______

    C. ______

    D. ______

    E. ______

    F. ______

    G. ______

    H. ______

16. The classic sign of AD is ______.

17. What is the purpose of the Alzheimer's Association's Safe Return Program?

    ______

    ______

    ______

18. List 3 possible causes of sundowning.

A. ____________________

____

B. ____________________

____

C. ____________________

____

19. Briefly describe catastrophic reactions.

____

____

____

20. Catastrophic reactions are common from

____________________.

21. List 5 common causes of agitation and restlessness.

A. ____________________

B. ____________________

C. ____________________

D. ____________________

E. ____________________

22. Sexual behaviors are labeled abnormal because of ____________________.

23. Persons with AD are not oriented to person, place, and time. Therefore sexual behaviors may involve ____________________

____

____________________.

24. What are some nonsexual reasons a person with dementia may touch or rub the genitals?

A. ____________________

B. ____________________

C. ____________________

25. Mr. John Kane has AD. He is a resident at Valley View Nursing Center. Why is it important to report any changes in his usual behavior to the nurse?

____

____

26. Some nursing centers have special secured units for persons with AD and other dementias. What is the purpose of these units?

____

____

27. Persons in the early stages of AD may live at home with family. Long-term care is needed when:

A. ____________________

B. ____________________

C. ____________________

D. ____________________

E. ____________________

28. List 2 organizations that provide support to persons with AD and their families.

A. ____________________

B. ____________________

Multiple Choice

Circle the BEST answer.

29. Which statement about acute confusion is *false?*
    A. Treatment is aimed at the cause.
    B. It occurs suddenly.
    C. It usually is permanent.
    D. It can occur postoperatively.

30. Delirium is an emergency.
    A. True
    B. False

31. A person in stage 1 of AD
    A. Is disoriented to time and place.
    B. Has fecal and urinary incontinence.
    C. Has problems with movement and gait.
    D. Cannot swallow.

32. Mr. Jones is confused. Which of the following measures is *not* helpful?
    A. Provide care in a calm, relaxed manner.
    B. Explain everything in great detail.
    C. Use touch to communicate.
    D. Tell him the date and time each morning.

33. Mrs. Adams has AD. You promote her safety by
    A. Keeping her restrained.
    B. Explaining safety rules to her.
    C. Changing her room frequently.
    D. Placing safety plugs in electrical outlets.

34. You are caring for a person with AD. Which action causes increased agitation?
    A. Rushing the person
    B. Keeping noise levels low
    C. Speaking in a calm, gentle voice
    D. Using touch to calm the person

35. Mrs. Adams is screaming. You can help by:
    A. Firmly asking her to stop.
    B. Taking her to her room and closing the door.
    C. Turning on loud music.
    D. Having a favorite caregiver comfort and calm her.

36. Repetitive behaviors are usually harmless.
    A. True
    B. False

37. The person with AD
    A. Chooses to be incontinent.
    B. Needs your support and understanding.
    C. Has control over his or her actions.
    D. Can understand and follow instructions.

38. The right to privacy and confidentiality is *not* important for persons with dementia.
    A. True
    B. False

39. Restraints can make confusion and demented behaviors worse.
    A. True
    B. False

ADDITIONAL LEARNING ACTIVITIES

1. Compare the signs and symptoms of delirium, depression, and early Alzheimer's disease. Answer the following questions.
   A. How are the signs and symptoms similar?
   B. How are the signs and symptoms different?
   C. Why is a correct diagnosis needed?

2. Read the vignette. Then answer the questions that follow.
Mrs. Lynn Abbott has AD. She has been living in her daughter's home. Her daughter works full time. She has been able to meet her mother's needs with the following in-home services:
   - *A home care aide to assist with Mrs. Abbott's bath twice a week.*
   - *Her mother attends an adult day care program 3 days a week.*
   - *A volunteer from Mrs. Abbott's church visits 1 day a week.*
   - *Mrs. Abbott and her daughter belong to an Alzheimer's support group.*

   During the past 2 weeks Mrs. Abbott has left her daughter's home 3 times. Twice a neighbor brought her home, and once she was found wandering in a grocery store 5 blocks from her daughter's home. Often Mrs. Abbott refuses to get dressed in the morning. She has also been incontinent of bladder several times in the past few days. She is becoming less interested in her personal hygiene. She has started to resist efforts to bathe her. Mrs. Abbott's daughter is afraid to leave her alone for even short periods of time. When Mrs. Abbott is not at the adult day care program, her daughter comes home during her lunch hour to check on her. If her daughter wants to go out in the evening, she gets a sitter to stay with Mrs. Abbott. She is looking for an assisted living facility or a nursing center for her mother. This is very difficult, as she feels she should care for her mother herself.

   A. What behaviors might be causing Mrs. Abbott's daughter to consider placement in an assisted living facility or a nursing center?
   B. What health and safety risks does Mrs. Abbott have?
   C. What effect does Mrs. Abbott's AD have on her daughter's daily life?
   D. What financial impact does Mrs. Abbott's AD have?
   E. What support systems is Mrs. Abbott's daughter using? Are there other support systems she might try? Explain.
   F. What physical needs does Mrs. Abbott have? Are Mrs. Abbott's physical needs likely to increase? Explain.
   G. What psychosocial needs does Mrs. Abbott have? Are her psychosocial needs likely to increase? Explain.
   H. What needs does Mrs. Abbott's daughter have?
   I. What fears might Mrs. Abbott's daughter have about placing her mother in an assisted living facility or a nursing center?
   J. If Mrs. Abbott's daughter admits her mother to an assisted living facility or a nursing center, what programs and services will help meet:
      (1) Mrs. Abbott's needs?
      (2) The daughter's needs?

36 Developmental Disabilities

OBJECTIVES

The questions and student activities in this chapter will help you meet these objectives.

- Define the key terms listed in Chapter 36
- Identify the areas of function limited by a developmental disability
- Explain how a developmental disability affects the child and family across the life span
- Explain when developmental disabilities occur
- Describe the causes of developmental disabilities
- Explain how the various developmental disabilities affect a person's function

STUDY QUESTIONS

Matching

Match the following terms with the correct definitions.

A. Developmental disability
B. Seizure
C. Convulsion
D. Diplegia
E. Spastic

1. _______ A seizure
2. _______ A disability occurring before 22 years of age
3. _______ Similar body parts are affected on both sides of the body
4. _______ The violent and sudden contractions or tremors of muscle groups
5. _______ Uncontrolled contractions of skeletal muscles

Fill in the Blanks

6. Congenital means ______________________

______________________.

7. A developmental disability can be a

______________________,

______________________,

______________________,

______________________,

or ______________________ disability.

8. With a development disability, function is limited in 3 or more of the following life skills:

   A. ______________________
   B. ______________________
   C. ______________________
   D. ______________________
   E. ______________________
   F. ______________________
   G. ______________________

9. Mental retardation involves low intellectual functioning and impaired adaptive behavior.

   A. Intellectual function relates to ____________

   ______________________.

   B. Adapt means to ______________________

   ______________________.

10. According to the ARC, mental retardation involves:

   A. ______________________
   B. ______________________
   C. ______________________

11. List 7 causes of mental retardation that occurs during pregnancy.

   A. ______________________
   B. ______________________
   C. ______________________
   D. ______________________
   E. ______________________
   F. ______________________
   G. ______________________

12. After age 35, persons with Down syndrome (DS) are at risk for ______________________.

13. Persons with DS have some level of

______________________.

14. Persons with DS need ______________________,

______________________,

______________________,

and ______________________ therapies.

15. ______________________ is a term applied to a group of disorders involving muscle weakness or poor muscle control.

16. Infants at risk for CP are those who:

   A. ______________________
   B. ______________________
   C. ______________________
   D. ______________________
   E. ______________________
   F. ______________________
   G. ______________________
   H. ______________________
   I. ______________________

17. Describe the following types of CP:

A. Spastic cerebral palsy ______________________

____

____

____

____

B. Athetoid cerebral palsy ______________________

____

____

____

____

C. Hemiplegia ______________________

____

____

____

____

D. Diplegia ______________________

____

____

____

____

E. Quadriplegia ______________________

____

____

____

____

____

18. The Epilepsy Foundation of America describes epilepsy as ______________________

____

______________________.

19. A seizure involving the whole brain is called ______________________.

20. ______________________ is a defect in the spinal column.

21. ______________________ often occurs with spina bifida.

22. Briefly describe these types of spina bifida:

A. Spina bifida occulta ______________________

____

____

____

____

B. Spina bifida cystica ______________________

____

____

____

____

23. Describe the 2 types of spina bifida cystica.

A. Meningocele ______________________

____

____

____

____

B. Myelomeningocele ____________________

____

____

____

____

24. With ______________________________, cerebrospinal fluid collects in and around the brain.

25. How is hydrocephalus treated?

____

____

Multiple Choice

Circle the BEST answer.

26. Persons with mental retardation do *not* develop sexually and do not have sexual urges.
    A. True
    B. False

27. The ARC believes that
    A. Children with mental retardation should live in nursing centers.
    B. Adults with mental retardation should not marry.
    C. Persons with mental retardation cannot have meaningful jobs.
    D. Persons with mental retardation should learn about sex, sexual abuse, safe sex, and other sexuality issues.

28. Down syndrome is caused by
    A. Injury during birth.
    B. Poor nutrition during pregnancy.
    C. An extra 21st chromosome.
    D. Lack of oxygen to the brain during birth.

29. Which statement about autism is *false?*
    A. Autism begins between 18 months and 3 years of age.
    B. Boys are affected more than girls.
    C. Social skills and communication skills are impaired.
    D. Persons with autism cannot develop social and work skills.

30. When controlled, epilepsy usually does *not* affect learning and activities of daily living.
    A. True
    B. False

31. Persons with epilepsy have higher rates of accidental deaths.
    A. True
    B. False

ADDITIONAL LEARNING ACTIVITIES

1. Use the yellow pages of the telephone book and the Internet (if available) to identify agencies and programs available in your community for persons with developmental disabilities. Answer these questions about each agency or program:
   A. What population is served?
   B. What services are provided?
   C. How is the agency or program funded?
   D. How do those in need of services access the agency or program?

2. Contact the school system in your community. Ask the following questions:
   A. How does the school system help meet the needs of persons with developmental disabilities?
   B. What special programs are available to meet special needs?
   C. Are all areas of the schools handicap-accessible?

3. How does your community meet the transportation needs of persons with developmental disabilities?

4. Are there appropriate housing options available in your community for persons with development disabilities?

5. Which businesses in your community hire persons with developmental disabilities?

37

Rehabilitation and Restorative Care

OBJECTIVES

The questions and student activities in this chapter will help you meet these objectives.

- Define the key terms listed in Chapter 37
- Describe how rehabilitation involves the whole person
- Identify the complications to prevent
- Identify the common reactions to rehabilitation
- Describe how rehabilitation can help a person work
- List the common rehabilitation services
- Explain your role in rehabilitation and restorative care
- Explain how to promote quality of life

STUDY QUESTIONS

Matching

Match the following terms with the correct definitions.

A. Prosthesis
B. Restorative nursing care
C. Activities of daily living (ADL)
D. Rehabilitation
E. Disability
F. Restorative aide

1. _______ The activities usually done during a normal day in a person's life
2. _______ Any lost, absent, or impaired physical or mental function
3. _______ An artificial replacement for a missing body part
4. _______ The process of restoring the person to the highest possible level of physical, psychological, social, and economic functioning
5. _______ An assistive person with special training in restorative nursing and rehabilitation skills
6. _______ Care that helps persons regain their health, strength, and independence

Fill in the Blanks

7. Explain the difference between an acute problem and a chronic problem.

____

____

____

____

8. The focus of rehabilitation is on _______________ _______________. When improved function is not possible, the goal is to _______________.

9. Restorative nursing programs do the following:

   A. _______________

   B. _______________

10. Illness, injury, or disability has _______________, _______________, and _______________ effects.

11. Disabilities in children can affect normal _______________.

12. Why does rehabilitation usually take longer in older persons?

____

____

____

13. Some persons need bladder training. The method depends on the person's _______________, _______________, and _______________.

14. What are the goals of bowel training?

   A. _______________

   B. _______________

15. Mr. Adams needs an artificial arm. What is the goal of this prosthesis?

____

____

16. List 4 possible psychological reactions to disability.

   A. _______________

   ____

   B. _______________

   ____

   C. _______________

   ____

   D. _______________

   ____

17. Successful rehabilitation depends on the person's _______________.

18. Who is the key member of the rehabilitation team?

____

19. What is the role of the family in the person's rehabilitation?

____

____

20. Every part of your job focuses on

____

____.

21. Successful rehabilitation and restorative care improve the person's quality of life. To promote the person's quality of life, you must:

A. ____________________________________

B. ____________________________________

C. ____________________________________

D. ____________________________________

E. ____________________________________

F. ____________________________________

G. ____________________________________

22. You are assisting Mr. Clark to apply a leg brace. Why should you practice applying the brace yourself?

____

____

Multiple Choice

Circle the BEST answer.

23. When does rehabilitation begin?
    A. When the person enters a rehabilitation hospital
    B. When the person goes home with home care
    C. When the person seeks health care
    D. When it is ordered by the doctor

24. Rehabilitation starts with
    A. Exercises.
    B. Bladder training.
    C. Preventing complications.
    D. Self-care activities.

25. You promote a person's rehabilitation by
    A. Doing as much as possible for the person.
    B. Helping the person focus on remaining abilities.
    C. Feeling sorry for the person.
    D. Focusing on what the person cannot do.

26. Mr. Clark is receiving physical therapy. You hear a caregiver shouting at him in an angry voice. You must
    A. Report what you heard to the nurse at once.
    B. Tell the caregiver to stop shouting.
    C. Tell Mr. Clark's family what you heard.
    D. Do nothing. It is none of your business.

27. Persons in nursing centers are *not* able to receive rehabilitation services.
    A. True
    B. False

28. Federal laws require that schools provide needed therapies.
    A. True
    B. False

29. Mr. Clark is making slow progress learning how to use a transfer board. He says he is tired and is not going to work today. You feel yourself getting impatient. You should:
    A. Tell Mr. Clark that he will never get better if he does not keep trying.
    B. Ask a co-worker to work with Mr. Clark today.
    C. Leave the room and come back when you are less impatient.
    D. Discuss your feelings with the nurse.

30. Which action is *not* helpful when assisting the person with rehabilitation?
    A. Keeping the person in good alignment at all times
    B. Practicing measures to prevent pressure ulcers
    C. Giving the person pity and sympathy
    D. Giving praise when a little progress is made

ADDITIONAL LEARNING ACTIVITIES

1. Do you have a family member or a friend with a physical disability? Interview the person if he or she is willing.
   A. Discuss how the disability affects activities of daily living.
   B. Is the person involved in rehabilitation?
   C. Are community programs available when needed?
   D. Does the person use self-help devices?
   E. Have any changes been made in the person's home to help maintain independence?
   F. Has the person's job been affected by the disability?

2. Read the vignette. Then answer the questions that follow.
   Mrs. *Barbara Brown is 60 years old. She is a widow. She works as a secretary for a lawyer. Mrs. Brown had a stroke. Her right side is paralyzed. She has facial drooping. Her speech is affected. She has trouble expressing herself. She needs assistance with all ADL. She is receiving rehabilitation in a skilled nursing center. Her goal is to learn to walk and to care for herself, so she can go home. She is afraid she will never be able to work as a secretary again.*

   Mrs. Brown is motivated and works hard with the rehabilitation team. She tells you that she is embarrassed by her appearance. She wants to eat in her room as she feels she is messy. She told the nurse that she does not want visitors until she is doing better.
   A. How does Mrs. Brown's stroke affect her physically, psychologically, socially, and financially?
   B. What effect does the stroke have on Mrs. Brown's self-image?
   C. What health team members might be involved in Mrs. Brown's rehabilitation?
   D. How can the health team promote Mrs. Brown's right to:
      (1) Privacy?
      (2) Personal choice?
      (3) Be free from abuse and mistreatment?
   E. What measures will promote her safety?

   After 8 weeks in the skilled nursing center, Mrs. Brown is going home with home care. She is doing most ADL herself. She uses a walker. She needs help with bathing. Someone will assist with shopping and transportation needs.

   Mrs. Brown has asked the lawyer she worked for if there are tasks she might do at home. The occupational therapist is working with her to help her regain job skills.
   A. What factors must be considered during the home assessment?
   B. What health team members might be involved in the home assessment?
   C. How might Mrs. Brown's rehabilitation continue in the home setting?

38

Caring for Mothers and Newborns

OBJECTIVES

The questions and student activities in this chapter will help you meet these objectives.

- Define the key terms listed in Chapter 38
- Describe how to meet an infant's safety and security needs
- Identify the signs and symptoms of illness in infants
- Explain how to help mothers with breast-feeding
- Describe three forms of baby formulas
- Explain how to bottle-feed babies
- Explain how to burp a baby
- Describe how to give cord care
- Describe the purposes of circumcision, needed observations, and the required care
- Explain how to bathe infants
- Explain why infants are weighed
- Describe the care needed by mothers after childbirth
- Perform the procedures described in Chapter 38

STUDY QUESTIONS

Complete the Crossword

Across

3. The vaginal discharge that occurs after childbirth
4. The surgical removal of foreskin from the penis
5. Prefix meaning "after"
6. Word element meaning "childbirth"

Down

1. Incision into the perineum
2. The cord that carries blood, oxygen, and nutrients from the mother to the fetus

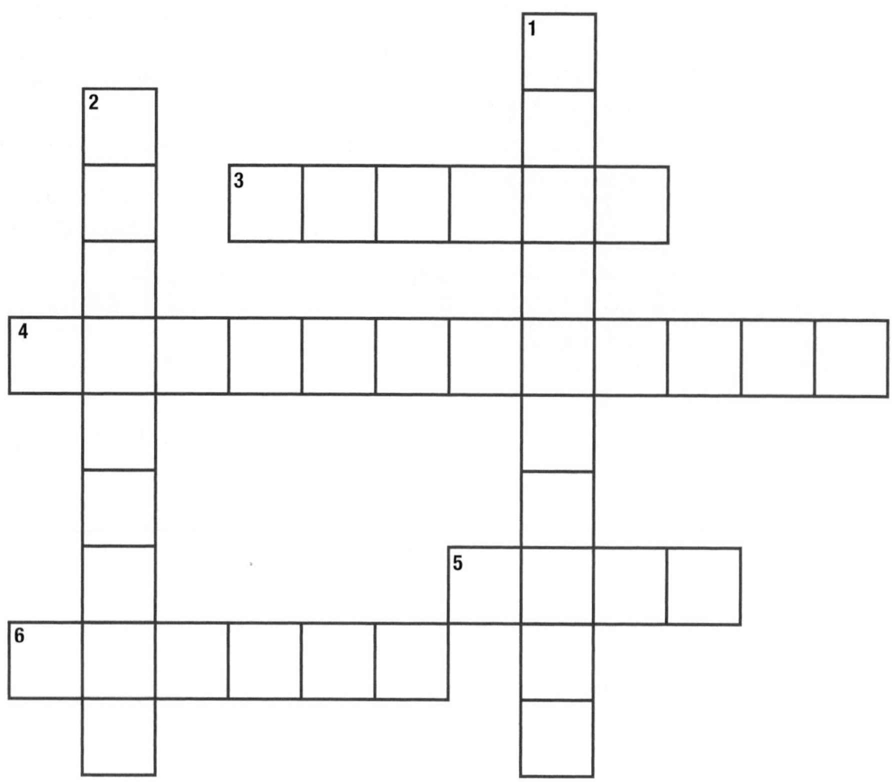

Fill in the Blanks

1. List 4 reasons that home care may be needed after childbirth.

   A. ____________________

   B. ____________________

   C. ____________________

   D. ____________________

2. Babies cry to ____________________.

3. Both hands are used to lift a newborn. Use one hand to support the ____________________.

   Use your other hand to support the ____________________.

4. What are the risks of laying an infant on an adult's or child's bed, water bed, or bunk bed?

   A. ____________________

   B. ____________________

   C. ____________________

5. Breast-fed babies are fed ____________________.

6. Mrs. Hart is breast-feeding her baby. Why does she use her nipple to stroke the baby's cheek or lower lip?

   ____

7. How should Mrs. Hart remove the baby from her breast?

   ____

8. Mrs. Hart and her baby have been discharged to home with home care services. You will be grocery shopping for her and planning meals. It is important for you to remember the following:

   A. ______________________________________

   ____

   B. ______________________________________

   ____

   C. ______________________________________

   ____

   D. ______________________________________

   ____

   E. ______________________________________

   ____

9. Formula comes in these 3 forms:

   A. ______________________________________

   B. ______________________________________

   C. ______________________________________

10. Test the temperature of the formula by

    ______________________________________.

11. Describe 2 ways to position a baby for burping.

    A. ______________________________________

    ____

    B. ______________________________________

    ____

12. To properly care for cloth diapers you need to:

    A. ______________________________________

    B. ______________________________________

    C. ______________________________________

    D. ______________________________________

    E. ______________________________________

    F. ______________________________________

    G. ______________________________________

13. You have changed Lisa Moore's diaper. What observations do you need to report and record?

    A. ______________________________________

    B. ______________________________________

    C. ______________________________________

    D. ______________________________________

14. What measures are practiced to keep babies safe during diapering?

    A. ______________________________________

    ____

    B. ______________________________________

    ____

    C. ______________________________________

    ____

    D. ______________________________________

    ____

15. You are giving cord care to Matthew Reed. What observations do you need to report to the nurse?

    A. ______________________________________

    ____

    B. ______________________________________

    ____

16. After circumcision, the penis will look

    ______________________________________,

    ______________________________________,

    and ______________________________________.

17. List 5 reasons that baths are important for babies.

    A. ______________________

    B. ______________________

    C. ______________________

    D. ______________________

    E. ______________________

18. What type of bath is given until the cord stump falls off and the umbilicus and circumcision heal?

    ____

19. What information do you need from the nurse and the care plan before bathing an infant?

    A. ______________________

    B. ______________________

    C. ______________________

    D. ______________________

    E. ______________________

20. The nurse tells you to weigh a baby. How do you meet the baby's safety needs?

    A. ______________________

    ____

    B. ______________________

    ____

21. The postpartum period starts with ______________________

    ______________________. It ends ______________________.

22. Involution of the uterus means ______________________

    ____

    ______________________.

23. A new mother has foul-smelling vaginal discharge 4 days after childbirth. This is a sign of

    ______________________.

24. How are sanitary pads applied and removed?

    ____

    ____

25. What is the purpose of an episiotomy?

    ____

    ____

26. A baby is delivered through an abdominal incision. This is called ______________________.

27. A C-section is done when:

    A. ______________________

    ____

    B. ______________________

    ____

    C. ______________________

    ____

    D. ______________________

    ____

Multiple Choice

Circle the BEST answer.

28. Infant safety is promoted by
    A. Putting pillows and soft toys in the crib.
    B. Laying babies on their stomachs for sleep.
    C. Allowing babies to cry until they fall asleep.
    D. Supporting the baby's neck when lifting or holding the baby.

29. Which action will *not* promote infant safety?
    A. Keeping your fingernails short
    B. Keeping pins and small objects out of the baby's reach
    C. Using the safety straps to keep the baby on the changing table if you need to get something
    D. Responding to the baby's cries

30. It is necessary to support the infant's head and neck for the first 3 months after birth.
    A. True
    B. False

31. Which is *not* a sign of illness in an infant?
    A. The baby cries when hungry.
    B. The baby is limp and slow to respond.
    C. The baby is flushed, pale, or perspiring.
    D. The baby has red or irritated eyes.

32. Mrs. Hart is breast-feeding her baby. Which is *false?*
    A. A nursing bra supports the breasts and provides comfort.
    B. Nursing pads are placed in the bra to absorb leaking milk.
    C. Warm water and soap are used to wash the breasts after each feeding.
    D. Nipples are air dried after washing to prevent cracking and soreness.

33. Mrs. Andrews is preparing formula for the entire day. Extra bottles are capped and stored in the refrigerator. These bottles are used within
    A. 12 hours.
    B. 24 hours.
    C. 2 days.
    D. 3 days.

34. Mrs. Andrews uses reusable bottle-feeding equipment for her baby. Which is *incorrect?*
    A. Use hot soapy water to wash bottle feeding equipment.
    B. Squeeze hot soapy water through the nipples.
    C. Rinse all items thoroughly in hot water.
    D. Use a clean towel to dry bottles and nipples.

35. Which action is correct when bottle feeding a baby?
    A. Warm the bottle in a container of lukewarm water or hold it under warm running tap water.
    B. Warm the bottle by setting it out at room temperature.
    C. Warm the bottle in the microwave.
    D. Give the formula cold out of the refrigerator.

36. You are bottle-feeding a baby. Which is *incorrect?*
    A. Prop the bottle and lay the baby down.
    B. Tilt the bottle so that the neck of the bottle and nipple are always full.
    C. Burp the baby when he or she has taken half the formula and at the end of the feeding.
    D. Discard any remaining formula.

37. Babies should wet at least
    A. 2 to 4 times a day.
    B. 4 to 6 times a day.
    C. 6 to 8 times a day.
    D. 10 to 12 times a day.

38. A baby's diaper is changed
    A. Every two hours.
    B. Before each feeding.
    C. When it is wet or soiled.
    D. When the baby cries.

39. If diaper pins are used for cloth diapers, the pins must point toward the abdomen.
    A. True
    B. False

40. Cord care involves all of the following *except*
    A. Keep the diaper below the cord.
    B. Give a sponge bath until the cord falls off.
    C. Pull the cord off when it looks ready to fall off.
    D. Keep the cord stump dry.

41. Which statement about circumcision is *false?*
    A. The area should be healed in 5 days.
    B. You must check for signs of bleeding and infection.
    C. There should be no odor or drainage.
    D. The penis is cleaned at each diaper change.

42. Which does *not* promote safety when bathing a baby?
    A. Always keep one hand on the baby.
    B. Never leave the baby alone.
    C. Water temperature is 110° F.
    D. Room temperature is kept at 75° to 80° F.

43. A baby's nails are best cut when the baby is sleeping.
    A. True
    B. False

44. Very fine fingernail scissors are used to cut a baby's fingernails.
    A. True
    B. False

45. Which is *not* a sign or symptom of postpartum complications?
   A. Burning on urination
   B. Lochia rubra during the first 3 to 4 days
   C. Fever of 100.4° F or greater
   D. Breast pain, tenderness, or swelling

46. A new mother expresses feelings of sadness and depression. You should report this to the nurse at once.
   A. True
   B. False

ADDITIONAL LEARNING ACTIVITIES

1. Carefully review the rules for infant safety (Box 38-1, pages 743 through 744 in the textbook). Using a doll, practice the following:
   A. Holding the baby using the cradle hold, the football hold, and the shoulder hold.
   B. Positioning the baby correctly in the crib.
   C. Applying powder to the baby.

2. List the factors that might affect a mother's emotional reactions after childbirth.

3. List measures that might help the new mother meet her physical and emotional needs.

4. If you are a mother, list the measures you used to meet your physical and emotional needs after childbirth. Answers these questions:
   A. How did members of the health care team provide support?
   B. What other support systems did you have?
   C. What did people say and do that was not helpful?
   D. How will your experience affect the care you provide to new mothers?

5. Review and practice the procedures in Chapter 38. Use the procedure checklists on pages 489 through 495 as a guide. Use a doll for the baby.

39

Basic Emergency Care

OBJECTIVES

The questions and student activities in this chapter will help you meet these objectives.

- Define the key terms listed in Chapter 39
- Describe the general rules of emergency care
- Identify the signs of cardiac arrest and obstructed airway
- Describe the signs, symptoms, and emergency care for hemorrhage
- Identify the signs, symptoms, and emergency care for shock
- Describe the types of seizures and how to care for a person during a seizure
- Describe the causes, types, and emergency care for burns
- Identify the common causes and emergency care for fainting
- Describe the signs, symptoms, and emergency care for stroke
- Perform the procedures described in Chapter 39

STUDY QUESTIONS

Complete the Crossword

Across

4. A life-threatening sensitivity to an antigen
5. Violent and sudden contractions or tremors of muscle groups
8. The excessive loss of blood in a short period of time

Down

1. Breathing stops but heart action continues for several minutes
2. A seizure
3. The sudden loss of consciousness from an inadequate blood supply to the brain
6. Emergency care given to an ill or injured person before medical help arrives
7. Results when organs and tissues do not get enough blood

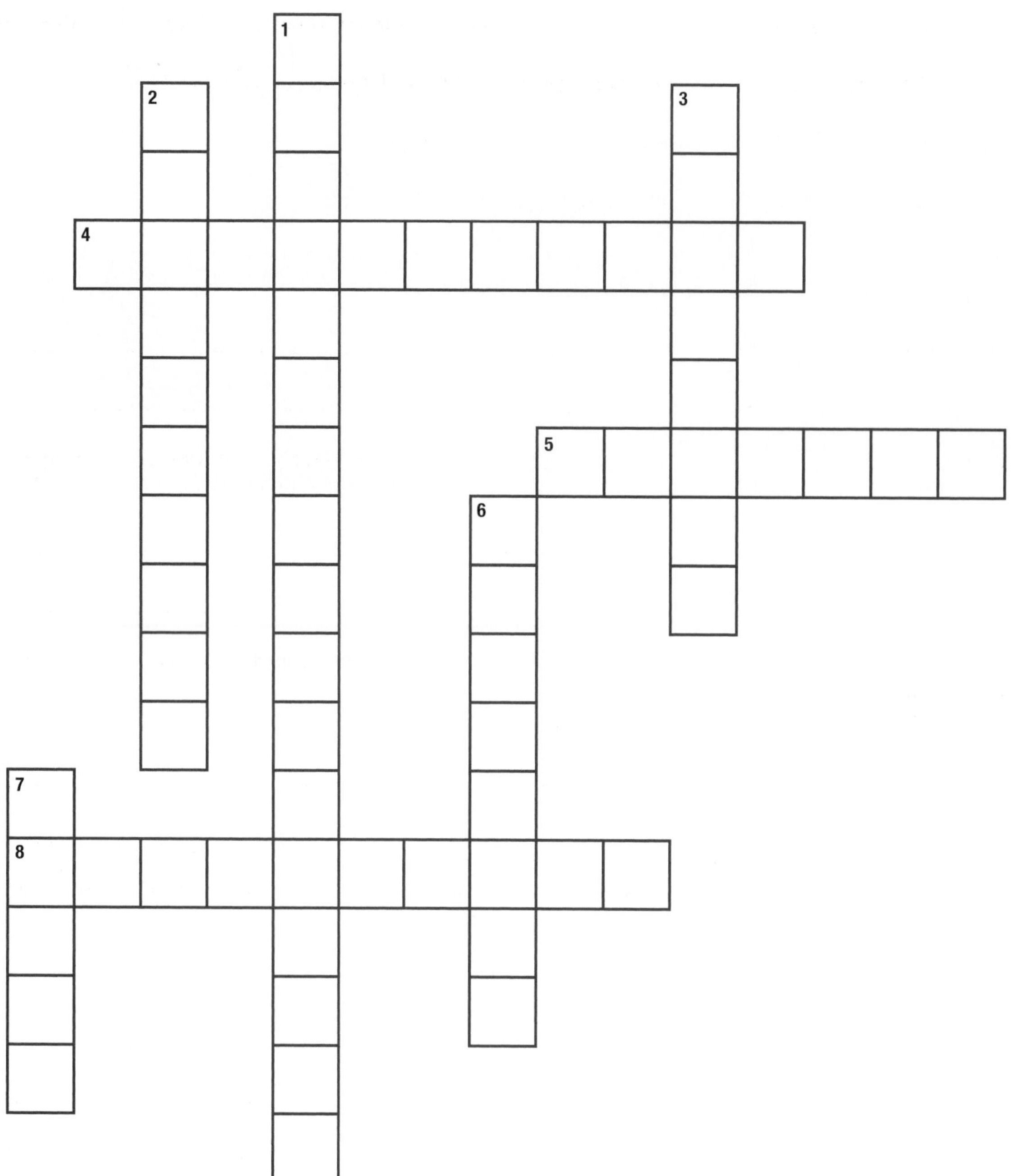

Matching

Match the following terms with the correct definitions.

A. Partial airway obstruction
B. Emergency Medical Services (EMS) system
C. Full thickness burns
D. Heimlich maneuver
E. Rescue breathing
F. Basic life support
G. Cardiac arrest

1. _______ The heart and breathing stop suddenly and without warning

2. _______ This system involves emergency personnel who are trained and educated to give emergency care

3. _______ Procedures which support breathing and circulation

4. _______ Breathing is done for the person (mouth-to-mouth, mouth-to-barrier device, or mouth-to-stoma)

5. _______ The person moves some air in and out of the lungs; the person is conscious

6. _______ Used to relieve a foreign-body airway obstruction (FBAO)

7. _______ Burns involving the dermis and the entire epidermis

Fill in the Blanks

8. The goals of first aid are to:

   A. ______________________

   B. ______________________

   C. ______________________

   D. ______________________

9. How do you activate the EMS system?

   ____

   ____

10. You have activated the EMS system. What information do you need to give the operator?

    A. ______________________

    B. ______________________

    C. ______________________

    D. ______________________

    E. ______________________

    F. ______________________

11. When the heart and breathing stops, the person is ______________________.

12. Mr. Brown is in respiratory arrest. If breathing in not restored, ______________________ will occur.

13. The American Heart Association's basic life support courses teach the adult Chain of Survival. Chain of Survival actions are:

    A. ______________________

    B. ______________________

    C. ______________________

    D. ______________________

14. What is the most common cause of death in infants from 2 weeks to 6 months of age?

    ____

    ____

15. What are the 3 major signs of cardiac arrest?

    A. ______________________

    B. ______________________

    C. ______________________

16. What are the 3 basic parts of cardiopulmonary resuscitation (CPR)?

    A. ______________________

    B. ______________________

    C. ______________________

17. Describe how to perform the head-tilt/chin-lift maneuver.

    A. ______________________

    ____

    B. ______________________

    ____

    C. ______________________

    ____

    D. ______________________

    ____

E. ______________________

____

F. ______________________

____

18. Describe how to check for adequate breathing.

A. ______________________

B. ______________________

C. ______________________

D. ______________________

E. ______________________

F. ______________________

19. What is the purpose of the barrier device used in mouth-to-barrier device rescue breathing?

____

____

20. When is mouth-to-nose breathing used?

A. ______________________

B. ______________________

C. ______________________

D. ______________________

E. ______________________

21. Before giving mouth-to-mouth or mouth-to-nose rescue breathing, always check to see of the person has a ______________________.

22. During CPR, ______________________ breaths are given after every ______________________ chest compressions.

23. Before starting chest compressions, check for ______________________.

24. CPR is done when the person ______________________, ______________________, and ______________________.

25. How far is the sternum depressed when doing chest compressions on an adult?

____

26. What should you do if you are alone and a child (8 years old or younger) is not responding?

A. ______________________

B. ______________________

C. ______________________

27. How will you perform rescue breathing on an infant?

____

____

28. Which pulse is used to check circulation in infants?

____

29. What is the most common cause of FBAO in adults?

____

____

30. The Heimlich maneuver is not effective for:

A. ______________________

B. ______________________

31. Abby Lewis is 2 years old. She is cyanotic and has problems breathing. She also has a fever, hoarseness, and respiratory congestion. What should you do?

____

____

32. The recovery position is ____________________

____________________. It is used when

____

____________________.

33. You should not use the recovery position if

____________________.

34. What is the purpose of an automated external defibrillator (AED)?

____

____

35. List 5 signs and symptoms of internal hemorrhage.

A. ____________________

B. ____________________

C. ____________________

D. ____________________

E. ____________________

36. Bleeding from ____________________

____________________ occurs in spurts.

37. What should you do if direct pressure over the bleeding site does not control external bleeding?

____

____

38. List the signs and symptoms of shock.

A. ____________________

B. ____________________

C. ____________________

D. ____________________

E. ____________________

F. ____________________

G. ____________________

39. List 8 signs and symptoms of anaphylactic shock.

A. ____________________

B. ____________________

C. ____________________

D. ____________________

E. ____________________

F. ____________________

G. ____________________

H. ____________________

40. List and briefly describe the 2 major types of seizures.

A. ____________________

____

B. ____________________

____

41. Describe the 2 phases of a generalized tonic-clonic seizure (grand mal seizure).

A. ____________________

____

B. ____________________

____

42. Where do most burns occur?

____

43. Describe the 2 types of burns.

A. Partial-thickness burns ____________________

____

____

B. Full-thickness burns ______________________

____

____

44. The severity of a burn depends on

______________________,

______________________,

and ______________________.

45. Emergency care of burns includes covering burn with ______________________

____

______________________.

46. ______________________,

______________________,

and ______________________

are warning signals of fainting.

47. Stroke occurs when ______________________

______________________.

48. Signs of stroke depend on ______________________

______________________.

49. Emergency care for stroke includes the following:

A. ______________________

B. ______________________

C. ______________________

D. ______________________

E. ______________________

F. ______________________

G. ______________________

H. ______________________

Multiple Choice

Circle the BEST answer.

50. When providing emergency care, it is important to do all of the following *except*
    A. Check for signs of life threatening problems.
    B. Move the person to a comfortable position.
    C. Call for help.
    D. Keep the person warm.

51. The airway is opened by
    A. Turning the head to the side.
    B. Lifting the head up and tilting forward.
    C. Sitting the person up.
    D. The head-tilt/chin-lift maneuver.

52. During two-person adult cardiopulmonary resuscitation, which is *correct?*
    A. Give 1 breath after every 10 chest compressions.
    B. Give 2 breaths after every 15 chest compressions.
    C. Give 1 breath after every 5 chest compressions.
    D. Give 1 breath at the same rate as chest compressions.

53. Which artery is used to check for a pulse before starting chest compressions?
    A. The radial artery
    B. The carotid artery
    C. The brachial artery
    D. The femoral artery

54. For chest compressions to be effective, the person
    A. Must be in a sitting position.
    B. Must be flat and on a soft surface.
    C. Must be supine and on a hard, flat surface.
    D. Is positioned with pillows.

55. You determine unresponsiveness in an adult by
    A. Observing the person's color.
    B. Feeling for a pulse.
    C. Taking the person's blood pressure.
    D. Tapping or gently shaking the person and asking, "Are you OK?"

56. When giving CPR to a child, give 5 chest compressions followed by 1 slow breath. Give 100 chest compressions per minute and 20 rescue breaths per minute.
    A. True
    B. False

57. A person has a complete airway obstruction. Which is *false?*
    A. The conscious person clutches at the throat.
    B. The person appears pale and cyanotic.
    C. The person can talk.
    D. The conscious person is very frightened.

58. The Heimlich maneuver can be performed with the person standing, sitting, or lying down.
    A. True
    B. False

59. If you find a person unconscious, you can assume the person is choking.
    A. True
    B. False

60. Back blows and chest thrusts are used to relieve FBAO in infants.
    A. True
    B. False

61. Mr. Jones is in ventricular fibrillation. Defibrillation as soon as possible increases his chance of survival.
    A. True
    B. False

62. Internal hemorrhage is suspected. Which is *correct?*
    A. Keep the person cool and in the semi-Fowler's position.
    B. Give the person cool water to drink.
    C. Apply pressure to the area.
    D. Activate the EMS system.

63. To control external hemorrhage, do all of the following *except*
    A. Have the person lie down.
    B. Remove any objects that have pierced or stabbed the person.
    C. Place a sterile dressing directly over the wound.
    D. Apply pressure with your hand directly over the bleeding site.

64. To prevent or treat shock, do all of the following *except*
    A. Maintain an open airway.
    B. Control hemorrhage.
    C. Keep the person warm.
    D. Keep the person in Fowler's position.

65. Anaphylactic shock is an emergency. The EMS system must be activated.
    A. True
    B. False

66. Which action will protect the person from injury during a generalized tonic-clonic seizure?
    A. Lower the person to the floor.
    B. Turn the person on his or her back.
    C. Restrain body movements during the seizure.
    D. Give the person water to drink.

67. Generalized absence seizures are more common in older adults than in other age-groups.
    A. True
    B. False

68. Emergency care for burns includes
    A. Removing the person from the fire or burn source.
    B. Removing burned clothing.
    C. Putting oil, butter, salve, or ointments on the burns.
    D. Keeping the person uncovered and the burn areas open to the air.

69. Emergency care for fainting includes all of the following *except*
    A. Have the person sit or lie down.
    B. Loosen clothing.
    C. If the person is lying down, elevate the legs.
    D. Give the person sips of cool water.

70. There is no need to protect the person's right to privacy and confidentiality during an emergency.
    A. True
    B. False

ADDITIONAL LEARNING ACTIVITIES

1. Identify the EMS system in your community.
   A. Check the yellow pages of the telephone book.
   B. Do you know how to activate the EMS system in an emergency?
   C. If you have children, do they know how to activate the EMS system in your community?

2. Are you and your family prepared to respond to emergency situations in your home?
   A. Are emergency phone numbers easily found?
   B. Do members of your family know what information to give the operator in an emergency?
   C. Do you and your family know basic life support procedures?

3. Do you know which agencies in your community offer classes in basic life support procedures and first aid? The list below may be helpful.
   A. Hospitals
   B. Nursing centers
   C. Community colleges
   D. The American Heart Association
   E. The American Red Cross
   F. The National Safety Council

4. If possible, enroll in a basic life support class. Your instructor can help you with this process.

40 The Dying Person

OBJECTIVES

The questions and student activities in this chapter will help you meet these objectives.

- Define the key terms listed in Chapter 40
- Describe terminal illness
- Explain the factors that affect attitudes about death
- Describe how different age-groups view death
- Describe the five stages of dying
- Explain how to meet the needs of the dying person and family
- Describe hospice care
- Explain the importance of the Patient Self-Determination Act
- Explain what is meant by a "Do-Not-Resuscitate" order
- Identify the signs of approaching death and the signs of death
- Explain how to assist with postmortem care
- Perform the procedure described in Chapter 40

STUDY QUESTIONS

Matching

Match the following terms with the correct definitions.

A. Postmortem
B. Rigor mortis
C. Hospice care
D. Durable power of attorney
E. Living will
F. Advance directive
G. Terminal illness
H. Reincarnation

1. _______ A document stating a person's wishes about health care when that person cannot make his or her own decisions

2. _______ After death

3. _______ The belief that the spirit or soul is reborn in another human body or in another form of life

4. _______ A document about measures that support or maintain life when death is likely

5. _______ The stiffness or rigidity of skeletal muscles that occurs after death

6. _______ An illness or injury for which there is no reasonable expectation of recovery

7. _______ An option for the terminally ill; care focuses on physical, emotional, social, and spiritual needs of dying persons and their families

8. _______ Gives the power to make health care decisions to another person

Fill in the Blanks

9. ______________________________ and ______________________________ strongly influence living and dying.

10. ______________________________, ______________________________, ______________________________, and ______________________________ influence attitudes about death.

11. In ______________________________ quality of life is more important than length of life because of beliefs in reincarnation.

12. List 5 things adults may fear when facing death.
    A. ______________________________
    B. ______________________________
    C. ______________________________
    D. ______________________________
    E. ______________________________

13. Adults often resent death because it affects ______________________________, ______________________________, ______________________________, and ______________________________.

14. Why might some older people welcome death?
    ____
    ____
    ____

15. List the 5 stages of dying described by Dr. Elizabeth Kübler-Ross.
    A. ______________________________
    B. ______________________________
    C. ______________________________
    D. ______________________________
    E. ______________________________

16. How can you use listening and touch to help meet the dying person's psychological, social, and spiritual needs?
    A. Listening: ______________________________
    ____
    ____
    ____
    B. Touch: ______________________________
    ____
    ____
    ____

17. ______________________________ is one of the last functions lost. Always assume that the person can ______________________________.

18. ______________________,

______________________,

______________________,

______________________,

and ______________ promote

comfort when caring for the dying person.

19. Which position is usually best for breathing problems?

____

20. The goal of hospice care is to ______________

______________________.

21. The Patient Self-Determination Act and OBRA

give persons the right to ______________

______________________.

They also give the right to make ______________

______________________.

22. A living will instructs doctors:

A. ______________________

B. ______________________

23. The doctor has written a "Do-Not-Resuscitate" (DNR) order for Miss Lake. What does this mean?

____

____

24. What should you do if you do not agree with a person's care or resuscitation decisions?

____

____

25. List 6 signs that signal death is near.

A. ______________________

____

B. ______________________

____

C. ______________________

____

D. ______________________

____

E. ______________________

____

F. ______________________

____

26. Mr. Dorian died in his home. What legal requirements do you need to be aware of when there is a death in the home?

____

____

____

27. The signs of death include:

A. ______________________

B. ______________________

28. What information do you need from the nurse when assisting with postmortem care?

A. ______________________

B. ______________________

C. ______________________

D. ______________________

Multiple Choice

Circle the BEST answer.

29. Attitudes and beliefs about death usually stay the same throughout a person's life.
   A. True
   B. False

30. Children between the ages of 3 and 5
   A. Know that death is final.
   B. Often think they will die.
   C. Often blame themselves when someone dies.
   D. Are not curious about death.

31. The person in the bargaining stage of dying
   A. Is very sad.
   B. Makes promises in exchange for more time.
   C. Is calm and at peace.
   D. Feels anger and rage.

32. Mary is dying. She asks you to stay and talk in the middle of the night. Which is *correct?*
   A. Tell Mary that she needs to sleep.
   B. Call Mary's family to stay with her.
   C. Call a pastor to talk with Mary.
   D. Being there and listening help meet Mary's psychological and social needs.

33. You promote comfort when caring for a dying person by
   A. Playing cheerful music.
   B. Whispering when in the person's presence.
   C. Avoiding touch.
   D. Providing good skin care and personal hygiene.

34. A darkened room is comforting to the dying person.
   A. True
   B. False

35. Health care agencies must inform all persons of the right to advance directives on admission.
   A. True
   B. False

36. Freedom from restraint does not apply to the dying person.
   A. True
   B. False

37. The dying person has the right to receive kind and respectful care before and after death.
   A. True
   B. False

38. Postmortem care involves all of the following except
   A. Pronouncing the person dead.
   B. Positioning the body in normal alignment before rigor mortis sets in.
   C. Preparing the body for viewing by the family.
   D. Bathing soiled areas.

39. It is not necessary to provide privacy when doing postmortem care because the person is dead.
   A. True
   B. False

40. When providing postmortem care, you must practice Standard Precautions and follow the Bloodborne Pathogen Standard.
   A. True
   B. False

ADDITIONAL LEARNING ACTIVITIES

1. List your thoughts and feelings about death and dying. Answer these questions:
   A. How do your religion, culture, and age affect your feelings about death?
   B. Have you had experience with the death of a family member or friend that affects your feelings about death and dying? Explain.
   C. How do you feel about living wills?

2. Review the Dying Person's Bill of Rights (Box 40-1 on page 794 in the textbook). List measures you can use to promote these rights when caring for the dying person.

3. List ways you can help the family and friends of a dying person.
   A. What needs might they have?
   B. What fears might they have?
   C. What support systems are available?
   D. What are the roles of various members of the health care team in providing support and comfort?

4. Do you have fears about caring for dying persons? Discuss them with your instructor.
   A. How can you deal with your feelings and fears?

Procedure Checklists

Using a Fire Extinguisher

Name: ______________________

Date: ______________________

Procedure	S	U	Comments
1. Pulled the fire alarm.			
2. Got the nearest fire extinguisher.			
3. Carried it upright.			
4. Took it to the fire.			
5. Removed the safety pin.			
6. Directed the hose at the base of the fire.			
7. Pushed the top handle down.			
8. Swept the hose slowly back and forth at the base of the fire.			

Date of Satisfactory Completion ______________ Instructor's Initials ______________

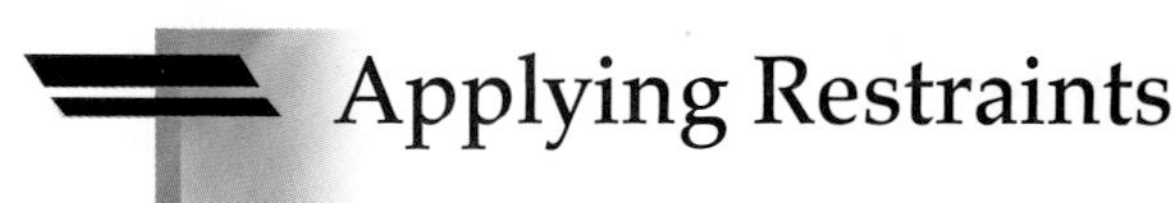

Applying Restraints

Name: ____________________

Date: ____________________

Pre-Procedure	S	U	Comments
• Knocked before entering the person's room.			
• Addressed the person by name.			
• Introduced yourself by name and title.			
1. Followed Delegation Guidelines. Reviewed Safety Alert.			
2. Collected the following:			
• Correct type and size of restraints			
• Padding for bony areas			
• Bed rail pads or gap protectors			
3. Practiced hand hygiene.			
4. Identified the person. Checked the ID bracelet against the assignment sheet. Called the person by name.			
5. Explained the procedure to the person.			
6. Provided for privacy.			

Procedure	S	U	Comments
7. Made sure the person was comfortable and in good body alignment.			
8. Put the bed rail pads or gap protectors on the bed if the person was in bed, if needed. Followed the manufacturer's instructions.			
9. Padded bony areas according to the nurse's instructions.			
10. Read the manufacturer's instructions. Noted the front and back of the restraint.			
11. For wrist restraints:			
a. Applied the restraint following the manufacturer's instructions. Placed the soft part toward the skin.			
b. Secured the restraint so it was snug but not tight. Made sure you could slide one or two fingers under the restraint. Followed the manufacturer's instructions.			
c. Tied the straps to the movable part of the bed frame out of the person's reach. Used an agency-approved tie. Left 1 to 2 inches of slack in the straps.			
d. Repeated steps 11a, 11b, and 11c for the other wrist.			
12. For mitt restraints:			
a. Made sure the person's hands were clean and dry.			
b. Applied the mitt restraint. Followed the manufacturer's instructions.			
c. Tied the straps to the movable part of the bed frame. Used an agency-approved tie. Left 1 to 2 inches of slack in the straps.			

Procedure—cont'd	S	U	Comments
d. Made sure the restraint was snug. Slid fingers between the restraint and the wrist. Adjusted the straps if it was too loose or too tight. Checked for snugness again.	______	______	______
e. Repeated steps 12b, 12c, and 12d for the other hand.	______	______	______
13. For a belt restraint:			
a. Assisted the person to a sitting position.	______	______	______
b. Applied the restraint with your free hand. Followed the manufacturer's instructions.	______	______	______
c. Removed wrinkles or creases from the front and back of the restraint.	______	______	______
d. Brought the ties through the slots in the belt.	______	______	______
e. Helped the person lie down if he or she was in bed.	______	______	______
f. Made sure the person was comfortable and in good body alignment.	______	______	______
g. Secured the straps to the movable part of the bed frame out of the person's reach or to the chair or wheelchair. Used an agency-approved tie. Left 1 to 2 inches of slack in the straps.	______	______	______
14. For a vest restraint:			
a. Assisted the person to a sitting position.	______	______	______
b. Applied the restraint with your free hand. The V-part of the vest crossed in front. Followed the manufacturer's instructions.	______	______	______
c. Made sure the vest was free of wrinkles in the front and back.	______	______	______
d. Helped the person lie down if he or she was in bed.	______	______	______
e. Brought the straps through the slots.	______	______	______
f. Made sure the person was comfortable and in good body alignment.	______	______	______
g. Secured the straps to the chair or to the movable part of the bed frame. If secured to the bed frame, the straps were secured at waist level out of the person's reach. Used an agency-approved tie. Left 1 to 2 inches of slack in the straps.	______	______	______
h. Made sure the vest was snug. Slid an open hand between the restraint and the person. Adjusted the restraint if it was too loose or too tight. Checked for snugness again.	______	______	______
15. For a jacket restraint:			
a. Assisted the person to a sitting position.	______	______	______
b. Applied the restraint with your free hand. Followed the manufacturer's instructions. The jacket opening was in back.	______	______	______
c. Closed the back with the zipper, ties, or hook and loop closures.	______	______	______
d. Made sure the side seams were under the arms. Removed any wrinkles in the front and back.	______	______	______
e. Helped the person lie down if he or she was in bed.	______	______	______

Procedure—cont'd

	S	U	Comments
f. Made sure the person was comfortable and in good body alignment.			
g. Secured the straps to the chair or to the movable part of the bed frame. If secured to the bed frame, the straps were secured at waist level out of the person's reach. Used an agency-approved knot. Left 1 to 2 inches of slack in the straps.			
h. Made sure the jacket was snug. Slid an open hand between the restraint and the person. Adjusted the restraint if it was too loose or too tight. Checked for snugness again.			
16. For elbow restraints:			
a. Wrapped the restraint around the child's elbow. Followed the manufacturer's instructions.			
b. Secured the restraint. Followed the manufacturer's instructions. Left 1 to 2 inches of slack in the straps.			
c. Repeated steps 16a and 16b for the other arm.			

Post-Procedure

	S	U	Comments
17. Positioned the person as the nurse directed.			
18. Placed the signal light within the person's reach.			
19. Raised or lowered bed rails. Followed the care plan and the manufacturer's instructions for the restraint.			
20. Unscreened the person.			
21. Decontaminated hands.			
22. Checked the person and the restraints at least every 15 minutes. Reported and recorded observations.			
a. For wrist and mitt restraints: checked the pulse, color, and temperature of the restrained parts.			
b. For vest, jacket, and belt restraints: checked the person's breathing. Called the nurse if the person was not breathing or was having difficulty breathing. Made sure the restraint was properly positioned in the front and back.			
23. Did the following at least every 2 hours:			
• Removed the restraint.			
• Repositioned the person.			
• Met food, fluid, hygiene, and elimination needs.			
• Gave skin care.			
• Performed range-of-motion exercises or ambulated the person. Followed the care plan.			
• Reapplied the restraints.			
24. Reported and recorded observations and the care given.			

Date of Satisfactory Completion ____________________ Instructor's Initials ____________________

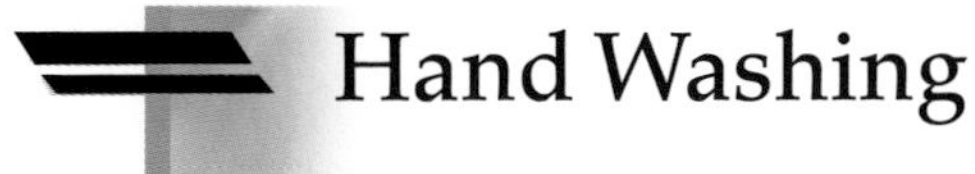

Hand Washing

Name: ______________________

Date: ______________________

Procedure	S	U	Comments
1. Reviewed Safety Alert.	____	____	____________
2. Made sure to have soap, paper towels, orange stick or nail file, and a wastebasket. Collected missing items.	____	____	____________
3. Pushed watch up 4 to 5 inches. Also pushed up uniform sleeves.	____	____	____________
4. Stood away from the sink so that clothes did not touch the sink. Stood so the soap and faucet were easy to reach.	____	____	____________
5. Turned on and adjusted the water until it felt warm.	____	____	____________
6. Wet wrists and hands. Kept hands lower than elbows.	____	____	____________
7. Applied about 1 teaspoon of soap to hands.	____	____	____________
8. Rubbed palms together and interlaced fingers to work up a good lather for at least 15 seconds.	____	____	____________
9. Washed each hand and wrist thoroughly. Cleaned well between the fingers.	____	____	____________
10. Cleaned under the fingernails. Rubbed the finger tips against the palms.	____	____	____________
11. Cleaned under fingernails with a nail file or orange stick.	____	____	____________
12. Rinsed wrists and hands well. Water flowed from the arms to the hands.	____	____	____________
13. Repeated steps 7 through 12, if needed.	____	____	____________
14. Dried wrists and hands with paper towels. Patted dry starting at the fingertips.	____	____	____________
15. Discarded the paper towels.	____	____	____________
16. Turned off faucets with clean paper towels. Used a clean paper towel for each faucet.	____	____	____________
17. Discarded paper towels.	____	____	____________

Date of Satisfactory Completion ______________ Instructor's Initials ______________

Removing Gloves

Name: ____________________

Date: ____________________

Procedure	S	U	Comments
1. Made sure that glove only touched glove.	______	______	____________
2. Grasped a glove just below the cuff. Grasped it on the outside.	______	______	____________
3. Pulled the glove down over the hand so it was inside out.	______	______	____________
4. Held the removed glove with the other gloved hand.	______	______	____________
5. Reached inside the other glove. Used the first two fingers of the ungloved hand.	______	______	____________
6. Pulled the glove down (inside out) over the hand and the other glove.	______	______	____________
7. Discarded the gloves. Followed agency policy.	______	______	____________
8. Decontaminated hands.	______	______	____________

Date of Satisfactory Completion ____________________ Instructor's Initials ____________________

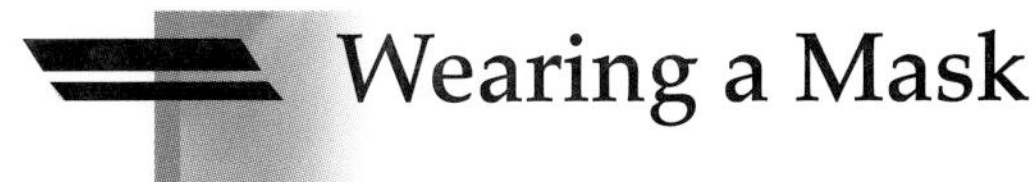

Wearing a Mask

Name: ______________________

Date: ______________________

Procedure	S	U	Comments
1. Practiced hand hygiene.	____	____	____________
2. Picked up the mask by its upper ties. Did not touch the part that will cover the face.	____	____	____________
3. Placed the mask over the nose and mouth.	____	____	____________
4. Placed the upper strings above the ears. Tied them at the back of the head.	____	____	____________
5. Tied the lower strings at the back of the neck. The lower part of the mask was under the chin.	____	____	____________
6. Pinched the metal band around the nose. The top of the mask was snug over the nose. If glasses were worn, the mask was snug under the bottom of the glasses.	____	____	____________
7. Decontaminated hands. Put on gloves.	____	____	____________
8. Provided care.	____	____	____________
9. Changed the mask if it became moist or contaminated.	____	____	____________
10. Removed the mask as follows:			
a. Removed the gloves.	____	____	____________
b. Decontaminated hands.	____	____	____________
c. Untied the lower strings.	____	____	____________
d. Untied the top strings.	____	____	____________
e. Held the top strings. Removed the mask.	____	____	____________
f. Brought the strings together. The inside of the mask folded together. Did not touch the inside of the mask.	____	____	____________
11. Discarded the mask. Followed agency policy.	____	____	____________
12. Decontaminated hands.	____	____	____________

Date of Satisfactory Completion ______________________ Instructor's Initials ______________________

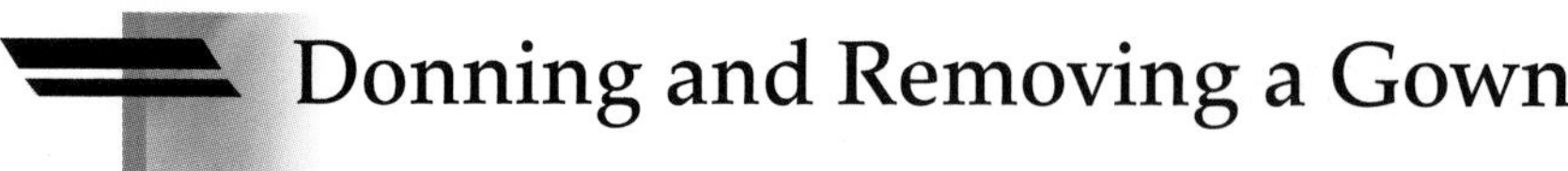

Donning and Removing a Gown

Name: ______________________

Date: ______________________

Procedure	S	U	Comments
1. Removed the watch and all jewelry.	______	______	______________
2. Rolled up uniform sleeves.	______	______	______________
3. Practiced hand hygiene.	______	______	______________
4. Put on a facemask if required.	______	______	______________
5. Held a clean gown out in front of you. Let it unfold. Did not shake the gown.	______	______	______________
6. Put the hands and arms through the sleeves.	______	______	______________
7. Made sure the gown covered the front of the uniform. It was snug at the neck.	______	______	______________
8. Tied the strings at the back of the neck.	______	______	______________
9. Overlapped the back of the gown. Made sure it covered the uniform. The gown was snug, not loose.	______	______	______________
10. Tied the waist strings at the back.	______	______	______________
11. Put on the gloves.	______	______	______________
12. Provided care.	______	______	______________
13. Removed and discarded the gloves. Decontaminated hands.	______	______	______________
14. Removed the gown:			
a. Untied the waist strings.	______	______	______________
b. Decontaminated hands.	______	______	______________
c. Untied the neck strings. Did not touch the outside of the gown.	______	______	______________
d. Pulled the gown down from the shoulder.	______	______	______________
e. Turned the gown inside out as it was removed. Held it at the inside shoulder seams and brought hands together.	______	______	______________
15. Rolled up the gown away from you. Kept it inside out.	______	______	______________
16. Discarded the gown. Followed agency policy.	______	______	______________
17. Decontaminated hands.	______	______	______________
18. Removed the facemask. Discarded it following agency policy.	______	______	______________
19. Decontaminated hands.	______	______	______________
20. Opened the door using a paper towel. Discarded it as you left.	______	______	______________

Date of Satisfactory Completion ______________ Instructor's Initials ______________

Double Bagging

Name: ____________________

Date: ____________________

Procedure	S	U	Comments
1. Asked a co-worker to help. The co-worker stood outside the room.	____	____	____________
2. Placed soiled linen, reusable items, disposable supplies, and trash in the right containers. Containers were lined with leakproof biohazard bags.	____	____	____________
3. Sealed the bags securely with ties.	____	____	____________
4. Asked the co-worker to make a wide cuff on the clean bag. It was held wide open.	____	____	____________
5. Placed the contaminated bag into the clean bag. Did not touch the outside of the clean bag.	____	____	____________
6. Asked the co-worker to seal the bag. Had the bag labeled according to agency policy.	____	____	____________
7. Repeated steps 4, 5, and 6 as needed for other contaminated bags.	____	____	____________
8. Asked the co-worker to take or send the bags to the appropriate department for disposal, disinfection, or sterilization.	____	____	____________

Date of Satisfactory Completion ____________________ Instructor's Initials ____________________

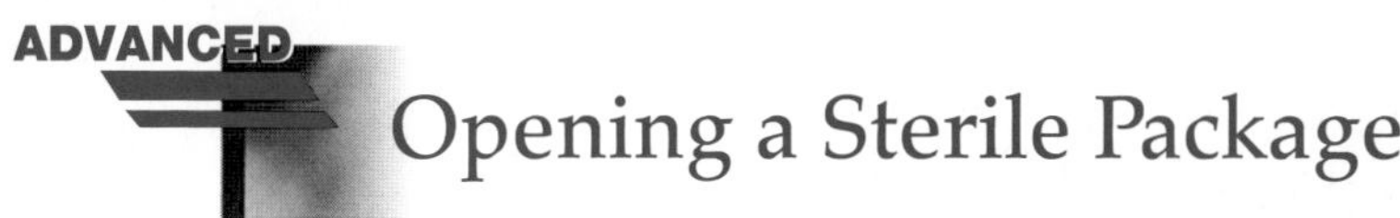

Opening a Sterile Package

Name: ______________________

Date: ______________________

Pre-Procedure	S	U	Comments
1. Followed Delegation Guidelines. Reviewed Safety Alerts.			
2. Explained the procedure to the person.			
3. Practiced hand hygiene.			
4. Collected all needed supplies and equipment.			
5. Inspected the package for sterility:			
a. Checked the label and chemical tape.			
b. Checked the expiration date.			
c. Saw if the package was dry.			
d. Checked for tears, holes, punctures, and watermarks.			
6. Identified the person. Checked the ID bracelet against the assignment sheet. Called the person by name.			
7. Provided for privacy.			
8. Provided for elimination needs. Practiced hand hygiene.			

Procedure

Procedure	S	U	Comments
9. Draped the person as directed.			
10. Arranged a work surface:			
a. Made sure there was enough room.			
b. Arranged the work surface at waist level and within vision.			
c. Cleaned and dried the work surface.			
d. Did not reach over or turn your back on the work surface.			
11. Opening a wrapped sterile package on a surface:			
a. Placed the package in the center of the work surface.			
b. Positioned the package so the top flap pointed toward you.			
c. Reached around the package. Grasped the outside of the top flap with the thumb and index finger.			
d. Pulled the flap open and laid it flat.			
e. Grasped the outside of the first side flap with the thumb and index finger. Used the right hand if the flap is on the right and the left hand if it is on the left. Pulled the flap open and laid it flat.			
f. Repeated step 11e for the other side flap.			
g. Grasped the outside of the fourth flap. Stood back and away from the package and pulled the flap back. Let the flap lie flat. Did not let the flap touch your uniform or any contaminated surface.			

Procedure—cont'd	S	U	Comments
h. Used the inside of the wrapper as a sterile field, if needed. Did not let any contaminated item touch the sterile area.			
12. Opening a wrapped sterile package while holding it:			
a. Held the package in the left hand if right-handed. Held it in the right hand if left-handed.			
b. Held the package so that the top flap pointed toward you.			
c. Reached behind the top flap. Opened it away from you.			
d. Opened each side flap away from the package.			
e. Opened the fourth flap toward you.			
f. Did not touch the inside wrapper or the package contents.			
g. Held the package so the nurse could grasp the contents.			
h. To transfer the package contents to a sterile field:			
(1) Held the wrapper back and away from the sterile field.			
(2) Dropped the contents onto the sterile field.			
13. Opening a peel-back package:			
a. Read the package instructions.			
b. Two flaps: grasped the two flaps and gently peeled the flaps back.			
c. One flap: held the package and pulled back the flap.			

Date of Satisfactory Completion ____________ Instructor's Initials ____________

ADVANCED

Opening and Pouring a Sterile Solution

Name: ______________________

Date: ______________________

Pre-Procedure	S	U	Comments
1. Reviewed Safety Alert.	_____	_____	____________
2. Obtained the correct solution.	_____	_____	____________
3. Inspected the container for cracks and breaks.	_____	_____	____________
4. Checked the seal. It was intact.	_____	_____	____________
Procedure			
5. Twisted off the cap to break the seal.	_____	_____	____________
6. Placed the cap, inside up, on a clean surface.	_____	_____	____________
7. Held the container 4 to 6 inches over the sterile bowl. Did not let the container touch the sterile bowl.	_____	_____	____________
8. Poured the solution into the sterile bowl. Poured slowly to avoid spills and splashes.	_____	_____	____________

Date of Satisfactory Completion ______________ Instructor's Initials ______________

ADVANCED

Setting Up a Sterile Field

Name: ______________________

Date: ______________________

Procedure	S	U	Comments
1. Followed Pre-Procedure steps listed in procedure: *Opening a Sterile Package.*	____	____	____________
2. Opened the sterile package.	____	____	____________
3. Picked up the folded top edge of the drape. Used the thumb and index finger.	____	____	____________
4. Removed the drape from the package. Lifted it away from you and let it unfold. Discarded the package.	____	____	____________
5. Did not let the drape touch the uniform or any other object or surface.	____	____	____________
6. Picked up the other corner of the drape. Held the drape away from you and other surfaces.	____	____	____________
7. Laid the drape on the work surface. Started with the bottom half.	____	____	____________
8. Added other sterile items to the sterile field:			
a. Opened each sterile package.	____	____	____________
b. Held the package wrapper back and away from the sterile field.	____	____	____________
c. Dropped the contents onto the sterile field or used a transfer forceps.	____	____	____________

Date of Satisfactory Completion ______________ Instructor's Initials ______________

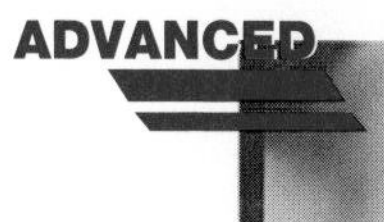

Donning and Removing Sterile Gloves

Name: ____________________

Date: ____________________

Procedure	S	U	Comments
1. Followed Delegation Guidelines. Reviewed Safety Alerts.			
2. Practiced hand hygiene.			
3. Set up a sterile field.			
4. Inspected the package for sterility:			
a. Checked the expiration date.			
b. Saw if the package was dry.			
c. Checked for tears, holes, punctures, and watermarks.			
5. Opened the package using the peel-back method.			
6. Placed the inner package on the work surface. Did not place it on the sterile field.			
7. Read the manufacturer's instructions on the inner package.			
8. Arranged the inner package for left, right, up, and down. The left glove was on the left. The right glove was on the right. The cuffs were near you with the fingers pointing away.			
9. Grasped the folded edges of the inner package. Used the thumb and index finger of each hand.			
10. Folded back the inner package to expose the gloves. Did not touch or otherwise contaminate the inside of the package or the gloves.			
11. Noted that each glove has a cuff about 2 to 3 inches wide.			
12. Put on the right glove if right-handed. Put on the left glove if left-handed:			
a. Picked up the glove with the other hand. Used the thumb and index and middle fingers.			
b. Touched only the cuff and the inside of the glove.			
c. Turned the hand to be gloved palm side up.			
d. Lifted the cuff up. Slid the fingers and hand into the glove.			
e. Pulled the glove up over the hand. If some fingers got stuck, left them that way until the other glove was on. Did not let the outside of the glove touch any non-sterile surface.			
f. Left the cuff turned down.			
13. Put on the other glove. Used the gloved hand:			
a. Reached under the cuff of the second glove. Used the four fingers of the gloved hand. Kept the gloved thumb close to the gloved palm.			

Procedure—cont'd	S	U	Comments
b. Pulled on the second glove. The gloved hand did not touch the cuff or any surface. Held the thumb of the first gloved hand away from the gloved palm.	______	______	______
14. Adjusted each glove with the other hand. The gloves were smooth and comfortable.	______	______	______
15. Slid the fingers under the cuffs to pull them up.	______	______	______
16. Touched only sterile items.	______	______	______
17. Removed the gloves.	______	______	______
18. Decontaminated hands.	______	______	______

Date of Satisfactory Completion ______________ Instructor's Initials ______________

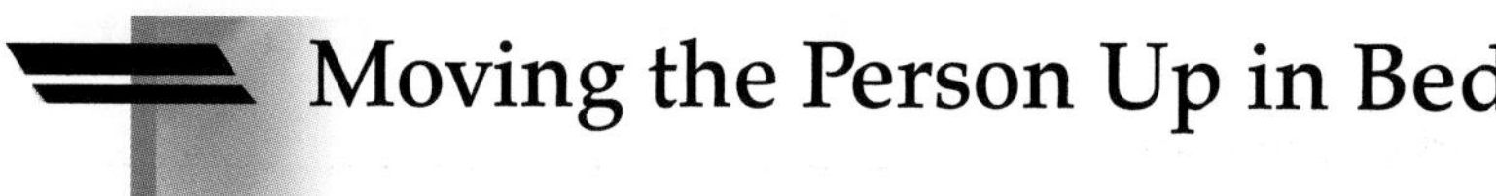

Moving the Person Up in Bed

Name: ______________________

Date: ______________________

Pre-Procedure	S	U	Comments
• Knocked before entering the person's room.			
• Addressed the person by name.			
• Introduced yourself by name and title.			
1. Followed Delegation Guidelines. Reviewed Safety Alert.			
2. Asked a co-worker to assist if needed.			
3. Practiced hand hygiene.			
4. Identified the person. Checked the ID bracelet against the assignment sheet. Called the person by name.			
5. Explained the procedure to the person.			
6. Provided for privacy.			
7. Locked the bed wheels.			
8. Raised the bed for body mechanics. Bed rails were up if used.			

Procedure	S	U	Comments
9. Lowered the head of the bed to a level appropriate for the person. It was as flat as possible.			
10. Stood on one side of the bed. The co-worker stood on the other side.			
11. Lowered the bed rail near you. The co-worker did the same.			
12. Placed the pillow against the headboard if the person could be without it.			
13. Stood with a wide base of support. Pointed the foot near the head of the bed toward the head of the bed. Faced the head of the bed.			
14. Bent the hips and knees. Kept the back straight.			
15. Placed one arm under the person's shoulder and one arm under the thighs. The co-worker did the same. Grasped each other's forearms.			
16. Asked the person to grasp the trapeze if he or she had one.			
17. Had the person flex both knees.			
18. Explained that you would move on the count of "3." The person pushed against the bed with the feet if able.			
19. Moved the person to the head of the bed on the count of "3." Shifted weight from the rear leg to the front leg.			
20. Repeated steps 13 through 19 if necessary.			

Post-Procedure	S	U	Comments
21. Put the pillow under the person's head and shoulders. Straightened linens.	______	______	______
22. Provided for comfort. Positioned the person in good alignment.	______	______	______
23. Placed the signal light within reach.	______	______	______
24. Raised or lowered bed rails. Followed the care plan.	______	______	______
25. Raised the head of the bed to a level appropriate for the person.	______	______	______
26. Lowered the bed to its lowest position.	______	______	______
27. Unscreened the person.	______	______	______
28. Decontaminated hands.	______	______	______
29. Reported and recorded observations.	______	______	______

Date of Satisfactory Completion ______________________ Instructor's Initials ______________________

Moving the Person Up in Bed With a Lift Sheet

Name: ____________________

Date: ____________________

Pre-Procedure	S	U	Comments
• Knocked before entering the person's room.			
• Addressed the person by name.			
• Introduced yourself by name and title.			
1. Followed Delegation Guidelines. Reviewed Safety Alert.			
2. Asked a co-worker to help.			
3. Practiced hand hygiene.			
4. Identified the person. Checked the ID bracelet against the assignment sheet. Called the person by name.			
5. Explained the procedure to the person.			
6. Provided for privacy.			
7. Locked the bed wheels.			
8. Raised the bed for body mechanics. Bed rails were up if used.			

Procedure

	S	U	Comments
9. Lowered the head of the bed to a level appropriate for the person. It was as flat as possible.			
10. Stood on one side of the bed. The co-worker stood on the other side.			
11. Lowered the bed rails if up.			
12. Placed the pillow against the headboard if the person could be without it.			
13. Stood with a broad base of support. Pointed the foot near the head of the bed toward the head of the bed. Faced that direction.			
14. Rolled the sides of the lift sheet up close to the person.			
15. Grasped the rolled up lift sheet firmly near the person's shoulders and buttocks. Supported the head.			
16. Bent the hips and knees.			
17. Moved the person up in bed on the count of "3." Shifted weight from the rear leg to the front leg.			
18. Repeated steps 13 through 17 if necessary.			
19. Unrolled the lift sheet.			

Post-Procedure	S	U	Comments
20. Put the pillow under the person's head and shoulders. Straightened linens.	______	______	______
21. Provided for comfort. Positioned the person in good alignment.	______	______	______
22. Placed the signal light within reach.	______	______	______
23. Raised or lowered bed rails. Followed the care plan.	______	______	______
24. Raised the head of the bed to a level appropriate for the person.	______	______	______
25. Lowered the bed to its lowest position.	______	______	______
26. Unscreened the person.	______	______	______
27. Decontaminated hands.	______	______	______
28. Reported and recorded observations.	______	______	______

Date of Satisfactory Completion ______________________ Instructor's Initials ____________________

Moving the Person to the Side of the Bed

Name: ______________________

Date: ______________________

Pre-Procedure

	S	U	Comments
• Knocked before entering the person's room.	____	____	____________
• Addressed the person by name.	____	____	____________
• Introduced yourself by name and title.	____	____	____________
1. Followed Delegation Guidelines. Reviewed Safety Alert.	____	____	____________
2. Asked a co-worker to help if using a lift sheet.	____	____	____________
3. Practiced hand hygiene.	____	____	____________
4. Identified the person. Checked the ID bracelet against the assignment sheet. Called the person by name.	____	____	____________
5. Explained the procedure to the person.	____	____	____________
6. Provided for privacy.	____	____	____________
7. Locked the bed wheels.	____	____	____________
8. Raised the bed for body mechanics. Bed rails were up if used.	____	____	____________

Procedure

	S	U	Comments
9. Lowered the head of the bed to a level appropriate for the person. It was as flat as possible.	____	____	____________
10. Stood on the side of the bed to which you moved the person.	____	____	____________
11. Lowered the bed rail near you if bed rails were used.	____	____	____________
12. Stood with the feet about 12 inches apart. One foot was in front of the other. Flexed the knees.	____	____	____________
13. Crossed the person's arms over the person's chest.	____	____	____________
14. Method 1: Moving the person in segments:			
a. Placed your arm under the person's neck and shoulders. Grasped the far shoulder.	____	____	____________
b. Placed the other arm under the mid-back.	____	____	____________
c. Moved the upper part of the person's body toward you. Rocked backward and shifted weight to your rear leg.	____	____	____________
d. Placed one arm under the person's waist and one under the thighs.	____	____	____________
e. Rocked backward to move the lower part of the person toward you.	____	____	____________
f. Repeated the procedure for the legs and feet. Your arms were under the person's thighs and calves.	____	____	____________

Procedure—cont'd	S	U	Comments
15. Method 2: Moving the person with a lift sheet:			
a. Rolled the lift sheet up close to the person.	____	____	____
b. Grasped the rolled up lift sheet near the person's shoulders and buttocks. The co-worker did the same. Supported the head.	____	____	____
c. Rocked backward on the count of "3," moving the person toward you. The co-worker rocked backward slightly and then forward toward you while keeping the arms straight.	____	____	____
d. Unrolled the lift sheet. Removed any wrinkles.	____	____	____

Post-Procedure

16. Provided for comfort.	____	____	____
17. Positioned the person in good alignment. Followed the nurse's directions and the care plan.	____	____	____
18. Placed the signal light within reach.	____	____	____
19. Raised or lowered bed rails. Followed the care plan.	____	____	____
20. Lowered the bed to its lowest position.	____	____	____
21. Unscreened the person.	____	____	____
22. Decontaminated hands.	____	____	____
23. Reported and recorded observations.	____	____	____

Date of Satisfactory Completion ______________________ Instructor's Initials ____________________

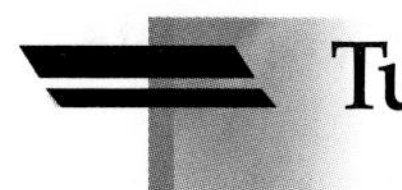

Turning and Positioning a Person

Name: ______________________

Date: ______________________

Pre-Procedure	S	U	Comments
• Knocked before entering the person's room.			
• Addressed the person by name.			
• Introduced yourself by name and title.			
1. Followed Delegation Guidelines. Reviewed Safety Alert.			
2. Practiced hand hygiene.			
3. Identified the person. Checked the ID bracelet against the assignment sheet. Called the person by name.			
4. Explained the procedure to the person.			
5. Provided for privacy.			
6. Locked the bed wheels.			
7. Raised the bed for body mechanics. Bed rails were up if used.			

Procedure	S	U	Comments
8. Lowered the head of the bed to a level appropriate for the person. It was as flat as possible.			
9. Stood on the side of the bed opposite to where you turned the person. The far bed rail was up if used.			
10. Lowered the bed rail near you.			
11. Moved the person to the side near you.			
12. Crossed the person's arms over the person's chest. Crossed the leg near you over the far leg.			
13. Moving the person away from you:			
a. Stood with a wide base of support. Flexed the knees.			
b. Placed one hand on the person's shoulder. Placed the other on the buttock near you.			
c. Pushed the person gently toward the other side of the bed. Shifted weight from the rear leg to the front leg.			
14. Moving the person toward you:			
a. Raised the bed rail.			
b. Went to the other side. Lowered the bed rail if used.			
c. Stood with a wide base of support. Flexed the knees.			
d. Placed one hand on the person's far shoulder. Placed the other on the far hip.			
e. Rolled the person toward you gently.			

Procedure—cont'd	S	U	Comments
15. Positioned the person. Followed the nurse's directions and the care plan. The following is common:	______	______	______
a. Placed a pillow under the head and neck.	______	______	______
b. Adjusted the shoulder. The person should not lie on an arm.	______	______	______
c. Placed a small pillow under the upper hand and arm.	______	______	______
d. Positioned a pillow against the back.	______	______	______
e. Flexed the upper knee. Positioned the upper leg in front of the lower leg.	______	______	______
f. Supported the upper leg and thigh on pillows.	______	______	______

Post-Procedure

	S	U	Comments
16. Provided for comfort.	______	______	______
17. Placed the signal light within reach.	______	______	______
18. Raised or lowered bed rails. Followed the care plan.	______	______	______
19. Lowered the bed to its lowest position.	______	______	______
20. Unscreened the person.	______	______	______
21. Decontaminated hands.	______	______	______
22. Reported and recorded observations.	______	______	______

Date of Satisfactory Completion ______________ Instructor's Initials ______________

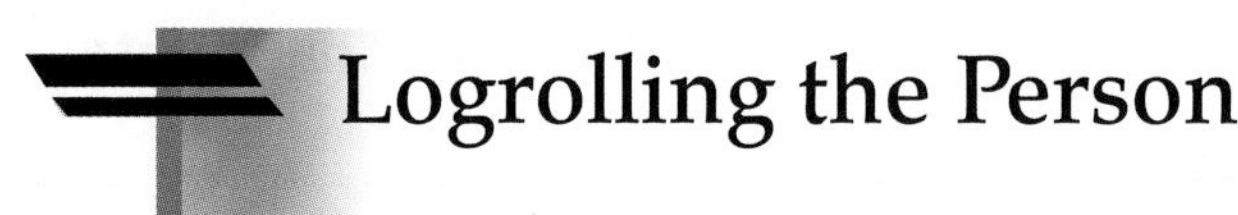

Logrolling the Person

Name: ______________________

Date: ______________________

Pre-Procedure	S	U	Comments
• Knocked before entering the person's room.	___	___	___
• Addressed the person by name.	___	___	___
• Introduced yourself by name and title.	___	___	___
1. Followed Delegation Guidelines. Reviewed Safety Alert.	___	___	___
2. Asked a co-worker to help.	___	___	___
3. Practiced hand hygiene.	___	___	___
4. Identified the person. Checked the ID bracelet against the assignment sheet. Called the person by name.	___	___	___
5. Explained the procedure to the person.	___	___	___
6. Provided for privacy.	___	___	___
7. Locked the bed wheels.	___	___	___
8. Raised the bed for body mechanics. Bed rails were up if used.	___	___	___

Procedure

	S	U	Comments
9. Made sure the bed was flat.	___	___	___
10. Stood on the side opposite to which you turned the person. The co-worker stood on the other side.	___	___	___
11. Lowered the bed rails if used.	___	___	___
12. Moved the person as a unit to the side of the bed near you. Used the turn sheet.	___	___	___
13. Placed the person's arms across the chest. Placed a pillow between the knees.	___	___	___
14. Raised the bed rail if used.	___	___	___
15. Went to the other side.	___	___	___
16. Stood near the shoulders and chest. The co-worker stood near the buttocks and thighs.	___	___	___
17. Stood with a broad base of support. One foot was in front of the other.	___	___	___
18. Asked the person to hold his or her body rigid.	___	___	___
19. Rolled the person toward you or used a turn sheet. Turned the person as a unit.	___	___	___

Post-Procedure	S	U	Comments
20. Provided for comfort. Positioned the person in good alignment. Used pillows as directed by the nurse and care plan:			
a. One pillow against the back for support.			
b. One pillow under the head and neck if allowed.			
c. One pillow or folded bath blanket between the legs.			
d. A small pillow under the arm and hand.			
21. Placed the signal light within reach.			
22. Raised or lowered bed rails. Followed the care plan.			
23. Lowered the bed to its lowest position.			
24. Unscreened the person.			
25. Decontaminated hands.			
26. Reported and recorded observations.			

Date of Satisfactory Completion ________________ Instructor's Initials ________________

Helping the Person Sit on the Side of the Bed (Dangle)

Name: ______________________

Date: ______________________

Pre-Procedure	S	U	Comments
• Knocked before entering the person's room.			
• Addressed the person by name.			
• Introduced yourself by name and title.			
1. Followed Delegation Guidelines. Reviewed Safety Alert.			
2. Explained the procedure to the person.			
3. Practiced hand hygiene.			
4. Identified the person. Checked the ID bracelet against the assignment sheet. Called the person by name.			
5. Decided what side of the bed to use.			
6. Moved furniture to provide moving space.			
7. Provided for privacy.			
8. Positioned the person in the side-lying position facing you. The person laid on the strong side.			
9. Locked the bed wheels.			
10. Raised the bed for body mechanics. Bed rails were up if used.			

Procedure

	S	U	Comments
11. Raised the head of the bed to a sitting position.			
12. Lowered the bed rail if up.			
13. Stood by the person's hips. Faced the foot of the bed.			
14. Stood with the feet apart. The foot near the head of the bed was in front of the other foot.			
15. Slid one arm under the person's neck and shoulders. Grasped the far shoulder. Placed the other hand over the thighs near the knees.			
16. Pivoted toward the foot of the bed while moving the person's legs and feet over the side of the bed. As the legs went over the edge of the mattress, the trunk was upright.			
17. Asked the person to hold onto the edge of the mattress. This supported the person in the sitting position.			
18. Did not leave the person alone. Provided support if necessary.			
19. Checked the person's condition:			
a. Asked how the person felt. Asked if the person felt dizzy or lightheaded.			
b. Checked pulse and respirations.			
c. Checked for difficulty breathing.			
d. Noted if the skin is pale or bluish in color.			

Procedure—cont'd	S	U	Comments
20. Helped the person lie down if necessary.			
21. Reversed the procedure to return the person to bed.			
22. Lowered the head of the bed after the person returned to bed. Helped him or her move to the center of the bed.			

Post-Procedure	S	U	Comments
23. Provided for comfort. Positioned the person in good alignment.			
24. Placed the signal light within reach.			
25. Lowered the bed to its lowest position.			
26. Raised or lowered bed rails. Followed the care plan.			
27. Returned furniture to its proper place.			
28. Unscreened the person.			
29. Decontaminated hands.			
30. Reported and recorded observations.			

Date of Satisfactory Completion ______________________ Instructor's Initials ______________________

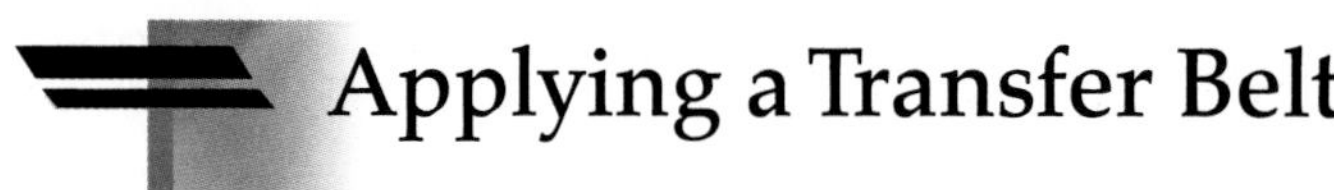

Applying a Transfer Belt

Name: ______________________

Date: ______________________

Pre-Procedure	S	U	Comments
• Knocked before entering the person's room.			
• Addressed the person by name.			
• Introduced yourself by name and title.			

Procedure	S	U	Comments
1. Reviewed Safety Alert.			
2. Practiced hand hygiene.			
3. Identified the person. Checked the ID bracelet against the assignment sheet. Called the person by name.			
4. Explained the procedure to the person.			
5. Provided for privacy.			
6. Assisted the person to a sitting position.			
7. Applied the belt around the person's waist over clothing. Did not apply it over bare skin.			
8. Tightened the belt so it was snug. It did not cause discomfort or impair breathing. You were able to slide 4 fingers under the belt.			
9. Made sure that a woman's breasts were not caught under the belt.			
10. Placed the buckle off center in the front or in the back for the person's comfort. The buckle was not over the spine.			

Date of Satisfactory Completion ______________ Instructor's Initials ______________

Transferring the Person to a Chair or Wheelchair

Name: ______________________

Date: ______________________

Pre-Procedure	**S**	**U**	**Comments**
• Knocked before entering the person's room.	____	____	____________
• Addressed the person by name.	____	____	____________
• Introduced yourself by name and title.	____	____	____________
1. Followed Delegation Guidelines. Reviewed Safety Alerts.	____	____	____________
2. Explained the procedure to the person.	____	____	____________
3. Collected the following:			
• Wheelchair or arm chair	____	____	____________
• Bath blanket	____	____	____________
• Lap blanket	____	____	____________
• Robe and nonskid footwear	____	____	____________
• Paper or sheet	____	____	____________
• Transfer belt if needed	____	____	____________
• Seat cushion if needed	____	____	____________
4. Practiced hand hygiene.	____	____	____________
5. Identified the person. Checked the ID bracelet against the assignment sheet. Called the person by name.	____	____	____________
6. Provided for privacy.	____	____	____________
7. Decided which side of the bed to use. Moved furniture for moving space.	____	____	____________

Procedure			
8. Placed the chair at the head of the bed. The chair was even with the headboard.	____	____	____________
9. Placed a folded bath blanket or cushion on the seat (if needed).	____	____	____________
10. Locked wheelchair wheels. Raised the footplates. Removed or swung the front rigging out of the way.	____	____	____________
11. Lowered the bed to its lowest position. Locked the bed wheels.	____	____	____________
12. Fanfolded top linens to the foot of the bed.	____	____	____________
13. Placed the paper or sheet under the person's feet. Put footwear on the person.	____	____	____________
14. Helped the person sit on the side of the bed. His or her feet touched the floor.	____	____	____________
15. Helped the person put on a robe.	____	____	____________
16. Applied the transfer belt if needed.	____	____	____________

Procedure—cont'd	S	U	Comments
17. Method 1: Using a transfer belt:			
a. Stood in front of the person.			
b. Had the person hold onto the mattress.			
c. Made sure the person's feet were flat on the floor.			
d. Had the person lean forward.			
e. Grasped the transfer belt at each side. Grasped the belt from underneath.			
f. Braced your knees against the person's knees. Blocked the person's feet with your feet or used the knee and foot of one leg to block the person's weak foot. Placed the other foot slightly behind you for balance.			
g. Asked the person to push down on the mattress and to stand on the count of "3." Pulled the person into a standing position as you straightened your knees.			
18. Method 2: No transfer belt:			
a. Followed steps 17a through 17c.			
b. Placed your hands under the person's arms. The hands were around the person's shoulder blades.			
c. Had the person lean forward.			
d. Braced your knees against the person's knees. Blocked the person's feet with your feet or used the knee and foot of one leg to block the person's weak foot. Placed the other foot slightly behind you for balance.			
e. Asked the person to push down on the mattress and to stand on the count of "3." Pulled the person up into a standing position as you straightened the knees.			
19. Supported the person in the standing position. Held the transfer belt or kept the hands around the person's shoulder blades. Continued to block the person's feet and knees with your feet and knees.			
20. Turned the person so he or she could grasp the far arm of the chair. The legs touched the edge of the chair.			
21. Continued to turn the person until the other armrest was grasped.			
22. Lowered the person into the chair as you bent your hips and knees. The person assisted by leaning forward and bending the elbows and knees.			
23. Made sure the buttocks were to the back of the seat. Positioned the person in good alignment.			
24. Attached the wheelchair front rigging. Positioned the person's feet on the wheelchair footplates.			
25. Covered the person's lap and legs with a lap blanket. Kept the blanket off the floor and the wheels.			
26. Removed the transfer belt if used.			
27. Positioned the chair as the person preferred. Locked the wheelchair wheels.			

Post-Procedure	S	U	Comments
28. Placed the signal light and other needed items within reach.	______	______	____________________
29. Unscreened the person.	______	______	____________________
30. Decontaminated hands.	______	______	____________________
31. Reported and recorded observations.	______	______	____________________

Date of Satisfactory Completion ____________________ Instructor's Initials ____________________

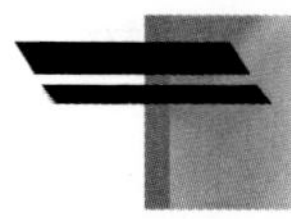

Transferring the Person from the Chair or Wheelchair to Bed

Name: ______________________

Date: ______________________

Pre-Procedure	S	U	Comments
• Knocked before entering the person's room.			
• Addressed the person by name.			
• Introduced yourself by name and title.			
1. Followed Delegation Guidelines. Reviewed Safety Alerts.			
2. Explained the procedure to the person.			
3. Collected paper or sheet and a transfer belt if needed.			
4. Practiced hand hygiene.			
5. Identified the person. Checked the ID bracelet against the assignment sheet. Called the person by name.			
6. Provided for privacy.			

Procedure	S	U	Comments
7. Moved furniture for moving space.			
8. Raised the head of the bed to a sitting position. The bed was in the lowest position.			
9. Moved the signal light so it was on the strong side when the person was in bed.			
10. Positioned the chair or wheelchair so the person's strong side was next to the bed. Had a co-worker help if necessary.			
11. Locked the wheelchair and bed wheels.			
12. Removed and folded the lap blanket.			
13. Removed the person's feet from the footplates. Raised the footplates. Removed or swung the front rigging out of the way.			
14. Applied the transfer belt if needed.			
15. Made sure the person's feet were flat on the floor.			
16. Stood in front of the person.			
17. Asked the person to hold onto the armrests or placed your arms under the person's arms. The hands were around the shoulder blades.			
18. Had the person lean forward.			
19. Grasped the transfer belt on each side if using it. Grasped underneath the belt.			
20. Braced your knees against the person's knees. Blocked the person's feet with your feet or used the knee and foot of one leg to block the person's weak foot. Placed the other foot slightly behind for balance.			

Procedure—cont'd

	S	U	Comments
21. Asked the person to push down on the armrests on the count of "3." Pulled the person into a standing position as you straightened your knees.			
22. Supported the person in the standing position. Held the transfer belt or kept your hands around the person's shoulder blades. Continued to block the person's knees and feet with your knees and feet.			
23. Turned the person so he or she could reach the edge of the mattress. The legs touched the mattress.			
24. Continued to turn the person until he or she could reach the mattress with both hands.			
25. Lowered the person onto the bed as you bent your hips and knees. The person assisted by leaning forward and bending the elbows and knees.			
26. Removed the transfer belt.			
27. Removed the robe and footwear.			
28. Helped the person lie down.			

Post-Procedure

	S	U	Comments
29. Provided for comfort. Covered the person as needed.			
30. Placed the signal light and other needed items within reach.			
31. Arranged furniture to meet the person's needs.			
32. Unscreened the person.			
33. Decontaminated hands.			
34. Reported and recorded observations.			

Date of Satisfactory Completion ______________ Instructor's Initials ______________

Transferring the Person to a Wheelchair With Assistance

Name: ____________________

Date: ____________________

Pre-Procedure

	S	U	Comments
• Knocked before entering the person's room.	___	___	___
• Addressed the person by name.	___	___	___
• Introduced yourself by name and title.	___	___	___
1. Followed Delegation Guidelines. Reviewed Safety Alerts.	___	___	___
2. Asked a co-worker to help.	___	___	___
3. Explained the procedure to the person.	___	___	___
4. Collected the following:			
• Wheelchair with removable arm rests	___	___	___
• Bath blanket	___	___	___
• Lap blanket	___	___	___
• Nonskid footwear	___	___	___
• Cushion if used	___	___	___
5. Decontaminated your hands.	___	___	___
6. Identified the person. Checked the ID bracelet against the assignment sheet. Called the person by name.	___	___	___
7. Provided for privacy.	___	___	___
8. Decided which side of the bed to use. Moved furniture for moving space.	___	___	___

Procedure

	S	U	Comments
9. Fanfolded top linens to the foot of the bed.	___	___	___
10. Assisted the person to the side of the bed near you. Raised the head of the bed to help the person to a sitting position.	___	___	___
11. Placed the wheelchair at the side of the bed even with the person's hips.	___	___	___
12. Removed the front rigging.	___	___	___
13. Removed the armrest near the bed.	___	___	___
14. Put the cushion or a folded bath blanket on the seat.	___	___	___
15. Locked wheelchair and bed wheels.	___	___	___
16. Stood behind the wheelchair. Put your arms under the person's arms and grasped the person's forearms.	___	___	___
17. Had the co-worker grasp the person's thighs and calves.	___	___	___
18. Brought the person toward the chair on the count of "3." Lowered the person into the chair.	___	___	___
19. Made sure the person's buttocks were to the back of the seat. Positioned the person in good alignment.	___	___	___
20. Put the armrest and front rigging on the wheelchair.	___	___	___

Procedure—cont'd	S	U	Comments
21. Put footwear on the person. Positioned the person's feet on the footplates.	______	______	______________
22. Covered the person's lap and legs with a lap blanket. Kept the blanket off the floor and wheels.	______	______	______________
23. Positioned the chair as the person preferred. Locked the wheelchair wheels.	______	______	______________
Post-Procedure			
24. Placed the signal light and other needed items within reach.	______	______	______________
25. Unscreened the person.	______	______	______________
26. Decontaminated hands.	______	______	______________
27. Reported and recorded observations.	______	______	______________

Date of Satisfactory Completion ______________________ Instructor's Initials ______________________

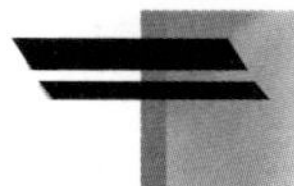

Transferring the Person Using a Mechanical Lift

Name: ______________________

Date: ______________________

Pre-Procedure	**S**	**U**	**Comments**
• Knocked before entering the person's room.			
• Addressed the person by name.			
• Introduced yourself by name and title.			
1. Followed Delegation Guidelines. Reviewed Safety Alert.			
2. Asked a co-worker to help.			
3. Explained the procedure to the person.			
4. Collected the following:			
• Mechanical lift			
• Arm chair or wheelchair			
• Footwear			
• Bath blanket or cushion			
• Lap blanket			
5. Practiced hand hygiene.			
6. Identified the person. Checked the ID bracelet against the assignment sheet. Called the person by name.			
7. Provided for privacy.			

Procedure

	S	U	Comments
8. Centered the sling under the person. Positioned the sling according to the manufacturer's instructions.			
9. Placed the chair at the head of the bed. It was even with the headboard and about 1 foot away from the bed. Placed a folded bath blanket or cushion in the chair.			
10. Locked the bed wheels. Lowered the bed to its lowest position.			
11. Raised the lift so it could be positioned over the person.			
12. Positioned the lift over the person.			
13. Locked the lift wheels in position.			
14. Attached the sling to the swivel bar			
15. Raised the head of the bed to a sitting position.			
16. Crossed the person's arms over the chest. The person held onto the straps or chains but not the swivel bar.			
17. Raised the lift high enough until the person and sling were free of the bed.			
18. Had the co-worker support the person's legs as you moved the lift and person away from the bed.			

Procedure—cont'd

	S	U	Comments
19. Positioned the lift so that the person's back was toward the chair.			
20. Positioned the chair so the person could be lowered into it.			
21. Lowered and guided the person into the chair.			
22. Lowered the swivel bar to unhook the sling. Left the sling under the person unless otherwise indicated.			
23. Put footwear on the person. Positioned the person's feet on wheelchair footplates.			
24. Covered the person's lap and legs with a lap blanket. Kept it off the floor and wheels.			
25. Positioned the chair as the person preferred. Locked the wheelchair wheels.			

Post-Procedure

	S	U	Comments
26. Placed the signal light and other needed items within reach.			
27. Unscreened the person.			
28. Decontaminated hands.			
29. Reported and recorded observations.			

Date of Satisfactory Completion ______________________ Instructor's Initials ____________________

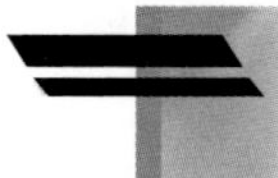

Transferring the Person To and From the Toilet

Name: ______________________

Date: ______________________

Pre-Procedure	S	U	Comments
• Knocked before entering the person's room.	____	____	______________
• Addressed the person by name.	____	____	______________
• Introduced yourself by name and title.	____	____	______________
1. Followed Delegation Guidelines. Reviewed Safety Alert.	____	____	______________
2. Practiced hand hygiene.	____	____	______________
3. Made sure the person had an elevated toilet seat. The toilet seat and wheelchair were at the same level.	____	____	______________
4. Checked the grab bars by the toilet. If they were loose, told the nurse. Did not transfer the person to the toilet if the grab bars were not secure.	____	____	______________

Procedure

Procedure	S	U	Comments
5. Had the person wear nonskid footwear.	____	____	______________
6. Positioned the wheelchair next to the toilet if there was enough room. If not, positioned the wheelchair at a right angle to the toilet.	____	____	______________
7. Locked the wheelchair wheels.	____	____	______________
8. Raised the footplates. Removed or swung front rigging out of the way.	____	____	______________
9. Applied the transfer belt.	____	____	______________
10. Helped the person unfasten clothing.	____	____	______________
11. Used the transfer belt to help the person stand and to turn to the toilet. The person used the grab bars to turn to the toilet.	____	____	______________
12. Supported the person with the transfer belt while he or she lowered clothing, or had the person hold onto the grab bars for support. Lowered the person's pants and undergarments.	____	____	______________
13. Used the transfer belt to lower the person onto the toilet seat.	____	____	______________
14. Removed the transfer belt.	____	____	______________
15. Told the person you would stay nearby. Reminded the person to use the signal light or call for help when needed.	____	____	______________
16. Closed the bathroom door to provide for privacy.	____	____	______________
17. Stayed near the bathroom. Completed other tasks in the person's room.	____	____	______________
18. Knocked on the bathroom door when the person called.	____	____	______________

Procedure—cont'd	S	U	Comments
19. Helped with wiping, perineal care, flushing, and hand-washing as needed.	______	______	______
20. Applied the transfer belt.	______	______	______
21. Used the transfer belt to help the person stand.	______	______	______
22. Helped the person raise and secure clothing.	______	______	______
23. Used the transfer belt to transfer the person to the wheelchair.	______	______	______
24. Made sure the person's buttocks were to the back of the seat. Positioned the person in good alignment.	______	______	______
25. Positioned the person's feet on the footplates.	______	______	______
26. Covered the person's lap and legs with a lap blanket. Kept the blanket off the floor and wheels.	______	______	______
27. Positioned the chair as the person preferred. Locked the wheelchair wheels.	______	______	______
Post-Procedure			
28. Placed the signal light and other needed items within reach.	______	______	______
29. Unscreened the person.	______	______	______
30. Practiced hand hygiene.	______	______	______
31. Reported and recorded observations.	______	______	______

Date of Satisfactory Completion ____________________ Instructor's Initials ____________________

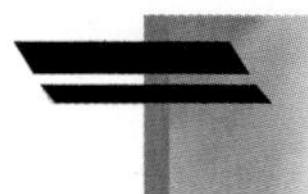

Transferring the Person to a Stretcher

Name: ____________________

Date: ____________________

Pre-Procedure	**S**	**U**	**Comments**
• Knocked before entering the person's room.	____	____	____________
• Addressed the person by name.	____	____	____________
• Introduced yourself by name and title.	____	____	____________
1. Followed Delegation Guidelines. Reviewed Safety Alert.	____	____	____________
2. Asked 2 co-workers to help.	____	____	____________
3. Explained the procedure to the person.	____	____	____________
4. Collected the following:			
• Stretcher covered with a sheet or bath blanket	____	____	____________
• Bath blanket	____	____	____________
• Pillow(s) if needed	____	____	____________
5. Practiced hand hygiene.	____	____	____________
6. Identified the person. Checked the ID bracelet against the assignment sheet. Called the person by name.	____	____	____________
7. Provided for privacy.	____	____	____________
8. Raised the bed to its highest level.	____	____	____________
Procedure			
9. Positioned yourself and co-workers. Two workers stood on the side of the bed where the stretcher would be. The third worker stood on the other side of the bed.	____	____	____________
10. Covered the person with a bath blanket. Fanfolded top linens to the foot of the bed.	____	____	____________
11. Loosened the cotton drawsheet on each side.	____	____	____________
12. Lowered the head of the bed. It was as flat as possible.	____	____	____________
13. Lowered the bed rails if used.	____	____	____________
14. Moved the person to the side of the bed.	____	____	____________
15. Protected the person from falling. Held the far arm and leg.	____	____	____________
16. Had the co-workers position the stretcher next to the bed. They stood behind the stretcher.	____	____	____________
17. Locked the bed and stretcher wheels.	____	____	____________
18. Rolled up and grasped the drawsheet. The entire length of the person's body was supported.	____	____	____________
19. Transferred the person to the stretcher on the count of "3" by lifting and pulling the person. The person was centered on the stretcher.	____	____	____________
20. Placed a pillow or pillows under the person's head and shoulders if allowed. Raised the head of the stretcher if allowed.	____	____	____________

Procedure—cont'd	S	U	Comments
21. Covered the person. Provided for comfort.	______	______	______________________
22. Fastened safety straps. Raised the side rails.	______	______	______________________
23. Unlocked the stretcher's wheels. Transported the person.	______	______	______________________

Post-Procedure

	S	U	Comments
24. Decontaminated hands.	______	______	______________________
25. Reported and recorded:			
• The time of the transport	______	______	______________________
• Where the person was transported to	______	______	______________________
• Who went with him or her	______	______	______________________
• How the transfer was tolerated	______	______	______________________

Date of Satisfactory Completion ______________________ Instructor's Initials ______________________

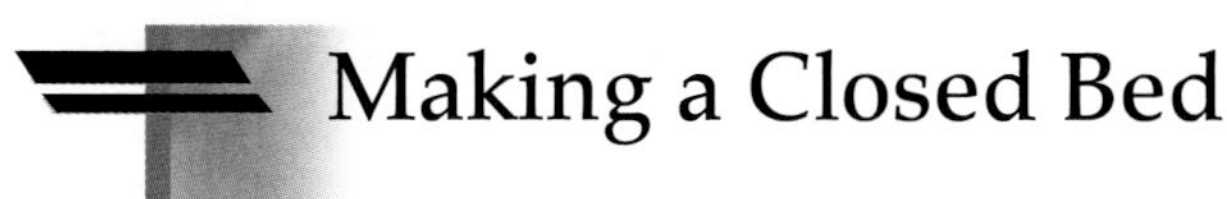

Making a Closed Bed

Name: ______________________

Date: ______________________

Pre-Procedure	S	U	Comments
• Knocked before entering the person's room.			
• Addressed the person by name.			
• Introduced yourself by name and title.			
1. Followed Delegation Guidelines. Reviewed Safety Alert.			
2. Practiced hand hygiene.			
3. Collected clean linen:			
• Mattress pad (if needed)			
• Bottom sheet (flat sheet or fitted sheet)			
• Plastic drawsheet or waterproof pad (if needed)			
• Cotton drawsheet (if needed)			
• Top sheet			
• Blanket			
• Bedspread			
• Two pillowcases			
• Bath towel(s)			
• Hand towel			
• Washcloth			
• Gown			
• Bath blanket			
• Gloves			
• Laundry bag			
4. Placed linen on a clean surface.			
5. Raised the bed for body mechanics.			

Procedure

	S	U	Comments
6. Put on the gloves.			
7. Removed linen. Rolled each piece away from you. Placed each piece in a laundry bag. Discarded disposable bed protectors in the trash.			
8. Cleaned the bed frame and mattress if this is part of your job.			
9. Removed and discarded the gloves. Decontaminated hands.			
10. Moved the mattress to the head of the bed.			
11. Put the mattress pad on the mattress. It was even with the top of the mattress.			

Procedure—cont'd	S	U	Comments
12. Placed the bottom sheet on the mattress pad:			
a. Unfolded it lengthwise.			
b. Placed the center crease in the middle of the bed.			
c. Positioned the lower edge even with the bottom of the mattress.			
d. Placed the large hem at the top and the small hem at the bottom.			
e. Faced hem-stitching downward, away from the person.			
13. Opened the sheet. Fanfolded it to the other side of the bed.			
14. Tucked the top of the sheet under the mattress. The sheet was tight and smooth.			
15. Made a mitered corner if using a flat sheet.			
16. Placed the plastic drawsheet on the bed.			
17. Opened the plastic drawsheet. Fanfolded it to the other side of the bed.			
18. Placed a cotton drawsheet over the plastic drawsheet. It covered the entire plastic drawsheet.			
19. Opened the cotton drawsheet. Fanfolded it to the other side of the bed.			
20. Tucked both drawsheets under the mattress or tucked each in separately.			
21. Went to the other side of the bed.			
22. Mitered the top corner of the flat bottom sheet.			
23. Pulled the bottom sheet tight so there were no wrinkles. Tucked in the sheet.			
24. Pulled the drawsheets tight so there were no wrinkles. Tucked both in together or separately.			
25. Went to the other side of the bed.			
26. Put the top sheet on the bed:			
a. Unfolded it lengthwise.			
b. Placed the center crease in the middle.			
c. Placed the large hem even with the top of the mattress.			
d. Opened the sheet. Fanfolded it to the other side.			
e. Faced hem-stitching outward away from the person.			
f. Did not tuck the bottom in yet.			
g. Did not tuck top linens in on the sides.			
27. Placed the blanket on the bed:			
a. Unfolded it so the center crease was in the middle.			
b. Put the upper hem about 6 to 8 inches from the top of the mattress. (Done if steps 33 and 34 *are not* done.)			
c. Opened the blanket. Fanfolded it to the other side.			
d. Turned the top sheet down over the blanket. Hem stitching was down, away from the person.			

Procedure—cont'd

	S	U	Comments
28. Placed the bedspread on the bed:			
a. Unfolded it so the center crease was in the middle.			
b. Placed the upper hem even with the top of the mattress.			
c. Opened and fanfolded the spread to the other side.			
d. Made sure the spread facing the door was even. It covered all top linens.			
29. Tucked in top linens together at the foot of the bed. They were smooth and tight. Made a mitered corner.			
30. Went to the other side.			
31. Straightened all top linen. Worked from the head of the bed to the foot.			
32. Tucked in the top linens together. Made a mitered corner.			
33. Turned the top hem of the spread under the blanket to make a cuff.			
34. Turned the top sheet down over the spread. Hem stitching was down.			
35. Put the pillowcase on the pillow. Folded extra material under the pillow at the seam end of the pillowcase.			
36. Placed the pillow on the bed. The open end was away from the door. The seam of the pillowcase was toward the head of the bed.			

Post-Procedure

	S	U	Comments
37. Attached the signal light to the bed.			
38. Lowered the bed to its lowest position. Locked the bed wheels.			
39. Put towels, washcloth, gown, and bath blanket in the bedside stand.			
40. Followed agency policy for dirty linen.			
41. Decontaminated hands.			

Date of Satisfactory Completion ____________________ Instructor's Initials ____________________

Making an Open Bed

Name: ______________________

Date: ______________________

Pre-Procedure	S	U	Comments
• Knocked before entering the person's room.	_____	_____	__________
• Addressed the person by name.	_____	_____	__________
• Introduced yourself by name and title.	_____	_____	__________

Procedure	S	U	Comments
1. Followed Delegation Guidelines. Reviewed Safety Alert.	_____	_____	__________
2. Practiced hand hygiene.	_____	_____	__________
3. Collected linen for a closed bed.	_____	_____	__________
4. Made a closed bed.	_____	_____	__________
5. Fanfolded top linens to the foot of the bed.	_____	_____	__________
6. Attached the signal light to the bed.	_____	_____	__________
7. Lowered the bed to its lowest position.	_____	_____	__________
8. Put towels, washcloth, gown, and bath blanket in the bedside stand.	_____	_____	__________
9. Followed agency policy for dirty linen.	_____	_____	__________
10. Decontaminated hands.	_____	_____	__________

Date of Satisfactory Completion ______________________ Instructor's Initials ______________________

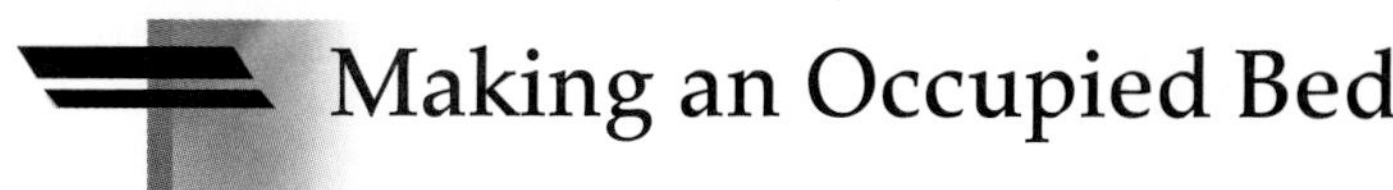

Making an Occupied Bed

Name: ______________________

Date: ______________________

Pre-Procedure	S	U	Comments
• Knocked before entering the person's room.	____	____	____________
• Addressed the person by name.	____	____	____________
• Introduced yourself by name and title.	____	____	____________
1. Followed Delegation Guidelines. Reviewed Safety Alerts.	____	____	____________
2. Explained the procedure to the person.	____	____	____________
3. Practiced hand hygiene.	____	____	____________
4. Collected the following:			
a. Gloves	____	____	____________
b. Laundry bag	____	____	____________
c. Clean linen	____	____	____________
5. Placed linen on a clean surface.	____	____	____________
6. Identified the person. Checked the ID bracelet against the assignment sheet. Called the person by name.	____	____	____________
7. Provided for privacy.	____	____	____________
8. Removed the signal light.	____	____	____________
9. Raised the bed for body mechanics. Bed rails were up if used.	____	____	____________
10. Lowered the head of the bed. It was as flat as possible.	____	____	____________

Procedure

11. Lowered the bed rail near you.	____	____	____________
12. Put on gloves.	____	____	____________
13. Loosened top linens at the foot of the bed.	____	____	____________
14. Removed the bedspread. Then removed the blanket. Placed each over the chair.	____	____	____________
15. Covered the person with a bath blanket:	____	____	____________
a. Unfolded a bath blanket over the top sheet.	____	____	____________
b. Asked the person to hold onto the bath blanket. If the person could not, tucked the top part under the person's shoulders.	____	____	____________
c. Grasped the top sheet under the bath blanket at the shoulders. Brought the sheet down to the foot of the bed. Removed the sheet from under the blanket.	____	____	____________
16. Moved the mattress to the head of the bed.	____	____	____________
17. Positioned the person on the side of the bed away from you. Adjusted the pillow for comfort.	____	____	____________

Procedure—cont'd	S	U	Comments
18. Loosened bottom linens from the head to the foot of the bed.			
19. Fanfolded bottom linens one at a time toward the person. Started with the cotton drawsheet.			
20. Placed a clean mattress pad on the bed. Unfolded it lengthwise. The center crease was in the middle. Fanfolded the top part toward the person.			
21. Placed the bottom sheet on the mattress pad. Hemstitching was away from the person. Unfolded the sheet so the crease was in the middle. The small hem was even with the bottom of the mattress. Fanfolded the top part toward the person.			
22. Made a mitered corner at the head of the bed. Tucked the sheet under the mattress from the head to the foot.			
23. Pulled the plastic drawsheet toward you over the bottom sheet. Tucked excess material under the mattress. Did the following for a clean plastic drawsheet.			
a. Placed the plastic drawsheet on the bed. It was about 14 inches from the mattress top.			
b. Fanfolded the top part toward the person.			
c. Tucked in the excess fabric			
24. Placed the cotton drawsheet over the plastic drawsheet. Fanfolded the top part toward the person. Tucked in excess fabric.			
25. Raised the bed rail if used. Went to the other side and lowered the bed rail.			
26. Explained to the person that he or she would roll over a bump. Assured the person that he or she would not fall.			
27. Helped the person turn to the other side. Adjusted the pillow for comfort.			
28. Loosened bottom linens. Removed one piece at a time. Placed each piece in the laundry bag. Discarded disposable bed protectors in the trash.			
29. Removed and discarded the gloves. Decontaminated your hands.			
30. Straightened and smoothed the mattress pad.			
31. Pulled the clean bottom sheet toward you. Made a mitered corner at the top. Tucked the sheet under the mattress from the head to the foot of the bed.			
32. Pulled the drawsheets tightly toward you. Tucked both under together or separately.			
33. Positioned the person supine in the center of the bed. Adjusted the pillow for comfort.			
34. Put the top sheet on the bed. Unfolded it lengthwise. The crease was in the middle. The large hem was even with the top of the mattress. Hem stitching was on the outside.			
35. Asked the person to hold onto the top sheet or tuck the top sheet under the person's shoulders. Removed the bath blanket.			

Procedure—cont'd	S	U	Comments
36. Placed the blanket on the bed. Unfolded it so the crease was in the middle and it covered the person. The upper hem was 6 to 8 inches from the top of the mattress.			
37. Placed the bedspread on the bed. Unfolded it so the center crease was in the middle and it covered the person. The top hem was even with the mattress top.			
38. Turned the top hem of the spread under the blanket to make a cuff.			
39. Brought the top sheet down over the spread to form a cuff.			
40. Went to the foot of the bed.			
41. Made a toe pleat about 6 to 8 inches from the foot of the bed.			
42. Lifted the mattress corner with one arm. Tucked all top linens under the mattress together. Made a mitered corner.			
43. Raised the bed rail if used. Went to the other side and lowered the bed rail if used.			
44. Straightened and smoothed top linens.			
45. Tucked the top linens under the mattress. Made a mitered corner.			
46. Changed the pillowcase(s).			

Post-Procedure

	S	U	Comments
47. Placed the signal light within reach.			
48. Raised or lowered bed rails. Followed the care plan.			
49. Raised the head of the bed to a level appropriate for the person. Provided for comfort.			
50. Lowered the bed to its lowest position. Locked the bed wheels.			
51. Put towels, washcloth, gown, and bath blanket in the bed-side stand.			
52. Unscreened the person. Thanked him or her for cooperating.			
53. Followed agency policy for dirty linen.			
54. Decontaminated hands.			

Date of Satisfactory Completion ____________ Instructor's Initials ____________

Making a Surgical Bed

Name: ____________________

Date: ____________________

Procedure	S	U	Comments
1. Followed Delegation Guidelines. Reviewed Safety Alerts.	___	___	___
2. Practiced hand hygiene.	___	___	___
3. Collected the following:			
• Clean linen	___	___	___
• Gloves	___	___	___
• Laundry bag	___	___	___
• Equipment requested by the nurse	___	___	___
4. Placed linen on a clean surface.	___	___	___
5. Removed the signal light.	___	___	___
6. Raised the bed for body mechanics.	___	___	___
7. Removed all linen from the bed. Wore gloves.	___	___	___
8. Made a closed bed. Did not tuck the top linens under the mattress.	___	___	___
9. Folded all top linens at the foot of the bed back onto the bed. The fold was even with the edge of the mattress.	___	___	___
10. Fanfolded linen lengthwise to the side of the bed farthest from the door.	___	___	___
11. Put the pillowcase(s) on the pillow(s).	___	___	___
12. Placed the pillow(s) on a clean surface.	___	___	___
13. Left the bed in its highest position.	___	___	___
14. Left both bed rails down.	___	___	___
15. Put the towels, washcloth, gown, and bath blanket in the bedside stand.	___	___	___
16. Moved furniture away from the bed. Allowed room for the stretcher and for the staff.	___	___	___
17. Did not attach the signal light to the bed.	___	___	___
18. Followed agency policy for soiled linen.	___	___	___
19. Decontaminated hands.	___	___	___

Date of Satisfactory Completion ____________________ Instructor's Initials ____________________

Assisting the Person to Brush the Teeth

Name: ____________________

Date: ____________________

Pre-Procedure

	S	U	Comments
• Knocked before entering the person's room.			
• Addressed the person by name.			
• Introduced yourself by name and title.			
1. Followed Delegation Guidelines. Reviewed Safety Alert.			
2. Explained the procedure to the person.			
3. Practiced hand hygiene.			
4. Collected the following:			
• Toothbrush			
• Toothpaste			
• Mouthwash (or solution noted on the care plan)			
• Dental floss (if used)			
• Water glass with cool water			
• Straw			
• Kidney basin			
• Hand towel			
• Paper towels			
5. Placed the paper towels on the overbed table. Arranged items on top of them.			
6. Identified the person. Checked the ID bracelet against the assignment sheet. Called the person by name.			
7. Provided for privacy.			
8. Positioned the person so he or she could brush with ease.			

Procedure

	S	U	Comments
9. Lowered the bed rail (if used).			
10. Placed the towel over the person's chest.			
11. Adjusted the overbed table in front of the person.			
12. Let the person perform oral hygiene.			
13. Removed the towel when the person was done.			
14. Adjusted the overbed table next to the bed.			

Post-Procedure

	S	U	Comments
15. Provided for comfort.			
16. Placed the signal light within reach.			
17. Raised or lowered bed rails. Followed the care plan.			

Post-Procedure—cont'd	S	U	Comments
18. Cleaned and returned items to their proper place. Wore gloves.			
19. Wiped off the overbed table with the paper towels. Discarded the paper towels.			
20. Removed the gloves. Decontaminated hands.			
21. Unscreened the person.			
22. Followed agency policy for dirty linen.			
23. Decontaminated hands.			
24. Reported and recorded observations.			

Date of Satisfactory Completion ______________ Instructor's Initials ______________

Brushing the Person's Teeth

Name: ______________________

Date: ______________________

Pre-Procedure	S	U	Comments
• Knocked before entering the person's room.	____	____	____________
• Addressed the person by name.	____	____	____________
• Introduced yourself by name and title.	____	____	____________
1. Followed Delegation Guidelines. Reviewed Safety Alert.	____	____	____________
2. Explained the procedure to the person.	____	____	____________
3. Practiced hand hygiene.	____	____	____________
4. Collected gloves and items listed in procedure: *Assisting the Person to Brush the Teeth.*	____	____	____________
5. Placed the paper towels on the overbed table. Arranged items on top of them.	____	____	____________
6. Identified the person. Checked the ID bracelet against the assignment sheet. Called the person by name.	____	____	____________
7. Provided for privacy.	____	____	____________
8. Raised the bed for body mechanics. Bed rails were up if used.	____	____	____________
Procedure			
9. Lowered the bed rail near you if up.	____	____	____________
10. Assisted the person to a sitting position or to a side-lying position near you.	____	____	____________
11. Placed the towel over the person's chest.	____	____	____________
12. Adjusted the overbed table so it could be reached with ease.	____	____	____________
13. Put on the gloves.	____	____	____________
14. Applied toothpaste to the toothbrush.	____	____	____________
15. Held the toothbrush over the kidney basin. Poured some water over the brush.	____	____	____________
16. Brushed the teeth gently.	____	____	____________
17. Brushed the tongue gently.	____	____	____________
18. Let the person rinse the mouth with water. Held the kidney basin under the person's chin. Repeated this step as needed.	____	____	____________
19. Flossed the person's teeth.	____	____	____________
20. Let the person use mouthwash or other solution. Held the kidney basin under the chin.	____	____	____________
21. Removed the towel when done.	____	____	____________
22. Removed and discarded the gloves. Decontaminated hands.	____	____	____________

Post-Procedure	S	U	Comments
23. Provided for comfort.	______	______	______________________
24. Placed the signal light within reach.	______	______	______________________
25. Lowered the bed to its lowest position.	______	______	______________________
26. Raised or lowered bed rails. Followed the care plan.	______	______	______________________
27. Cleaned and returned equipment to its proper place. Wore gloves.	______	______	______________________
28. Wiped off the overbed table with the paper towels. Discarded the paper towels.	______	______	______________________
29. Removed the gloves. Decontaminated hands.	______	______	______________________
30. Adjusted the overbed table for the person.	______	______	______________________
31. Unscreened the person.	______	______	______________________
32. Followed agency policy for dirty linen.	______	______	______________________
33. Decontaminated hands.	______	______	______________________
34. Reported and recorded observations.	______	______	______________________

Date of Satisfactory Completion ______________________ Instructor's Initials ____________________

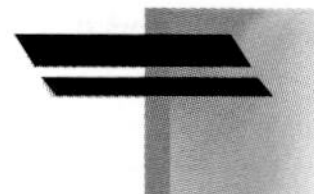

Flossing the Person's Teeth

Name: ______________________

Date: ______________________

Pre-Procedure	S	U	Comments
• Knocked before entering the person's room.			
• Addressed the person by name.			
• Introduced yourself by name and title.			
1. Followed Delegation Guidelines. Reviewed Safety Alert.			
2. Explained the procedure to the person.			
3. Practiced hand hygiene.			
4. Collected the following:			
• Kidney basin			
• Water glass with cool water			
• Floss			
• Hand towel			
• Paper towels			
• Gloves			
5. Placed the paper towels on the overbed table. Arranged items on top of them.			
6. Identified the person. Checked the ID bracelet against the assignment sheet. Called the person by name.			
7. Provided for privacy.			
8. Raised the bed for body mechanics. Bed rails were up if used.			

Procedure	S	U	Comments
9. Lowered the bed rail near you if up.			
10. Assisted the person to a sitting position or a side-lying position near you.			
11. Placed the towel over the person's chest.			
12. Adjusted the overbed table so it could be reached with ease.			
13. Put on the gloves.			
14. Broke off an 18-inch piece of floss from the dispenser.			
15. Held the floss between the middle fingers of each hand.			
16. Stretched the floss with the thumbs.			
17. Started at the upper back tooth on the right side. Worked around to the left side.			
18. Moved the floss gently up and down between the teeth. Moved floss up and down against the side of each tooth. Worked from the top of the crown to the gum line.			

Procedure—cont'd

	S	U	Comments
19. Moved to a new section of floss after every second tooth.			
20. Flossed the lower teeth. Held the floss with the index fingers. Used up- and down-motions as for the upper teeth. Started on the right side. Worked around to the left side.			
21. Let the person rinse his or her mouth. Held the kidney basin under the chin. Repeated rinsing as necessary.			
22. Removed the towel when done.			
23. Removed and discarded the gloves. Decontaminated hands.			

Post-Procedure

	S	U	Comments
24. Followed steps 23 through 34 for procedure: *Brushing the Person's Teeth.*			

Date of Satisfactory Completion ____________________ Instructor's Initials ____________________

Providing Mouth Care For an Unconscious Person

Name: ______________________

Date: ______________________

Pre-Procedure	S	U	Comments
• Knocked before entering the person's room.			
• Addressed the person by name.			
• Introduced yourself by name and title.			
1. Followed Delegation Guidelines. Reviewed Safety Alert.			
2. Practiced hand hygiene.			
3. Collected the following:			
• Cleaning agent			
• Sponge swabs			
• Padded tongue blade			
• Water glass with cool water			
• Hand towel			
• Kidney basin			
• Lip lubricant			
• Paper towels			
• Gloves			
4. Placed the paper towels on the overbed table. Arranged items on top of them.			
5. Identified the person. Checked the ID bracelet against the assignment sheet. Called the person by name.			
6. Explained the procedure to the person.			
7. Provided for privacy.			
8. Raised the bed for body mechanics. Bed rails were up if used.			
Procedure			
9. Lowered the bed rail near you if up.			
10. Put on the gloves.			
11. Positioned the person in a side-lying position near you. Turned the person's head well to the side.			
12. Placed the towel under the person's face.			
13. Placed the kidney basin under the chin.			
14. Adjusted the overbed table so it could be reached with ease.			
15. Separated the upper and lower teeth. Used the padded tongue blade. Did not use force.			

Procedure—cont'd	S	U	Comments
16. Cleaned the mouth using sponge swabs moistened with the cleaning agent:	______	______	____________________
a. Cleaned the chewing and inner surfaces of the teeth.	______	______	____________________
b. Cleaned the outer surfaces of the teeth.	______	______	____________________
c. Swabbed the roof of the mouth, inside of the cheeks, and the lips.	______	______	____________________
d. Swabbed the tongue.	______	______	____________________
e. Moistened a clean swab with water. Swabbed the mouth to rinse.	______	______	____________________
f. Placed used swabs in the kidney basin.	______	______	____________________
17. Applied lubricant to the lips.	______	______	____________________
18. Removed the towel.	______	______	____________________
19. Removed and discarded the gloves. Decontaminated hands.	______	______	____________________
20. Explained that the procedure is done. Explained that you would reposition the person.	______	______	____________________
21. Repositioned the person. Provided for comfort.	______	______	____________________
22. Raised or lowered bed rails. Followed the care plan.	______	______	____________________
Post-Procedure			
23. Placed the signal light within reach.	______	______	____________________
24. Lowered the bed to its lowest position.	______	______	____________________
25. Cleaned and returned equipment to its proper place. Discarded disposable items. Wore gloves.	______	______	____________________
26. Wiped off the overbed table with paper towels. Discarded the paper towels.	______	______	____________________
27. Removed the gloves. Decontaminated hands.	______	______	____________________
28. Unscreened the person.	______	______	____________________
29. Told the person that you were leaving the room.	______	______	____________________
30. Followed agency policy for dirty linen.	______	______	____________________
31. Decontaminated hands.	______	______	____________________
32. Reported and recorded observations.	______	______	____________________

Date of Satisfactory Completion ____________________ Instructor's Initials ____________________

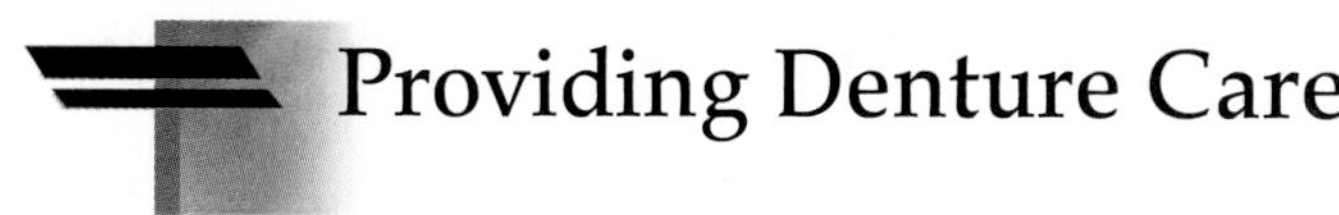

Providing Denture Care

Name: ______________________

Date: ______________________

Pre-Procedure	S	U	Comments
• Knocked before entering the person's room.	____	____	____________
• Addressed the person by name.	____	____	____________
• Introduced yourself by name and title.	____	____	____________
1. Followed Delegation Guidelines. Reviewed Safety Alerts.	____	____	____________
2. Explained the procedure to the person.	____	____	____________
3. Practiced hand hygiene.	____	____	____________
4. Collected the following:			
• Denture brush or soft-bristled toothbrush	____	____	____________
• Denture cup labeled with the person's name and room number	____	____	____________
• Cleaning agent	____	____	____________
• Water glass with cool water	____	____	____________
• Straw	____	____	____________
• Mouthwash (or other noted solution)	____	____	____________
• Kidney basin	____	____	____________
• Two hand towels	____	____	____________
• Gauze squares	____	____	____________
• Gloves	____	____	____________
5. Identified the person. Checked the ID bracelet against the assignment sheet. Called the person by name.	____	____	____________
6. Provided for privacy.	____	____	____________

Procedure

	S	U	Comments
7. Lowered the bed rail near you if used.	____	____	____________
8. Placed a towel over the person's chest.	____	____	____________
9. Put on the gloves.	____	____	____________
10. Asked the person to remove the dentures. Carefully placed them in the kidney basin.	____	____	____________
11. Removed the dentures if the person could not do so. Used gauze squares to get a good grip on the dentures.	____	____	____________
a. Grasped the upper denture with the thumb and index finger. Moved it up and down slightly to break the seal. Gently removed the denture. Placed it in the kidney basin.	____	____	____________
b. Grasped and removed the lower denture with the thumb and index finger. Turned it slightly and lifted it out of the mouth. Placed it in the kidney basin.	____	____	____________

Procedure—cont'd

	S	U	Comments
12. Followed the care plan for raising bed rails.			
13. Took the kidney basin, denture cup, brush, and cleaning agent to the sink.			
14. Lined the sink with a towel. Filled the sink with water.			
15. Rinsed each denture under warm running water. Rinsed out the denture cup.			
16. Returned dentures to the denture cup.			
17. Applied the cleaning agent to the brush.			
18. Brushed the dentures.			
19. Rinsed dentures under running water. Used warm or cool water as directed by the cleaning agent manufacturer.			
20. Placed dentures in the denture cup. Covered the dentures with cool water.			
21. Cleaned the kidney basin.			
22. Took the denture cup and kidney basin to the bedside table.			
23. Lowered the bed rail if up.			
24. Positioned the person for oral hygiene.			
25. Had the person use mouthwash or noted solution. Held the kidney basin under the chin.			
26. Asked the person to insert the dentures. Inserted them if the person could not.			
a. Held the upper denture firmly with the thumb and index finger. Raised the upper lip with the other hand. Inserted the denture. Gently pressed on the denture with the index fingers to make sure it was in place.			
b. Held the lower denture with the thumb and index finger. Pulled the lower lip down slightly. Inserted the denture. Gently pressed down on it to make sure it was in place.			
27. Placed the denture cup in the top drawer of the bedside stand if the dentures were not worn. The dentures must be in water or in a denture soaking solution.			
28. Removed the towel.			
29. Removed the gloves. Decontaminated hands.			

Post-Procedure

	S	U	Comments
30. Assisted with hand washing.			
31. Provided for comfort.			
32. Placed the signal light within reach.			
33. Raised or lowered bed rails. Followed the care plan.			
34. Unscreened the person.			
35. Cleaned and returned equipment to its proper place. Discarded disposable items. Wore gloves for this step.			
36. Followed agency policy for dirty linen.			
37. Decontaminated hands.			
38. Reported and recorded observations.			

Date of Satisfactory Completion ____________________ Instructor's Initials ____________________

Giving a Complete Bed Bath

Name: ____________________

Date: ____________________

Pre-Procedure	S	U	Comments
• Knocked before entering the person's room.			
• Addressed the person by name.			
• Introduced yourself by name and title.			
1. Followed Delegation Guidelines. Reviewed Safety Alert.			
2. Identified the person. Checked the ID bracelet against the assignment sheet. Called the person by name.			
3. Explained the procedure to the person.			
4. Offered the bedpan or urinal. Provided for privacy.			
5. Practiced hand hygiene.			
6. Collected clean linen for a closed bed. Placed linen on a clean surface.			
7. Collected the following:			
• Wash basin			
• Soap			
• Bath thermometer			
• Orange stick or nail file			
• Washcloth			
• Two bath towels and two hand towels			
• Bath blanket			
• Clothing, gown, or pajamas			
• Items for oral hygiene			
• Lotion			
• Powder			
• Deodorant or antiperspirant			
• Brush and comb			
• Other grooming items if requested			
• Paper towels			
• Gloves			
8. Arranged items on the overbed table. Adjusted the height as needed.			
9. Closed doors and windows to prevent drafts.			
10. Provided for privacy.			
11. Raised the bed for body mechanics. Bed rails were up if used.			

Procedure	S	U	Comments
12. Removed the signal light. Lowered the bed rail near you if up.			
13. Put on gloves.			
14. Provided oral hygiene.			
15. Covered the person with a bath blanket. Removed top linens. (See procedure: *Making an Occupied Bed.*)			
16. Lowered the head of the bed. It was as flat as possible. The person had at least one pillow			
17. Covered the overbed table with paper towels.			
18. Raised the bed rail near you if bed rails are used. Both bed rails must be up.			
19. Filled the wash basin 2/3 full with water. Measured water temperature. Used a bath thermometer or tested the water by dipping the elbow or inner wrist into the basin.			
20. Placed the basin on the overbed table.			
21. Lowered the bed rail if up.			
22. Placed a hand towel over the person's chest.			
23. Made a mitt with the washcloth. Used a mitt for the entire bath.			
24. Washed around the person's eyes with water. Did not use soap. Gently wiped from the inner to the outer aspect of the eye with a corner of the mitt. Cleaned the far eye first. Repeated this step for the near eye. Used a clean part of the washcloth for each stroke.			
25. Asked the person if you should use soap to wash the face.			
26. Washed the face, ears, and neck. Rinsed and patted dry with the towel on the chest.			
27. Helped the person move to the side of the bed near you.			
28. Removed the gown. Did not expose the person.			
29. Placed a bath towel lengthwise under the far arm.			
30. Supported the arm with the palm under the person's elbow. The person's forearm rested on your forearm.			
31. Washed the arm, shoulder, and underarm. Used long, firm strokes. Rinsed and patted dry.			
32. Placed the basin on the towel. Put the person's hand into the water. Washed it well. Cleaned under fingernails with an orange stick or nail file.			
33. Had the person exercise the hand and fingers.			
34. Removed the basin. Dried the hand well. Covered the arm with the bath blanket.			
35. Repeated steps 29 through 34 for the near arm.			
36. Placed a bath towel over the chest crosswise. Held the towel in place. Pulled the bath blanket from under the towel to the waist.			
37. Lifted the towel slightly and washed the chest. Did not expose the person. Rinsed and patted dry especially under breasts.			

Procedure—cont'd	S	U	Comments
38. Moved the towel lengthwise over the chest and abdomen. Did not expose the person. Pulled the bath blanket down to the pubic area.			
39. Lifted the towel slightly and washed the abdomen. Rinsed and patted dry.			
40. Pulled the bath blanket up to the shoulders covering both arms. Removed the towel.			
41. Changed soapy or cool water. Measured bath water as in step 19. If bed rails were used, raised the bed rail near you before leaving the bedside. Lowered it when you returned.			
42. Uncovered the far leg. Did not expose the genital area. Placed a towel lengthwise under the foot and leg.			
43. Bent the knee and supported the leg with your arm. Washed it with long, firm strokes. Rinsed and patted dry.			
44. Placed the basin on the towel near the foot.			
45. Lifted the leg slightly. Slid the basin under the foot.			
46. Placed the foot in the basin. Used an orange stick or nail file to clean under toenails if necessary. If the person could not bend the knees:			
a. Washed the foot. Carefully separated the toes. Rinsed and patted dry.			
b. Cleaned under the toenails with an orange stick or nail file if necessary.			
47. Removed the basin. Dried the leg and foot. Covered the leg with the bath blanket. Removed the towel.			
48. Repeated steps 42 through 47 for the near leg.			
49. Changed the water. Measured bath water as in step 19. If bed rails were used, raised the bed rail near you before leaving the bedside. Lowered it when you returned.			
50. Turned the person onto the side away from you. The person was covered with the bath blanket.			
51. Uncovered the back and buttocks. Did not expose the person. Placed a towel lengthwise on the bed along the back.			
52. Washed the back. Worked from the back of the neck to the lower end of the buttocks. Used long, firm, continuous strokes. Rinsed and dried well.			
53. Gave a back massage.			
54. Turned the person onto his or her back.			
55. Changed the water for perineal care. Measured bath water as in step 19. If bed rails were used, raised the bed rail near you before leaving the bedside. Lowered it when you returned.			
56. Let the person wash the genital area. Adjusted the overbed table so the person could reach the wash basin, soap, and towels with ease. Placed the signal light within reach. Asked the person to signal when finished. Made sure the person understood what to do.			

Procedure—cont'd	S	U	Comments
57. Removed the gloves. Decontaminated hands.	_____	_____	_____
58. Answered the signal light promptly. Provided perineal care if the person could not do so. Decontaminated hands and wore gloves for perineal care.	_____	_____	_____
59. Gave a back massage if you had not already done so.	_____	_____	_____
60. Applied deodorant or antiperspirant. Applied lotion and powder as requested.	_____	_____	_____
61. Put clean garments on the person.	_____	_____	_____
62. Combed and brushed the hair.	_____	_____	_____
63. Made the bed. Attached the signal light.	_____	_____	_____

Post-Procedure

	S	U	Comments
64. Provided for comfort.	_____	_____	_____
65. Lowered the bed to its lowest position.	_____	_____	_____
66. Raised or lower bed rails. Followed the care plan.	_____	_____	_____
67. Emptied and cleaned the wash basin. Returned it and other supplies to their proper place.	_____	_____	_____
68. Wiped off the overbed table with the paper towels. Discarded the paper towels.	_____	_____	_____
69. Unscreened the person.	_____	_____	_____
70. Followed agency policy for dirty linen.	_____	_____	_____
71. Decontaminated hands.	_____	_____	_____
72. Reported and recorded observations.	_____	_____	_____

Date of Satisfactory Completion _______________ Instructor's Initials _______________

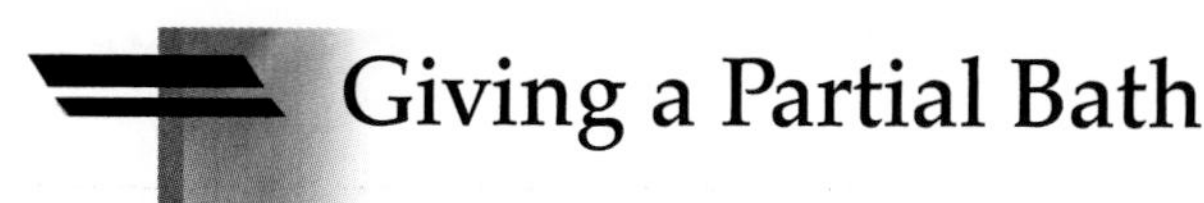

Giving a Partial Bath

Name: ______________________

Date: ______________________

Pre-Procedure	S	U	Comments
• Knocked before entering the person's room.	____	____	____________
• Addressed the person by name.	____	____	____________
• Introduced yourself by name and title.	____	____	____________
1. Followed Delegation Guidelines. Reviewed Safety Alert.	____	____	____________
2. Followed steps 2 through 10 in procedure: *Giving a Complete Bed Bath.*	____	____	____________

Procedure			
3. Made sure the bed was in the lowest position.	____	____	____________
4. Assisted with oral hygiene. Wore gloves. Adjusted the overbed table as needed.	____	____	____________
5. Removed top linen. Covered the person with a bath blanket.	____	____	____________
6. Covered the overbed table with paper towels.	____	____	____________
7. Filled the wash basin with water. Measured water temperature with the bath thermometer or tested bath water by dipping the elbow or inner wrist into the basin.	____	____	____________
8. Placed the basin on the overbed table.	____	____	____________
9. Positioned the person in Fowler's position or assisted the person to sit at the bedside.	____	____	____________
10. Adjusted the overbed table so the person could reach the basin and supplies.	____	____	____________
11. Helped the person undress.	____	____	____________
12. Asked the person to wash easy to reach body parts. Explained that you would wash the back and areas the person cannot reach.	____	____	____________
13. Placed the signal light within reach. Asked the person to signal when help was needed or bathing is complete.	____	____	____________
14. Left the room after decontaminating hands.	____	____	____________
15. Returned when the signal light is on. Knocked before entering. Decontaminated hands.	____	____	____________
16. Changed the bath water. Measured bath water temperature as in step 7.	____	____	____________
17. Raised the bed for body mechanics. The far bed rail was up if used.	____	____	____________
18. Asked what was washed. Put on gloves. Washed and dried areas the person could not reach. The face, hands, underarms, back, buttocks, and perineal area were washed for the partial bath.	____	____	____________

Procedure—cont'd

	S	U	Comments
19. Removed the gloves. Decontaminated hands.			
20. Gave a back massage.			
21. Applied lotion, powder, and deodorant or antiperspirant as requested.			
22. Helped the person put on clean garments.			
23. Assisted with hair care and other grooming needs.			
24. Assisted the person to a chair. (Lowered the bed if the person transfers to a chair.) Otherwise, turned the person onto the side away from you.			
25. Made the bed.			
26. Lowered the bed to its lowest position.			

Post-Procedure

	S	U	Comments
27. Provided for comfort.			
28. Placed the signal light within reach.			
29. Raised or lowered bed rails. Followed the care plan.			
30. Emptied and cleaned the basin. Returned the basin and supplies to their proper place.			
31. Wiped off the overbed table with the paper towels. Discarded the paper towels.			
32. Unscreened the person.			
33. Followed agency policy for dirty linen.			
34. Decontaminated hands.			
35. Reported and recorded observations.			

Date of Satisfactory Completion ____________________ Instructor's Initials ____________________

Assisting With a Tub Bath or Shower

Name: ______________________

Date: ______________________

Pre-Procedure	S	U	Comments
• Knocked before entering the person's room.			
• Addressed the person by name.			
• Introduced yourself by name and title.			
1. Followed Delegation Guidelines. Reviewed Safety Alert.			
2. Reserved the bathtub or shower.			
3. Identified the person. Checked the ID bracelet against the assignment sheet. Called the person by name.			
4. Explained the procedure to the person.			
5. Practiced hand hygiene.			
6. Collected the following:			
• Washcloth and two bath towels			
• Soap			
• Bath thermometer (for a tub bath)			
• Clothing, gown, or pajamas			
• Grooming items as requested			
• Robe and nonskid footwear			
• Rubber bath mat if needed			
• Disposable bath mat			
• Gloves			
• Wheelchair or shower chair			

Procedure	S	U	Comments
7. Placed items in the tub or shower room. Used the space provided or a chair.			
8. Cleaned the tub or shower.			
9. Placed a rubber bath mat in the tub or on the shower floor. Did not block the drain.			
10. Placed the disposable bath mat on the floor in front of the tub or shower.			
11. Put the "Occupied" sign on the door.			
12. Returned to the person's room. Provided for privacy.			
13. Helped the person sit on the side of the bed.			
14. Helped the person put on a robe and nonskid footwear.			
15. Assisted or transported the person to the tub or shower room.			

Procedure—cont'd

Procedure—cont'd	S	U	Comments
16. For a tub bath:			
a. Had the person sit on a chair.			
b. Filled the tub halfway with warm water (105° F; 41° C). Measured water temperature with the bath thermometer or checked the digital display.			
17. For a shower:			
a. Turned on the shower.			
b. Adjusted water temperature and pressure.			
18. Helped the person undress and remove footwear.			
19. Helped the person into the tub or shower. Positioned the shower chair, and locked the wheels.			
20. Assisted with washing if necessary. Wore gloves.			
21. Asked the person to use the signal light when done or when help was needed. Reminded the person that a tub bath lasts no longer than 20 minutes.			
22. Placed a towel across the chair.			
23. Left the room if the person could bathe unattended. If not, stayed in the room or remained nearby. Removed the gloves and decontaminated hands if you left the room.			
24. Checked the person every 5 minutes.			
25. Returned when the person signaled. Knocked before entering. Decontaminated hands.			
26. Turned off the shower or drained the tub. Covered the person while the tub drained.			
27. Helped the person out of the tub or shower and onto the chair.			
28. Helped the person dry off. Patted gently. Dried under breasts, between skin folds, in the perineal area, and between the toes.			
29. Assisted with lotion and other grooming items as needed.			
30. Helped the person dress and put on footwear.			
31. Helped the person return to the room. Provided for privacy.			
32. Assisted the person to a chair or into bed.			
33. Provided a back massage if the person returned to bed.			
34. Assisted with hair care and other grooming needs.			

Post-Procedure

Post-Procedure	S	U	Comments
35. Made the bed. Provided for comfort.			
36. Raised or lowered bed rails. Followed the care plan.			
37. Placed the signal light within reach.			
38. Unscreened the person.			
39. Cleaned the tub or shower. Removed soiled linen. Wore gloves for this step.			

Post-Procedure—cont'd	S	U	Comments
40. Discarded disposable items. Put the "Unoccupied" sign on the door. Returned supplies to their proper place.			
41. Followed agency policy for dirty linen.			
42. Decontaminated hands.			
43. Reported and recorded observations.			

Date of Satisfactory Completion ______________________ Instructor's Initials ______________________

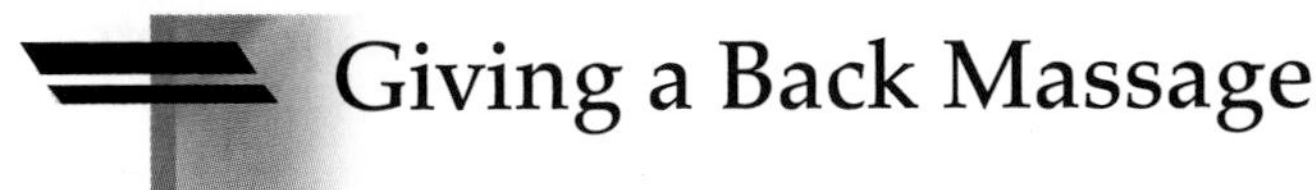

Giving a Back Massage

Name: ______________________

Date: ______________________

Pre-Procedure	S	U	Comments
• Knocked before entering the person's room.			
• Addressed the person by name.			
• Introduced yourself by name and title.			
1. Followed Delegation Guidelines. Reviewed Safety Alert.			
2. Identified the person. Checked the ID bracelet against the assignment sheet. Called the person by name.			
3. Explained the procedure to the person.			
4. Practiced hand hygiene.			
5. Collected the following:			
• Bath blanket			
• Bath towel			
• Lotion			
6. Provided for privacy.			
7. Raised the bed for body mechanics. Bed rails were up if used.			

Procedure	S	U	Comments
8. Lowered the bed rail near you if up.			
9. Positioned the person in the prone or side-lying position with the back toward you.			
10. Exposed the back, shoulders, upper arms, and buttocks. Covered the rest of the body with the bath blanket.			
11. Laid the towel on the bed along the back.			
12. Warmed the lotion.			
13. Explained that the lotion may feel cool and wet.			
14. Applied lotion to the lower back area.			
15. Stroked up from the buttocks to the shoulders. Then stroked down over the upper arms. Stroked up the upper arms, across the shoulders, and down the back to the buttocks. Used firm strokes. Kept hands in contact with the person's skin.			
16. Repeated step 15 for at least 3 minutes.			
17. Kneaded by grasping skin between the thumb and fingers. Kneaded half of the back. Started at the buttocks and moved up to the shoulder. Then kneaded down from the shoulder to the buttocks. Repeated on the other half of the back.			

Procedure—cont'd	S	U	Comments
18. Applied lotion to bony areas. Used circular motions with the tips of the index and middle fingers.	_____	_____	__________
19. Used fast movements to stimulate. Used slow movements to relax the person.	_____	_____	__________
20. Stroked with long, firm movements to end the massage. Told the person you were finishing.	_____	_____	__________
21. Covered the person. Removed the towel and bath blanket.	_____	_____	__________
Post-Procedure			
22. Provided for comfort.	_____	_____	__________
23. Lowered the bed to its lowest position.	_____	_____	__________
24. Raised or lowered bed rails. Followed the care plan.	_____	_____	__________
25. Placed the signal light within reach.	_____	_____	__________
26. Returned lotion to its proper place.	_____	_____	__________
27. Unscreened the person.	_____	_____	__________
28. Followed agency policy for dirty linen.	_____	_____	__________
29. Decontaminated hands.	_____	_____	__________
30. Reported and recorded observations.	_____	_____	__________

Date of Satisfactory Completion ____________________ Instructor's Initials ____________________

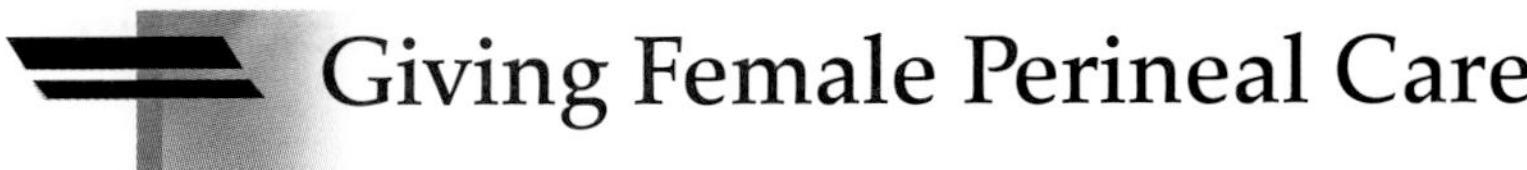

Giving Female Perineal Care

Name: ______________________

Date: ______________________

Pre-Procedure	S	U	Comments
• Knocked before entering the person's room.			
• Addressed the person by name.			
• Introduced yourself by name and title.			
1. Followed Delegation Guidelines. Reviewed Safety Alert.			
2. Explained the procedure to the person.			
3. Practiced hand hygiene.			
4. Collected the following:			
• Soap			
• At least 4 washcloths			
• Bath towel			
• Bath blanket			
• Bath thermometer			
• Washbasin			
• Waterproof pad			
• Gloves			
• Paper towels			
5. Covered the overbed table with paper towels. Arranged items on top of them.			
6. Identified the person. Checked the ID bracelet against the assignment sheet. Called her by name.			
7. Provided for privacy.			
8. Raised the bed for body mechanics. Bed rails were up if used.			

Procedure	S	U	Comments
9. Lowered the bed rail near you if up.			
10. Covered the person with a bath blanket. Moved top linens to the foot of the bed.			
11. Positioned the person on her back.			
12. Draped her.			
13. Raised the bed rail if used.			
14. Filled the wash basin two-thirds full. Measured water temperature according to agency policy.			
15. Placed the basin on the overbed table.			
16. Lowered the bed rail if up.			
17. Put on the gloves.			

Procedure—cont'd	S	U	Comments
18. Helped the person flex her knees and spread her legs, or helped her spread her legs as much as possible with her knees straight.			
19. Placed a waterproof pad under her buttocks.			
20. Folded the corner of the bath blanket between her legs onto her abdomen.			
21. Wet the washcloths. Squeezed out excess water before using them.			
22. Applied soap to a washcloth.			
23. Separated the labia. Cleaned downward from front to back with one stroke.			
24. Repeated steps 22 and 23 until the area was clean. Used a clean part of the washcloth for each stroke. Used more than one washcloth if needed.			
25. Rinsed the perineum with a clean washcloth. Separated the labia. Stroked downward from front to back. Repeated as necessary. Used a clean part of the washcloth for each stroke. Used more than one washcloth if needed.			
26. Patted the area dry with the towel.			
27. Folded the blanket back between her legs.			
28. Helped the person lower her legs and turn onto her side away from you.			
29. Applied soap to a washcloth.			
30. Cleaned the rectal area. Cleaned from the vagina to the anus with one stroke.			
31. Repeated steps 29 and 30 until the area was clean. Used a clean part of the washcloth for each stroke. Used more than one washcloth if needed.			
32. Rinsed the rectal area with a washcloth. Stroked from the vagina to the anus. Repeated as necessary. Used a clean part of the washcloth for each stroke. Used more than one washcloth if needed.			
33. Patted the area dry with the towel.			
34. Removed the waterproof pad.			
35. Removed and discarded the gloves. Decontaminated hands.			

Post-Procedure

36. Provided for comfort.			
37. Covered the person. Removed the bath blanket.			
38. Lowered the bed to its lowest position.			
39. Raised or lowered bed rails. Followed the care plan.			
40. Placed the signal light within reach.			
41. Emptied and cleaned the wash basin. Wore gloves.			
42. Returned the basin and supplies to their proper place.			

Post-Procedure—cont'd	S	U	Comments
43. Wiped off the overbed table with the paper towels. Discarded the paper towels.	______	______	______________________
44. Removed the gloves. Decontaminated hands.	______	______	______________________
45. Unscreened the person.	______	______	______________________
46. Followed agency policy for dirty linen.	______	______	______________________
47. Decontaminated hands.	______	______	______________________
48. Reported and recorded observations.	______	______	______________________

Date of Satisfactory Completion ______________________ Instructor's Initials ____________________

Giving Male Perineal Care

Name: ____________________

Date: ____________________

Pre-Procedure	S	U	Comments
• Knocked before entering the person's room.			
• Addressed the person by name.			
• Introduced yourself by name and title.			

Procedure	S	U	Comments
1. Followed steps 1 through 22 in procedure: *Giving Female Perineal Care.*			
2. Retracted the foreskin if the person was uncircumcised.			
3. Grasped the penis.			
4. Cleaned the tip. Used a circular motion. Started at the meatus and worked outward. Repeated as needed. Used a clean part of the washcloth each time.			
5. Rinsed the area with another washcloth.			
6. Returned the foreskin to its natural position.			
7. Cleaned the shaft of the penis. Used firm downward strokes. Rinsed the area.			
8. Helped the person flex his knees and spread his legs, or helped him spread his legs as much as possible with his knees straight.			
9. Cleaned the scrotum. Rinsed well. Observed for redness and irritation in the skin folds.			
10. Patted the penis and scrotum dry.			
11. Folded the bath blanket back between his legs.			
12. Helped him lower his legs and turn onto his side away from you.			
13. Cleaned the rectal area. Rinsed and dried well.			
14. Removed the waterproof pad.			
15. Removed and discarded the gloves. Decontaminated hands.			

Post-Procedure	S	U	Comments
16. Followed steps 36 through 48 in procedure: *Giving Female Perineal Care.*			

Date of Satisfactory Completion ____________________ Instructor's Initials ____________________

Brushing and Combing a Person's Hair

Name: ______________________

Date: ______________________

Pre-Procedure	S	U	Comments
• Knocked before entering the person's room.	____	____	____________
• Addressed the person by name.	____	____	____________
• Introduced yourself by name and title.	____	____	____________
1. Followed Delegation Guidelines. Reviewed Safety Alert.	____	____	____________
2. Identified the person. Checked the ID bracelet against the assignment sheet. Called the person by name.	____	____	____________
3. Explained the procedure to the person. Asked the person how to style hair.	____	____	____________
4. Collected the following:			
• Comb and brush	____	____	____________
• Bath towel	____	____	____________
• Hair care items as requested	____	____	____________
5. Arranged items on the bedside stand.	____	____	____________
6. Practiced hand hygiene.	____	____	____________
7. Provided for privacy.	____	____	____________

Procedure

8. Lowered the bed rail if used.	____	____	____________
9. Helped the person to the chair. The person put on a robe and nonskid footwear. (If the person was in bed, raised the bed for body mechanics. Bed rails were up if used. Lowered the near bed rail. Assisted the person to semi-Fowler's position if allowed.)	____	____	____________
10. Placed a towel across the shoulders or across the pillow.	____	____	____________
11. Asked the person to remove eyeglasses. Put them in the eyeglass case. Put the case inside the bedside stand.	____	____	____________
12. Parted hair into 2 sections. Divided one side into 2 sections.	____	____	____________
13. Brushed the hair. Started at the scalp and brushed toward the hair ends. Repeated for each section.	____	____	____________
14. Styled the hair as the person preferred.	____	____	____________
15. Removed the towel.	____	____	____________
16. Let the person put on the eyeglasses.	____	____	____________

Post-Procedure	S	U	Comments
17. Provided for comfort.	______	______	______________________
18. Lowered the bed to its lowest position.	______	______	______________________
19. Raised or lowered bed rails. Followed the care plan.	______	______	______________________
20. Placed the signal light within reach.	______	______	______________________
21. Unscreened the person.	______	______	______________________
22. Cleaned and returned items to their proper place.	______	______	______________________
23. Followed agency policy for dirty linen.	______	______	______________________
24. Decontaminated hands.	______	______	______________________

Date of Satisfactory Completion ______________________ Instructor's Initials ______________________

Shampooing the Person's Hair

Name: ______________________

Date: ______________________

Pre-Procedure	S	U	Comments
• Knocked before entering the person's room.			
• Addressed the person by name.			
• Introduced yourself by name and title.			
1. Followed Delegation Guidelines. Reviewed Safety Alert.			
2. Explained the procedure to the person.			
3. Practiced hand hygiene.			
4. Collected the following:			
• Two bath towels			
• Hand towel or washcloth			
• Shampoo			
• Hair conditioner (if requested)			
• Bath thermometer			
• Pitcher or nozzle (if needed)			
• Shampoo tray (if needed)			
• Basin or pan (if needed)			
• Waterproof pad (if needed)			
• Gloves (if needed)			
• Comb and brush			
• Hair dryer			
5. Arranged items nearby.			
6. Identified the person. Checked the ID bracelet against the assignment sheet. Called the person by name.			
7. Provided for privacy.			
8. Raised the bed for body mechanics for a shampoo in bed. The far bed rail was up if bed rails were used.			

Procedure	S	U	Comments
9. Positioned the person for the method you used. Placed the waterproof pad and shampoo tray under the head and shoulders if needed.			
10. Placed a bath towel across the shoulders or across the pillow.			
11. Brushed and combed the hair to remove snarls and tangles.			
12. Raised the bed rail if used.			
13. Obtained water. Tested temperature according to agency policy.			

Procedure—cont'd	S	U	Comments
14. Lowered the bed rail if used.			
15. Put on gloves (if needed).			
16. Asked the person to hold a dampened hand towel or washcloth over the eyes. It did not cover the nose and mouth.			
17. Used the pitcher or nozzle to wet the hair.			
18. Applied a small amount of shampoo.			
19. Worked up a lather with both hands. Started at the hairline. Worked toward the back of the head.			
20. Massaged the scalp with the fingertips. Did not scratch the scalp.			
21. Rinsed the hair.			
22. Repeated steps 18 through 21.			
23. Applied conditioner. Followed directions on the container.			
24. Squeezed water from the person's hair.			
25. Covered hair with a bath towel.			
26. Dried the person's face with the towel or washcloth used to protect the eyes.			
27. Helped the person raise the head if appropriate.			
28. Rubbed the hair and scalp with the towel. Used the second towel if the first was wet.			
29. Combed the hair to remove snarls and tangles.			
30. Dried and styled hair as quickly as possible.			

Post-Procedure

31. Removed and discarded the gloves (if used). Decontaminated hands.			
32. Provided for comfort.			
33. Lowered the bed to its lowest position.			
34. Raised or lowered bed rails. Followed the care plan.			
35. Placed the signal light within reach.			
36. Unscreened the person.			
37. Cleaned and returned equipment to its proper place. Discarded disposable items.			
38. Followed agency policy for dirty linen.			
39. Decontaminated hands.			

Date of Satisfactory Completion ____________________ Instructor's Initials ____________________

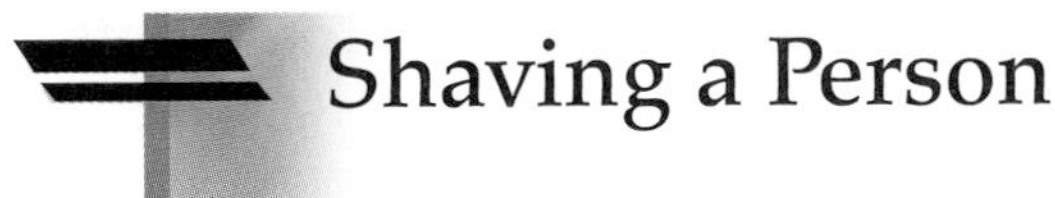

Shaving a Person

Name: ______________________

Date: ______________________

Pre-Procedure	S	U	Comments
• Knocked before entering the person's room.			
• Addressed the person by name.			
• Introduced yourself by name and title.			
1. Followed Delegation Guidelines. Reviewed Safety Alert.			
2. Explained the procedure to the person.			
3. Practiced hand hygiene.			
4. Collected the following:			
• Wash basin			
• Bath towel			
• Hand towel			
• Washcloth			
• Safety razor			
• Mirror			
• Shaving cream, soap, or lotion			
• Shaving brush			
• After-shave lotion (men only)			
• Tissues or paper towels			
• Gloves			
5. Arranged paper towels and supplies on the overbed table.			
6. Identified the person. Checked the ID bracelet against the assignment sheet. Called the person by name.			
7. Provided for privacy.			
8. Raised the bed for body mechanics. Bed rails were up if used.			
Procedure			
9. Filled the basin two-thirds full with warm water.			
10. Placed the basin on the overbed table.			
11. Lowered the bed rail near you if up.			
12. Assisted the person to semi-Fowler's position if allowed or to the supine position.			
13. Adjusted lighting to clearly see the person's face.			
14. Placed the bath towel over the chest.			
15. Adjusted the overbed table for easy reach.			

Procedure—cont'd

	S	U	Comments
16. Tightened the razor blade to the shaver.			
17. Washed the person's face. Did not dry.			
18. Wet the washcloth or towel. Wrung it out.			
19. Applied the washcloth or towel to the face for a few minutes.			
20. Put on gloves.			
21. Applied shaving cream with hands, or used a shaving brush to apply lather.			
22. Held the skin taut with one hand.			
23. Shaved in the direction of hair growth. Used shorter strokes around the chin and lips.			
24. Rinsed the razor often. Wiped it with tissues or paper towels.			
25. Applied direct pressure to any bleeding areas.			
26. Washed off any remaining shaving cream or soap. Dried with a towel.			
27. Applied after-shave lotion if requested.			
28. Removed the towel and gloves. Decontaminated hands.			
29. Moved the overbed table to the side of the bed.			

Post-Procedure

	S	U	Comments
30. Provided for comfort.			
31. Placed the signal light within reach.			
32. Lowered the bed to its lowest position.			
33. Raised or lowered bed rails. Followed the care plan.			
34. Cleaned and returned equipment and supplies to their proper place. Discarded disposable items. Wore gloves.			
35. Wiped off the overbed table with the paper towels. Discarded the paper towels.			
36. Removed the gloves. Decontaminated hands.			
37. Positioned the table for the person.			
38. Unscreened the person.			
39. Followed agency policy for dirty linen.			
40. Decontaminated hands.			
41. Reported nicks, cuts, irritation, or bleeding to the nurse.			

Date of Satisfactory Completion ______________________ Instructor's Initials ______________________

Giving Nail and Foot Care

Name: ______________________

Date: ______________________

Pre-Procedure	S	U	Comments
• Knocked before entering the person's room.			
• Addressed the person by name.			
• Introduced yourself by name and title.			
1. Followed Delegation Guidelines. Reviewed Safety Alert.			
2. Explained the procedure to the person.			
3. Practiced hand hygiene.			
4. Collected the following:			
• Wash basin or whirlpool foot bath			
• Soap			
• Bath thermometer			
• Bath towel			
• Hand towel			
• Washcloth			
• Kidney basin			
• Nail clippers			
• Orange stick			
• Emery board or nail file			
• Lotion or petroleum jelly			
• Paper towels			
• Disposable bath mat			
• Gloves			
5. Arranged paper towels and other items on the overbed table.			
6. Identified the person. Checked the ID bracelet against the assignment sheet. Called the person by name.			
7. Provided for privacy.			
8. Assisted the person to the bedside chair. Placed the signal light within reach.			

Procedure	S	U	Comments
9. Placed the bath mat under the feet.			
10. Filled the wash basin or whirlpool foot bath two-thirds full with water. The nurse told you what water temperature to use. Measured water temperature with a bath thermometer or tested it by dipping the elbow or inner wrist into the basin.			
11. Placed the basin or foot bath on the bath mat			

Procedure—cont'd	S	U	Comments
12. Helped the person put the feet into the basin or foot bath.			
13. Adjusted the overbed table in front of the person.			
14. Filled the kidney basin. Measured water temperature.			
15. Placed the kidney basin on the overbed table.			
16. Placed the person's fingers into the basin. Positioned the arms for comfort.			
17. Let the fingers soak for 5 to 10 minutes. Let the feet soak for 15 to 20 minutes. Rewarmed water as needed.			
18. Put on gloves.			
19. Cleaned under the fingernails with the orange stick. Used a towel to wipe the orange stick after each nail.			
20. Removed the kidney basin. Dried the hands and between the fingers thoroughly.			
21. Clipped fingernails straight across with the nail clippers.			
22. Shaped nails with an emery board or nail file.			
23. Pushed cuticles back with the orange stick or a washcloth.			
24. Applied lotion to the hands.			
25. Moved the overbed table to the side.			
26. Washed the feet with soap and a washcloth. Washed between the toes.			
27. Removed the feet from the basin or foot bath. Dried thoroughly, especially between the toes.			
28. Applied lotion or petroleum jelly to the tops and soles of the feet. Did not apply between the toes. Warmed lotion before applying it.			
29. Removed and discarded the gloves. Decontaminated hands.			
30. Helped the person put on socks and nonskid footwear.			

Post-Procedure	S	U	Comments
31. Provided for comfort.			
32. Placed the signal light within reach.			
33. Raised or lowered bed rails. Followed the care plan.			
34. Cleaned and returned equipment and supplies to their proper place. Discarded disposable items. Wore gloves for this step.			
35. Removed the gloves. Decontaminated hands.			
36. Unscreened the person.			
37. Followed agency policy for dirty linen.			
38. Decontaminated hands.			
39. Reported and recorded observations.			

Date of Satisfactory Completion ____________________ Instructor's Initials ____________________

Changing the Gown of a Person With an IV

Name: ______________________

Date: ______________________

Pre-Procedure	S	U	Comments
• Knocked before entering the person's room.	____	____	____________
• Addressed the person by name.	____	____	____________
• Introduced yourself by name and title.	____	____	____________
1. Followed Delegation Guidelines. Reviewed Safety Alert.	____	____	____________
2. Explained the procedure to the person.	____	____	____________
3. Practiced hand hygiene.	____	____	____________
4. Got a clean gown and a bath blanket.	____	____	____________
5. Identified the person. Checked the ID bracelet against the assignment sheet. Called the person by name.	____	____	____________
6. Provided for privacy.	____	____	____________
7. Raised the bed for body mechanics. Bed rails were up if used.	____	____	____________

Procedure

8. Lowered the bed rail near you if up.	____	____	____________
9. Covered the person with a bath blanket. Fanfolded linens to the foot of the bed.	____	____	____________
10. Untied the gown. Freed parts that the person was lying on.	____	____	____________
11. Removed the gown from the arm with no IV.	____	____	____________
12. Gathered up the sleeve of the arm with the IV. Slid it over the IV site and tubing. Removed the arm and hand from the sleeve.	____	____	____________
13. Kept the sleeve gathered. Slid your arm along the tubing to the bag.	____	____	____________
14. Removed the bag from the pole. Slid the bag and tubing through the sleeve. Did not pull on the tubing. Kept the bag above the person.	____	____	____________
15. Hung the IV bag on the pole.	____	____	____________
16. Gathered the sleeve of the clean gown that would go on the arm with the IV infusion.	____	____	____________
17. Removed the bag from the pole. Slipped the sleeve over the bag at the shoulder part of the gown. Hung the bag.	____	____	____________
18. Slid the gathered sleeve over the tubing, hand, arm, and IV site. Then slid it onto the shoulder.	____	____	____________
19. Put the other side of the gown on the person. Fastened the gown.	____	____	____________
20. Covered the person. Removed the bath blanket.	____	____	____________

Post-Procedure	S	U	Comments
21. Provided for comfort.	______	______	____________________
22. Placed the signal light within reach.	______	______	____________________
23. Lowered the bed to its lowest position.	______	______	____________________
24. Raised or lowered bed rails. Followed the care plan.	______	______	____________________
25. Unscreened the person.	______	______	____________________
26. Followed agency policy for dirty linen.	______	______	____________________
27. Decontaminated hands.	______	______	____________________
28. Checked the flow rate, or asked the nurse to check it.	______	______	____________________

Date of Satisfactory Completion ____________________ Instructor's Initials ____________________

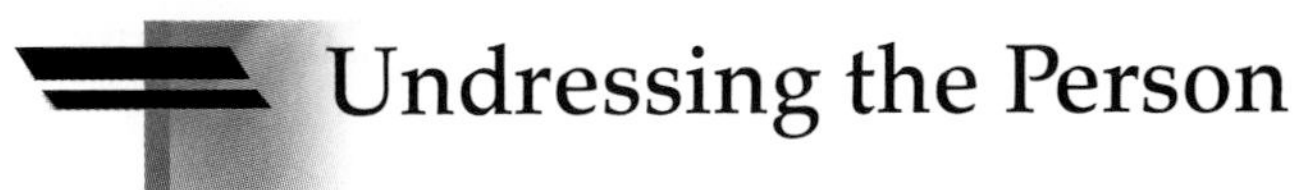

Undressing the Person

Name: ______________________

Date: ______________________

Pre-Procedure

	S	U	Comments
• Knocked before entering the person's room.	___	___	___
• Addressed the person by name.	___	___	___
• Introduced yourself by name and title.	___	___	___
1. Followed Delegation Guidelines.	___	___	___
2. Explained the procedure to the person.	___	___	___
3. Practiced hand hygiene.	___	___	___
4. Got a bath blanket.	___	___	___
5. Identified the person. Checked the ID bracelet against the assignment sheet. Called the person by name.	___	___	___
6. Provided for privacy.	___	___	___
7. Raised the bed for body mechanics. Bed rails were up if used.	___	___	___
8. Lowered the bed rail on the person's weak side.	___	___	___
9. Positioned the person supine.	___	___	___
10. Covered the person with the bath blanket. Fanfolded linens to the foot of the bed.	___	___	___

Procedure

	S	U	Comments
11. Removed garments that open in the back.	___	___	___
a. Raised the head and shoulders, or turned the person onto the side away from you.	___	___	___
b. Undid buttons, zippers, ties, or snaps.	___	___	___
c. Brought the sides of the garment to the sides of the person. If the person was in a side-lying position, tucked the far side under the person. Folded the near side onto the chest.	___	___	___
d. Positioned the person supine.	___	___	___
e. Slid the garment off the shoulder on the strong side. Removed it from the arm.	___	___	___
f. Repeated step 11e for the weak side.	___	___	___
12. Removed garments that open in the front.	___	___	___
a. Undid buttons, zippers, snaps, or ties.	___	___	___
b. Slid the garment off the shoulder and arm on the strong side.	___	___	___
c. Raised the head and shoulders. Brought the garment over to the weak side. Lowered the head and shoulders.	___	___	___
d. Removed the garment from the weak side.	___	___	___

Procedure—cont'd	S	U	Comments
e. If you could not raise the head and shoulders:			
(1) Turned the person toward you. Tucked the removed part under the person.			
(2) Turned the person onto the side away from you.			
(3) Pulled the side of the garment out from under the person. Made sure the person would not lie on it when supine.			
(4) Returned the person to the supine position.			
(5) Removed the garment from the weak side.			
13. Removed pullover garments.			
a. Undid any buttons, zippers, ties, or snaps.			
b. Removed the garment from the strong side.			
c. Raised the head and shoulders, or turned the person onto the side away from you. Brought the garment up to the person's neck.			
d. Removed the garment from the weak side.			
e. Brought the garment over the person's head.			
f. Positioned the person in the supine position.			
14. Removed pants or slacks.			
a. Removed footwear.			
b. Positioned the person supine.			
c. Undid buttons, zippers, ties, snaps, or buckles.			
d. Removed the belt.			
e. Asked the person to lift the buttocks off the bed. Slid the pants down over the hips and buttocks. Had the person lower the hips and buttocks.			
f. If the person could not raise the hips off the bed:			
(1) Turned the person toward you.			
(2) Slid the pants off the hip and buttock on the strong side.			
(3) Turned the person away from you.			
(4) Slid the pants off the hip and buttock on the weak side.			
g. Slid the pants down the legs and over the feet.			
15. Dressed the person.			
16. Helped the person get out of bed if he or she was to be up. If the person stayed in bed:			
a. Covered the person and removed the bath blanket.			
b. Provided for comfort.			
c. Lowered the bed to its lowest position.			
d. Raised or lowered bed rails. Followed the care plan.			

Post-Procedure	S	U	Comments
17. Placed the signal light within reach.			
18. Unscreened the person.			
19. Followed agency policy for soiled clothing.			
20. Decontaminated hands.			
21. Reported and recorded observations.			

Date of Satisfactory Completion ______________________ Instructor's Initials ____________________

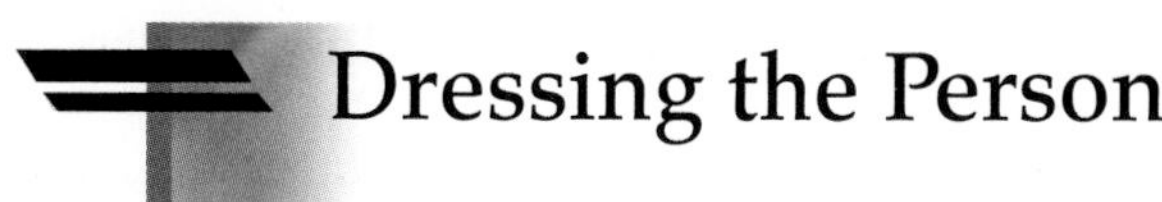

Dressing the Person

Name: ______________________

Date: ______________________

Pre-Procedure	S	U	Comments
• Knocked before entering the person's room.	______	______	______________
• Addressed the person by name.	______	______	______________
• Introduced yourself by name and title.	______	______	______________
1. Followed Delegation Guidelines.	______	______	______________
2. Explained the procedure to the person.	______	______	______________
3. Practiced hand hygiene.	______	______	______________
4. Got a bath blanket and clothing requested by the person.	______	______	______________
5. Identified the person. Checked the ID bracelet against the assignment sheet. Called the person by name.	______	______	______________
6. Provided for privacy.	______	______	______________
7. Raised the bed for body mechanics. Bed rails were up if used.	______	______	______________
8. Lowered the bed rail (if up) on the person's strong side.	______	______	______________
9. Undressed the person.	______	______	______________
10. Positioned the person supine.	______	______	______________
Procedure			
11. Covered the person with the bath blanket. Fanfolded linens to the foot of the bed.	______	______	______________
12. Put on garments that open in the back:	______	______	______________
a. Slid the garment onto the arm and shoulder of the weak side.	______	______	______________
b. Slid the garment onto the arm and shoulder of the strong side.	______	______	______________
c. Raised the person's head and shoulders.	______	______	______________
d. Brought the sides to the back.	______	______	______________
e. If the person was in a side-lying position:			
(1) Turned the person toward you.	______	______	______________
(2) Brought one side of the garment to the person's back.	______	______	______________
(3) Turned the person away from you.	______	______	______________
(4) Brought the other side to the person's back.	______	______	______________
f. Fastened buttons, snaps, ties, or zippers.	______	______	______________
g. Positioned the person supine.	______	______	______________
13. Put on garments that open in the front.	______	______	______________
a. Slid the garment onto the arm and shoulder on the weak side.	______	______	______________

Procedure—cont'd	S	U	Comments
b. Raised the head and shoulders. Brought the side of the garment around to the back. Lowered the person down. Slid the garment onto the arm and shoulder of the strong arm.			
c. If the person could not raise the head and shoulders:			
(1) Turned the person toward you.			
(2) Tucked the garment under the person.			
(3) Turned the person away from you.			
(4) Pulled the garment out from under the person.			
(5) Turned the person back to the supine position.			
(6) Slid the garment over the arm and shoulder of the strong arm.			
d. Fastened buttons, snaps, ties, or zippers.			
14. Put on pullover garments:			
a. Position the person supine.			
b. Brought the neck of the garment over the head.			
c. Slid the arm and shoulder of the garment onto the weak side.			
d. Raised the person's head and shoulders.			
e. Brought the garment down.			
f. Slid the arm and shoulder of the garment onto the strong side.			
g. If the person could not assume a semi-sitting position:			
(1) Turned the person toward you.			
(2) Tucked the garment under the person.			
(3) Turned the person away from you.			
(4) Pulled the garment out from under the person.			
(5) Positioned the person supine.			
(6) Slid the arm and shoulder of the garment onto the strong side.			
h. Fastened buttons, snaps, ties, or zippers.			
15. Put on pants or slacks:			
a. Slid the pants over the feet and up the legs.			
b. Asked the person to raise the hips and buttocks off the bed.			
c. Brought the pants up over the buttocks and hips.			
d. Asked the person to lower the hips and buttocks.			
e. If the person could not raise the hips and buttocks:			
(1) Turned person onto strong side.			
(2) Pulled the pants over the buttock and hip on the weak side.			
(3) Turned the person onto the weak side.			
(4) Pulled the pants over the buttock and hip on the strong side.			
(5) Positioned the person supine.			

Procedure—cont'd	S	U	Comments
f. Fastened buttons, ties, snaps, the zipper, and the belt buckle.	______	______	______________
16. Put socks and footwear on the person.	______	______	______________
17. Helped the person get out of bed. If the person stayed in bed:	______	______	______________
a. Covered the person and removed the bath blanket.	______	______	______________
b. Provided for comfort.	______	______	______________
c. Lowered the bed to its lowest position.	______	______	______________
d. Raised or lowered bed rails. Followed the care plan.	______	______	______________

Post-Procedure

18. Placed the signal light within reach.	______	______	______________
19. Unscreened the person.	______	______	______________
20. Followed agency policy for soiled clothing.	______	______	______________
21. Decontaminated hands.	______	______	______________
22. Reported and recorded observations.	______	______	______________

Date of Satisfactory Completion ______________ Instructor's Initials ______________

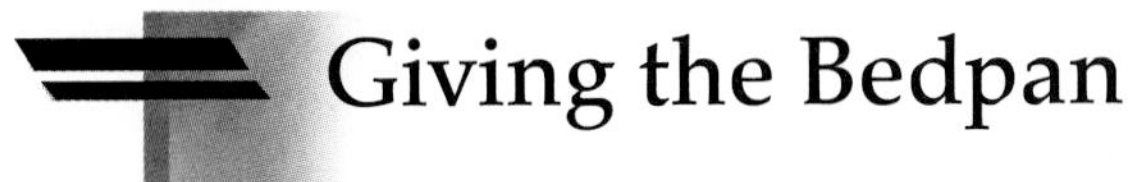

Giving the Bedpan

Name: ____________________

Date: ____________________

Pre-Procedure	S	U	Comments
• Knocked before entering the person's room.			
• Addressed the person by name.			
• Introduced yourself by name and title.			
1. Followed Delegation Guidelines. Reviewed Safety Alert.			
2. Provided for privacy.			
3. Practiced hand hygiene.			
4. Put on gloves.			
5. Collected the following:			
• Bedpan			
• Bedpan cover			
• Toilet tissue			
6. Arranged equipment on the chair or bed.			
7. Explained the procedure to the person.			

Procedure	S	U	Comments
8. Warmed and dried the bedpan if necessary.			
9. Lowered the bed rail near you if up.			
10. Positioned the person supine. Raised the head of the bed slightly.			
11. Folded the top linens and gown out of the way. Kept the lower body covered.			
12. Asked the person to flex the knees and raise the buttocks by pushing against the mattress with the feet.			
13. Slid your hand under the lower back. Helped raise the buttocks.			
14. Slid the bedpan under the person.			
15. If the person could not assist in getting on the bedpan:			
a. Turned the person onto the side away from you.			
b. Placed the bedpan firmly against the buttocks.			
c. Pushed the bedpan down and toward the person.			
d. Held the bedpan securely. Turned the person onto the back.			
e. Made sure the bedpan was centered under the person.			
16. Covered the person.			
17. Raised the head of the bed so the person was in a sitting position.			

Procedure—cont'd	S	U	Comments
18. Made sure the person was correctly positioned on the bedpan.			
19. Raised the bed rail if used.			
20. Placed the toilet tissue and signal light within reach.			
21. Asked the person to signal when done or when help was needed.			
22. Removed the gloves. Decontaminated hands.			
23. Left the room and closed the door.			
24. Returned when the person signaled. Knocked before entering.			
25. Decontaminated hands. Put on gloves.			
26. Raised the bed for body mechanics. Lowered the bed rail (if used) and the head of the bed.			
27. Asked the person to raise the buttocks. Removed the bedpan, or held the bedpan and turned the person onto the side away from you.			
28. Cleaned the genital area if the person could not do so. Cleaned from front to back with toilet tissue. Used fresh tissue for each wipe. Provided perineal care if needed.			
29. Covered the bedpan. Took it to the bathroom. Lowered the bed, and raised the bed rail (if used) before leaving the bedside.			
30. Noted the color, amount, and character of urine or feces.			
31. Emptied and rinsed the bedpan. Cleaned it with a disinfectant.			
32. Removed soiled gloves. Practiced hand hygiene and put on clean gloves.			
33. Returned the bedpan and clean cover to the bedside stand.			
34. Helped the person with handwashing.			
35. Removed the gloves. Decontaminated hands.			

Post-Procedure

	S	U	Comments
36. Provided for comfort.			
37. Placed the signal light within reach.			
38. Raised or lowered bed rails. Followed the care plan.			
39. Unscreened the person.			
40. Followed agency policy for soiled linen.			
41. Decontaminated hands.			
42. Reported and recorded observations.			

Date of Satisfactory Completion ____________________ Instructor's Initials ____________________

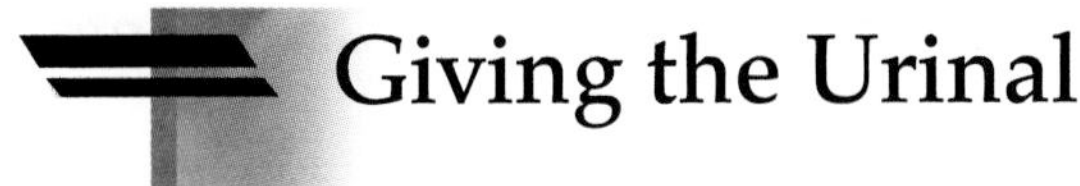

Giving the Urinal

Name: ______________________

Date: ______________________

Pre-Procedure	S	U	Comments
• Knocked before entering the person's room.			
• Addressed the person by name.			
• Introduced yourself by name and title.			
1. Followed Delegation Guidelines. Reviewed Safety Alert.			
2. Provided for privacy.			
3. Determined if the man would stand, sit, or lay in bed.			
4. Practiced hand hygiene.			
5. Put on gloves.			

Procedure

Procedure	S	U	Comments
6. Gave him the urinal if he was in bed. Reminded him to tilt the bottom down to prevent spills.			
7. If he was going to stand:			
a. Helped him sit on the side of the bed.			
b. Put nonskid footwear on him.			
c. Helped him stand. Provided support if he was unsteady.			
d. Gave him the urinal.			
8. Positioned the urinal if necessary. Positioned his penis in the urinal if he could not do so.			
9. Provided for privacy.			
10. Placed the signal light within reach. Asked him to signal when done or if he needs help.			
11. Removed the gloves. Decontaminated hands.			
12. Left the room and closed the door.			
13. Returned when he signaled. Knocked before entering.			
14. Decontaminated hands. Put on gloves.			
15. Closed the cap on the urinal. Took it to the bathroom.			
16. Noted the color, amount, and character of the urine.			
17. Emptied the urinal. Rinsed it with cold water. Cleaned it with a disinfectant.			
18. Returned the urinal to its proper place.			
19. Removed soiled gloves. Practiced hand hygiene and put on clean gloves.			
20. Assisted him with handwashing.			
21. Removed the gloves. Decontaminated hands.			

Post-Procedure	S	U	Comments
22. Provided for comfort.	______	______	____________________
23. Placed the signal light within reach.	______	______	____________________
24. Raised or lowered bed rails. Followed the care plan.	______	______	____________________
25. Unscreened him.	______	______	____________________
26. Followed agency policy for soiled linen.	______	______	____________________
27. Decontaminated hands.	______	______	____________________
28. Reported and recorded observations.	______	______	____________________

Date of Satisfactory Completion ____________________ Instructor's Initials ____________________

Helping the Person to the Commode

Name: ______________________

Date: ______________________

Pre-Procedure	S	U	Comments
• Knocked before entering the person's room.			
• Addressed the person by name.			
• Introduced yourself by name and title.			
1. Followed Delegation Guidelines. Reviewed Safety Alert.			
2. Explained the procedure to the person.			
3. Provided for privacy.			
4. Practiced hand hygiene.			
5. Put on gloves.			
6. Collected the following:			
• Commode			
• Toilet tissue			
• Bath blanket			
• Transfer belt			

Procedure

	S	U	Comments
7. Brought the commode next to the bed. Removed the chair seat and container lid.			
8. Helped the person sit on the side of the bed.			
9. Helped the person put on a robe and nonskid footwear.			
10. Assisted the person to the commode. Used the transfer belt.			
11. Covered the person with a bath blanket for warmth.			
12. Placed the toilet tissue and signal light within reach.			
13. Asked the person to signal when done or when help is needed. (Stayed with the person if necessary.)			
14. Removed the gloves. Decontaminated hands.			
15. Left the room. Closed the door.			
16. Returned when the person signaled. Knocked before entering.			
17. Decontaminated hands. Put on the gloves.			
18. Helped the person clean the genital area as needed. Removed the gloves, and practiced hand hygiene.			
19. Helped the person back to bed using the transfer belt. Removed the belt, robe, and footwear. Raised the bed rail if used.			
20. Put on clean gloves. Removed and covered the commode container. Cleaned the commode.			

Procedure—cont'd

Procedure—cont'd	S	U	Comments
21. Took the container to the bathroom.			
22. Checked urine and feces for color, amount, and character.			
23. Cleaned and disinfected the container.			
24. Returned the container to the commode. Returned other supplies to their proper place.			
25. Returned the commode to its proper place.			
26. Removed soiled gloves. Practiced hand hygiene and put on clean gloves.			
27. Assisted the person with handwashing.			
28. Removed the gloves. Decontaminated hands.			

Post-Procedure

Post-Procedure	S	U	Comments
29. Provided for comfort.			
30. Placed the signal light within reach.			
31. Raised or lowered bed rails. Followed the care plan.			
32. Unscreened the person.			
33. Followed agency policy for soiled linen.			
34. Decontaminated hands.			
35. Reported and recorded observations.			

Date of Satisfactory Completion ______________________ Instructor's Initials ______________________

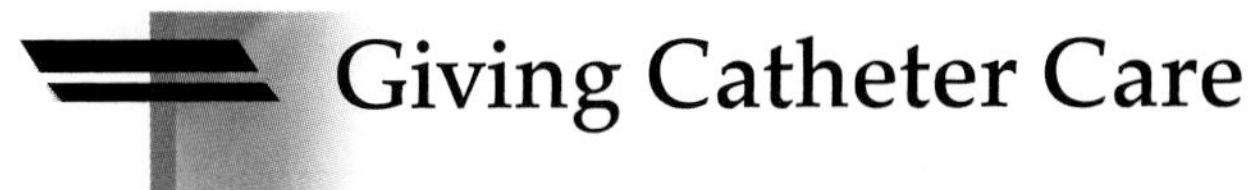

Giving Catheter Care

Name: ______________________

Date: ______________________

Pre-Procedure

	S	U	Comments
• Knocked before entering the person's room.			
• Addressed the person by name.			
• Introduced yourself by name and title.			
1. Followed Delegation Guidelines. Reviewed Safety Alert.			
2. Explained the procedure to the person.			
3. Practiced hand hygiene.			
4. Collected the following:			
• Items for perineal care			
• Gloves			
• Bed protector			
• Bath blanket			
5. Identified the person. Checked the ID bracelet against the assignment sheet. Called the person by name.			
6. Provided for privacy.			
7. Raised the bed for body mechanics. Bed rails were up if used.			

Procedure

	S	U	Comments
8. Lowered the bed rail near you if up.			
9. Put on the gloves.			
10. Covered the person with a bath blanket. Fanfolded top linens to the foot of the bed.			
11. Draped the person for perineal care.			
12. Folded back the bath blanket to expose the genital area.			
13. Placed the bed protector under the buttocks. Asked the person to flex the knees and raise the buttocks off the bed.			
14. Gave perineal care.			
15. Applied soap to a clean, wet washcloth.			
16. Separated the labia (female). In an uncircumcised male, retracted the foreskin. Checked for crusts, abnormal drainage, or secretions.			
17. Held the catheter near the meatus.			
18. Cleaned the catheter from the meatus down the catheter about 4 inches. Cleaned downward, away from the meatus with 1 stroke. Did not tug or pull on the catheter. Repeated as needed with a clean area of the washcloth. Used a clean washcloth if needed.			

Procedure—cont'd	S	U	Comments
19. Rinsed the catheter with a clean washcloth. Rinsed from the meatus down the catheter about 4 inches. Rinsed downward, away from the meatus with 1 stroke. Did not tug or pull on the catheter. Repeated as needed with a clean area of the washcloth. Used a clean washcloth if needed.			
20. Secured the catheter. Coiled and secured tubing.			
21. Removed the bed protector.			
22. Covered the person. Removed the bath blanket.			
23. Removed the gloves. Decontaminated hands.			

Post-Procedure

	S	U	Comments
24. Provided for comfort.			
25. Placed the signal light within reach.			
26. Raised or lowered bed rails. Followed the care plan.			
27. Lowered the bed to its lowest position.			
28. Cleaned and returned equipment to its proper place. Discarded disposable items. Wore gloves for this step.			
29. Removed the gloves. Decontaminated hands.			
30. Unscreened the person.			
31. Followed agency policy for soiled linen.			
32. Decontaminated hands.			
33. Reported and recorded observations.			

Date of Satisfactory Completion ____________________ Instructor's Initials ____________________

Changing a Leg Bag to a Drainage Bag

Name: ______________________

Date: ______________________

Pre-Procedure	S	U	Comments
• Knocked before entering the person's room.	___	___	___
• Addressed the person by name.	___	___	___
• Introduced yourself by name and title.	___	___	___
1. Followed Delegation Guidelines. Reviewed Safety Alert.	___	___	___
2. Explained the procedure to the person.	___	___	___
3. Practiced hand hygiene.	___	___	___
4. Collected the following:			
• Gloves	___	___	___
• Drainage bag and tubing	___	___	___
• Antiseptic wipes	___	___	___
• Bed protector	___	___	___
• Sterile cap and plug	___	___	___
• Catheter clamp	___	___	___
• Paper towels	___	___	___
• Bedpan	___	___	___
• Bath blanket	___	___	___
5. Arranged paper towels and equipment on the overbed table.	___	___	___
6. Identified the person. Checked the ID bracelet against the assignment sheet. Called the person by name.	___	___	___
7. Provided for privacy.	___	___	___

Procedure

	S	U	Comments
8. Had the person sit on the side of the bed.	___	___	___
9. Put on the gloves.	___	___	___
10. Exposed the catheter and leg bag.	___	___	___
11. Clamped the catheter.	___	___	___
12. Let urine drain from below the clamp site into the drainage tubing.	___	___	___
13. Helped the person lie down.	___	___	___
14. Raised the bed rails if used. Raised the bed for body mechanics.	___	___	___
15. Lowered the bed rail near you if up.	___	___	___
16. Covered the person with a bath blanket. Exposed the catheter and leg bag.	___	___	___
17. Placed the bed protector under the person's leg.	___	___	___

Procedure—cont'd	S	U	Comments
18. Opened the antiseptic wipes. Set them on the paper towels.			
19. Opened the package with the sterile cap and plug. Set the package on the paper towels. Did not let anything touch the sterile cap or plug.			
20. Opened the package with the drainage bag and tubing.			
21. Attached the drainage bag to the bed frame.			
22. Disconnected the catheter from the drainage tubing. Did not let anything touch the ends.			
23. Inserted the sterile plug into the catheter end. Only touched the end of the plug. Did not touch the part that goes inside the catheter. If the end of the catheter was contaminated, wiped the end with an antiseptic wipe before inserting the sterile plug.			
24. Placed the sterile cap on the end of the leg bag drainage tube. If the tubing end was contaminated, wiped the end with an antiseptic wipe before putting on the sterile cap.			
25. Removed the cap from the new drainage tubing.			
26. Removed the sterile plug from the catheter.			
27. Inserted the end for the drainage tubing into the catheter.			
28. Removed the clamp from the catheter.			
29. Looped drainage tubing on the bed. Secured tubing to the mattress.			
30. Removed the leg bag. Placed it in the bedpan.			
31. Removed and discarded the bed protector.			
32. Covered the person. Removed the bath blanket.			
33. Took the bedpan to the bathroom.			
34. Removed the gloves. Practiced hand hygiene.			

Post-Procedure

	S	U	Comments
35. Provided for comfort.			
36. Placed the signal light within reach.			
37. Raised or lowered bed rails. Followed the care plan.			
38. Lowered the bed to its lowest position.			
39. Unscreened the person.			
40. Put on clean gloves. Discarded disposable supplies.			
41. Emptied the drainage bag.			
42. Discarded the drainage tubing and bag following agency policy, or cleaned the bag following agency policy.			
43. Cleaned the bedpan. Placed it in a clean cover.			
44. Returned the bedpan and other supplies to their proper place.			
45. Removed the gloves. Decontaminated hands.			
46. Reported and recorded observations.			
47. Reversed the procedure to attach a leg bag to the catheter.			

Date of Satisfactory Completion ____________________ Instructor's Initials ____________________

Emptying a Urinary Drainage Bag

Name: ____________________

Date: ____________________

Pre-Procedure	S	U	Comments
• Knocked before entering the person's room.	___	___	___
• Addressed the person by name.	___	___	___
• Introduced yourself by name and title.	___	___	___
1. Followed Delegation Guidelines. Reviewed Safety Alert.	___	___	___
2. Collected equipment:			
• Graduate	___	___	___
• Gloves	___	___	___
• Paper towels	___	___	___
3. Practiced hand hygiene.	___	___	___
4. Explained the procedure to the person.	___	___	___
5. Identified the person. Checked the ID bracelet against the assignment sheet. Called the person by name.	___	___	___
6. Provided for privacy.	___	___	___
Procedure			
7. Put on the gloves.	___	___	___
8. Placed a paper towel on the floor. Placed the graduate on top of it.	___	___	___
9. Positioned the graduate under the collection bag.	___	___	___
10. Opened the clamp on the drain.	___	___	___
11. Let all urine drain into the graduate. Did not let the drain touch the graduate.	___	___	___
12. Closed and positioned the clamp.	___	___	___
13. Measured urine.	___	___	___
14. Removed and discarded the paper towel.	___	___	___
15. Rinsed the graduate. Returned it to its proper place.	___	___	___
16. Removed the gloves. Practiced hand hygiene.	___	___	___
17. Recorded the time and amount on the intake and output (I&O) record.	___	___	___
Post-Procedure			
18. Unscreened the person.	___	___	___
19. Reported and recorded the amount and other observations.	___	___	___

Date of Satisfactory Completion ____________________ Instructor's Initials ____________________

ADVANCED

Inserting a Straight Catheter

Name: ______________________

Date: ______________________

Pre-Procedure

	S	U	Comments
• Knocked before entering the person's room.			
• Addressed the person by name.			
• Introduced yourself by name and title.			
1. Followed Delegation Guidelines. Reviewed Safety Alert.			
2. Explained the procedure to the person.			
3. Practiced hand hygiene.			
4. Collected the following:			
• Straight catheterization kit			
• Flashlight or diagnostic lamp			
• Bath blanket			
• Soap			
• Wash basin with warm water			
• Washcloth and towel			
• Disposable gloves			
• Laboratory requisition slip (if a urine specimen is ordered)			
5. Identified the person. Checked the ID bracelet against the assignment sheet. Called the person by name.			
6. Provided for privacy.			
7. Raised the bed for body mechanics. Bed rails were up if used.			

Procedure

	S	U	Comments
8. Lowered the bed rail near you if up.			
9. Positioned the person supine. Covered the person with a bath blanket.			
10. Positioned and draped the person for perineal care.			
11. Put on the disposable gloves. Gave perineal care.			
12. Found the female meatus.			
13. Removed equipment and supplies used for perineal care. Removed the gloves, and decontaminated hands. (If you left the bedside, both bed rails were up if used. Lowered the bed rail near you when returning.)			
14. Positioned the flashlight or diagnostic lamp at the foot of the bed. Directed the light at the perineal area.			
15. Opened the plastic cover on the catheterization kit. Positioned the cover at the foot of the bed.			

Procedure—cont'd	S	U	Comments
16. Positioned the kit so it could be reached with ease. It was placed where it would not contaminate the sterile field.	______	______	______
17. Opened the kit. Followed directions on the package.	______	______	______
18. Put on the sterile gloves.	______	______	______
19. Organized the sterile field:	______	______	______
a. Opened sterile packages and containers (cotton balls, antiseptic solution, specimen container, lubricant).	______	______	______
b. Poured the antiseptic solution over the cotton balls.	______	______	______
c. Opened the specimen container.	______	______	______
20. Picked up the sterile waterproof pad. Stood back and let it unfold.	______	______	______
21. Positioned the waterproof pad:	______	______	______
a. For a female:			
(1) Held the pad with both hands.	______	______	______
(2) Did not touch anything but the pad.	______	______	______
(3) Cuffed the pad around the gloves.	______	______	______
(4) Asked the person to raise her buttocks off the bed.	______	______	______
(5) Slid the drape under her buttocks.	______	______	______
b. For a male:			
(1) Lifted the penis with the non-dominant hand.	______	______	______
(2) Laid the drape over the thighs.	______	______	______
(3) Laid the penis on the pad.	______	______	______
22. Draped the person:	______	______	______
a. For a female:			
(1) Picked up the fenestrated drape. Let it unfold.	______	______	______
(2) Draped it over the perineum. Exposed only the labia.	______	______	______
b. For a male:			
(1) Positioned the drape over the penis.	______	______	______
(2) Lifted the penis through the opening in the drape. Used the non-dominant hand. Laid the penis on the drape.	______	______	______
23. Placed the tray and its contents on the drape between the person's legs.	______	______	______
24. Lubricated the catheter:	______	______	______
a. Female—lubricated about 1 to 2 inches of the catheter tip.	______	______	______
b. Male—lubricated about 2 to 6 inches of the catheter tip.	______	______	______
25. Cleaned the meatus. Used a sterile cotton ball for each stroke. Discarded used cotton balls into the plastic cover. Did not let the forceps touch the cover.	______	______	______
a. For a female:			
(1) Separated the labia majora. Used the thumb and index finger of the non-dominant hand.	______	______	______
(2) Kept the labia separated until the catheter was inserted.	______	______	______

Procedure—cont'd	S	U	Comments
(3) Used the sterile gloved hand to pick up the forceps.			
(4) Picked up a cotton ball with the forceps.			
(5) Cleaned the labia minora on the side away from you. Wiped from the clitoris to the anus with one stroke. Discarded the cotton ball.			
(6) Picked up another cotton ball.			
(7) Cleaned the labia minora on the side near you. Wiped from the clitoris to the anus with one stroke. Discarded the cotton ball.			
(8) Picked up another cotton ball.			
(9) Cleaned the meatus. Wiped from the top down. Discarded the cotton ball.			
b. For a male:			
(1) Picked up the penis with the contaminated hand			
(2) Retracted the foreskin if the man was not circumcised.			
(3) Held the penis firmly behind the glans. Maintained this position until the catheter was inserted.			
(4) Picked up a cotton ball using sterile forceps.			
(5) Cleaned the meatus. Used a circular motion. Discarded the cotton ball.			
(6) Picked up another cotton ball.			
(7) Wiped around the meatus using a circular motion. Discarded the cotton ball.			
(8) Picked up another cotton ball.			
(9) Cleaned to where the fingers were holding the penis. Used a circular motion. Discarded the cotton ball.			
26. Placed the drainage end of the catheter into the urine basin.			
27. Picked up the catheter about 2 inches from the tip. Made sure the drainage end stayed in the urine basin.			
28. Inserted the catheter:			
a. Female:			
(1) Found the meatus and the vaginal opening.			
(2) Asked the person to take a deep breath.			
(3) Inserted the catheter into the meatus until urine flowed (about 3 inches). Inserted gently and slowly. (Did not force the catheter.)			
(4) Held the catheter in place with the contaminated hand.			
b. Male:			
(1) Held the penis so it is upright.			
(2) Asked the person to bear down as if voiding.			
(3) Inserted the catheter into the meatus. (Did not force the catheter.)			

Procedure—cont'd

Procedure—cont'd	S	U	Comments
(4) Advanced the catheter until urine flowed.			
(5) Laid the penis on the drape. Held the catheter in place with the contaminated hand.			
29. Collected a urine specimen if ordered. Continued to hold the catheter in place with the contaminated hand:			
a. Held the catheter over the specimen container with the sterile hand. Collected about 30 ml of urine.			
b. Pinched the catheter to stop the flow of urine.			
c. Covered the specimen container. Set it aside.			
30. Placed the end of the catheter into the urine basin.			
31. Let the bladder empty according to the nurse's instructions.			
32. Noted the amount of urine collected.			
33. Removed the catheter slowly. Discarded it into the cover.			
34. Returned foreskin to its natural position.			
35. Discarded equipment and supplies into the cover.			
36. Removed the gloves. Decontaminated hands.			
37. Covered the person. Removed the bath blanket.			

Post-Procedure

Post-Procedure	S	U	Comments
38. Provided for comfort.			
39. Placed the signal light within reach.			
40. Raised or lowered bed rails. Followed the care plan.			
41. Lowered the bed to its lowest position.			
42. Unscreened the person.			
43. Put on disposable gloves.			
44. Cleaned the wash basin. Returned usable supplies to their proper place.			
45. Followed agency policy for soiled linen.			
46. Decontaminated hands.			
47. Reported and recorded observations.			

Date of Satisfactory Completion ____________ Instructor's Initials ____________

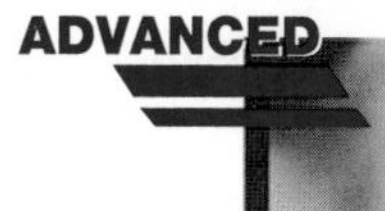

Inserting an Indwelling Catheter

Name: ______________________

Date: ______________________

Pre-Procedure	**S**	**U**	**Comments**
• Knocked before entering the person's room.			
• Addressed the person by name.			
• Introduced yourself by name and title.			
1. Followed Delegation Guidelines. Reviewed Safety Alert.			
2. Explained the procedure to the person.			
3. Practiced hand hygiene.			
4. Collected the following:			
• Indwelling catheterization kit			
• Flashlight or diagnostic lamp			
• Bath blanket			
• Soap			
• Wash basin with warm water			
• Washcloth and towel			
• Disposable gloves			
• Non-allergenic tape			
• Clip, tape, or safety pin and rubber band			
5. Identified the person. Checked the ID bracelet against the assignment sheet. Called the person by name.			
6. Provided for privacy.			
7. Raised the bed for body mechanics. Bed rails were up if used.			

Procedure	**S**	**U**	**Comments**
8. Followed steps 8 through 19 in procedure: *Inserting a Straight Catheter.*			
9. Checked the drainage system. Made sure that the:			
a. Catheter was attached to the drainage tubing.			
b. Drainage tubing was attached to the drainage bag.			
c. The drain was closed.			
10. Tested the balloon on the indwelling catheter. It inflated and did not leak:			
a. Attached the pre-filled syringe to the balloon port.			
b. Injected the water. The balloon inflated.			
c. Pulled back on the syringe to withdraw the fluid.			
d. Left the syringe attached to the balloon port.			

Procedure—cont'd	S	U	Comments
11. Positioned the waterproof pad.	______	______	______
12. Draped the person.	______	______	______
13. Placed the tray and its contents on the drape between the person's legs.	______	______	______
14. Lubricated the catheter.	______	______	______
15. Cleaned the meatus.	______	______	______
16. Inserted the catheter until urine appeared.	______	______	______
17. Advanced the catheter another 2 inches after urine appeared.	______	______	______
18. Held the catheter in place with the non-dominant hand.	______	______	______
19. Inflated the balloon by injecting the contents of the syringe. (Pulled back on the syringe if the person complained of pain. Inserted the catheter further and injected fluid again.	______	______	______
20. Removed the syringe from the balloon port.	______	______	______
21. Pulled back on the catheter gently and felt resistance.	______	______	______
22. Returned foreskin to its natural position.	______	______	______
23. Secured the catheter in place. Used the clip, tape, or safety pin and rubber band. Allowed enough slack so there was no pull on the catheter.	______	______	______
a. Female—taped the catheter to the inner thigh.	______	______	______
b. Male—taped the catheter to the thigh or lower abdomen.	______	______	______
24. Secured the drainage bag to the bed frame.	______	______	______
25. Coiled tubing on the bed.	______	______	______
26. Noted the amount of urine in the drainage bag.	______	______	______

Post-Procedure

	S	U	Comments
27. Followed steps 35 through 47 in procedure: *Inserting a Straight Catheter.*	______	______	______

Date of Satisfactory Completion ______________ Instructor's Initials ______________

ADVANCED

Removing an Indwelling Catheter

Name: ______________________

Date: ______________________

Pre-Procedure	S	U	Comments
• Knocked before entering the person's room.			
• Addressed the person by name.			
• Introduced yourself by name and title.			
1. Followed Delegation Guidelines. Reviewed Safety Alert.			
2. Explained the procedure to the person.			
3. Practiced hand hygiene.			
4. Collected the following:			
• Disposable towel			
• Syringe as directed by the nurse			
• Disposable bag			
• Gloves			
• Bath blanket			
5. Identified the person. Checked the ID bracelet against the assignment sheet. Called the person by name.			
6. Provided for privacy.			
7. Raised the bed for body mechanics. Bed rails were up if used.			

Procedure	S	U	Comments
8. Lowered the bed rail near you if up.			
9. Positioned the person as for a catheterization.			
10. Covered the person with a bath blanket.			
11. Put on the gloves.			
12. Removed the tape securing the catheter to the person.			
13. Positioned the towel:			
a. Female—between her legs.			
b. Male—over his thighs.			
14. Attached the syringe to the balloon port.			
15. Pulled back on the syringe slowly. Withdrew all water from the balloon. (Called for a nurse if could not remove all the water.)			
16. Removed the catheter gently.			
17. Discarded the catheter into the plastic bag.			
18. Dried the perineal area with the towel. Discarded the towel in the bag.			
19. Removed the gloves. Decontaminated hands.			
20. Covered the person. Removed the bath blanket.			

Post-Procedure	S	U	Comments
21. Provided for comfort.	______	______	______________________
22. Placed the signal light within reach.	______	______	______________________
23. Raised or lowered bed rails. Followed the care plan.	______	______	______________________
24. Lowered the bed to its lowest position.	______	______	______________________
25. Unscreened the person.	______	______	______________________
26. Put on gloves.	______	______	______________________
27. Took the drainage bag to the bathroom.	______	______	______________________
28. Measured the amount of urine in the drainage bag. Noted the amount.	______	______	______________________
29. Discarded the urine.	______	______	______________________
30. Placed the drainage bag in the plastic bag. Discarded the bag.	______	______	______________________
31. Removed the gloves. Decontaminated hands.	______	______	______________________
32. Reported and recorded observations.	______	______	______________________

Date of Satisfactory Completion ______________________ Instructor's Initials ____________________

Applying a Condom Catheter

Name: ____________________

Date: ____________________

Pre-Procedure	S	U	Comments
• Knocked before entering the person's room.	____	____	____________
• Addressed the person by name.	____	____	____________
• Introduced yourself by name and title.	____	____	____________
1. Followed Delegation Guidelines. Reviewed Safety Alert.	____	____	____________
2. Explained the procedure to the man.	____	____	____________
3. Practiced hand hygiene.	____	____	____________
4. Collected the following:			
• Condom catheter	____	____	____________
• Elastic tape	____	____	____________
• Drainage bag or leg bag	____	____	____________
• Cap for the drainage bag	____	____	____________
• Basin of warm water	____	____	____________
• Soap	____	____	____________
• Towel and washcloths	____	____	____________
• Bath blanket	____	____	____________
• Gloves	____	____	____________
• Bed protector	____	____	____________
• Paper towels	____	____	____________
5. Arranged paper towels and equipment on the overbed table.	____	____	____________
6. Provided for privacy.	____	____	____________
7. Identified the person. Checked the ID bracelet against the assignment sheet. Called the person by name.	____	____	____________
8. Raised the bed for body mechanics. Bed rails were up if used.	____	____	____________

Procedure	S	U	Comments
9. Lowered the bed rail near you if up.	____	____	____________
10. Covered the person with a bath blanket. Lowered top linens to the knees.	____	____	____________
11. Asked the person to raise his buttocks off the bed or turned him onto his side away from you.	____	____	____________
12. Slid the bed protector under his buttocks.	____	____	____________
13. Had the person lower his buttocks or turned him onto his back.	____	____	____________
14. Secured the drainage bag to the bed frame or had a leg bag ready. Closed the drain.	____	____	____________

Procedure—cont'd

	S	U	Comments
15. Exposed the genital area.			
16. Put on the gloves.			
17. Removed the condom catheter:			
a. Removed the tape. Rolled the sheath off the penis.			
b. Disconnected the drainage tubing from the condom. Capped the drainage tube.			
c. Discarded the tape and condom.			
18. Provided perineal care. Observed the penis for reddened areas and skin breakdown or irritation.			
19. Removed the protective backing from the condom.			
20. Held the penis firmly. Rolled the condom onto the penis. Left a 1-inch space between the penis and the end of the catheter.			
21. Secured the condom with elastic tape. Applied tape in a spiral. Did not apply tape completely around the penis.			
22. Connected the condom to the drainage tubing. Coiled excess tubing on the bed or attached a leg bag.			
23. Removed the bed protector and gloves. Discarded them. Practiced hand hygiene.			
24. Covered the person. Removed the bath blanket.			

Post-Procedure

	S	U	Comments
25. Provided for comfort.			
26. Placed the signal light within reach.			
27. Raised or lowered bed rails. Followed the care plan.			
28. Lowered the bed to its lowest position.			
29. Unscreened the person.			
30. Decontaminated hands. Put on clean gloves.			
31. Measured and recorded the amount of urine in the bag. Cleaned or discarded the collection bag.			
32. Cleaned and returned the wash basin and other equipment. Returned items to their proper place.			
33. Removed the gloves. Decontaminated hands.			
34. Reported and recorded observations.			

Date of Satisfactory Completion ____________ Instructor's Initials ____________

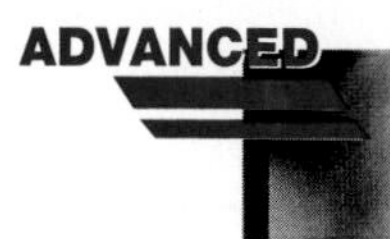

Checking for a Fecal Impaction

Name: ______________________

Date: ______________________

Pre-Procedure	S	U	Comments
• Knocked before entering the person's room.			
• Addressed the person by name.			
• Introduced yourself by name and title.			
1. Followed Delegation Guidelines. Reviewed Safety Alert.			
2. Explained the procedure to the person.			
3. Practiced hand hygiene.			
4. Collected the following:			
• Bedpan and cover			
• Bath blanket			
• Toilet tissue			
• Gloves			
• Lubricant			
• Waterproof pad			
• Basin of warm water			
• Soap			
• Washcloth			
• Bath towel			
5. Identified the person. Checked the ID bracelet against the assignment sheet. Called the person by name.			
6. Provided for privacy.			
7. Raised the bed for body mechanics. Bed rails were up if used.			

Procedure	S	U	Comments
8. Lowered the bed rail near you if up.			
9. Covered the person with a bath blanket. Fanfolded top linens to the foot of the bed.			
10. Positioned the person in Sins' position or in a left side-lying position.			
11. Put on the gloves.			
12. Placed the waterproof pad under the buttocks.			
13. Exposed the anal area.			
14. Lubricated the gloved index finger.			
15. Asked the person to take a deep breath through his or her mouth.			
16. Inserted the gloved finger while the person was taking a deep breath.			

Procedure—cont'd	S	U	Comments
17. Checked for a fecal mass.			
18. Removed the finger.			
19. Removed and discarded the gloves. Practiced hand hygiene.			
20. Put on clean gloves.			
21. Helped the person onto the bedpan or to the bathroom or commode if needed. Provided for privacy.			
22. Removed and discarded the gloves.			
23. Practiced hand hygiene.			
24. Washed the person's anal area with soap and water. Patted dry.			
25. Removed the waterproof pad and gloves. Decontaminated hands.			
26. Provided for comfort.			

Post-Procedure

	S	U	Comments
27. Covered the person. Removed the bath blanket.			
28. Placed the signal light within reach.			
29. Lowered the bed to its lowest position.			
30. Raised or lowered bed rails. Followed the care plan.			
31. Unscreened the person.			
32. Cleaned and returned equipment to its proper place. Discarded disposable items. Wore gloves.			
33. Followed agency policy for soiled linen.			
34. Removed the gloves. Practiced hand hygiene.			
35. Reported and recorded observations.			

Date of Satisfactory Completion ____________________ Instructor's Initials ____________________

ADVANCED

Removing a Fecal Impaction

Name: ______________________

Date: ______________________

Pre-Procedure	**S**	**U**	**Comments**
• Knocked before entering the person's room.	____	____	________________
• Addressed the person by name.	____	____	________________
• Introduced yourself by name and title.	____	____	________________

Procedure

1. Followed steps 1 through 12 in procedure: *Checking for a Fecal Impaction.*	____	____	________________
2. Checked the person's pulse. Noted the rate and rhythm.	____	____	________________
3. Exposed the anal area.	____	____	________________
4. Lubricated the gloved index finger.	____	____	________________
5. Asked the person to take a deep breath through the mouth.	____	____	________________
6. Inserted the lubricated, gloved index finger.	____	____	________________
7. Hooked the index finger around a small piece of feces.	____	____	________________
8. Removed the finger and the feces.	____	____	________________
9. Dropped the feces into the bedpan.	____	____	________________
10. Cleaned the finger with toilet tissue. Placed the toilet tissue in the bed pan.	____	____	________________
11. Reapplied lubricant as needed.	____	____	________________
12. Repeated steps 5 through 10 until feces was no longer felt.	____	____	________________
13. Checked the person's pulse at intervals. Used a clean gloved hand. Noted the rate and rhythm. Stopped the procedure if the pulse rate has slowed or if the rhythm was irregular.	____	____	________________
14. Wiped the anal area with toilet tissue.	____	____	________________
15. Covered the person with the bath blanket.	____	____	________________
16. Covered the bedpan.	____	____	________________
17. Removed and discarded the gloves. Practiced hand hygiene and put on clean gloves.	____	____	________________
18. Raised the bed rail if used. Took the bedpan to the bathroom.	____	____	________________
19. Emptied, cleaned, and disinfected the bedpan.	____	____	________________
20. Returned the bedpan to the bedside stand.	____	____	________________
21. Removed and discarded the gloves. Practiced hand hygiene.	____	____	________________
22. Filled the wash basin with warm water.	____	____	________________
23. Lowered the bed rail near you if up.	____	____	________________
24. Put on clean gloves.	____	____	________________

Procedure—cont'd	S	U	Comments
25. Washed the buttocks and gave perineal care.	_____	_____	_____
26. Removed the waterproof pad and the gloves. Practiced hand hygiene.	_____	_____	_____

Post-Procedure

27. Provided for comfort.	_____	_____	_____
28. Covered the person and removed the bath blanket.	_____	_____	_____
29. Placed the signal light within reach.	_____	_____	_____
30. Lowered the bed to its lowest position.	_____	_____	_____
31. Raised or lowered bed rails. Followed the care plan.	_____	_____	_____
32. Unscreened the person.	_____	_____	_____
33. Cleaned and returned equipment to its proper place. Discarded disposable items. Wore gloves.	_____	_____	_____
34. Followed agency policy for soiled linen.	_____	_____	_____
35. Removed the gloves. Decontaminated hands.	_____	_____	_____
36. Reported and recorded observations.	_____	_____	_____

Date of Satisfactory Completion _____ Instructor's Initials _____

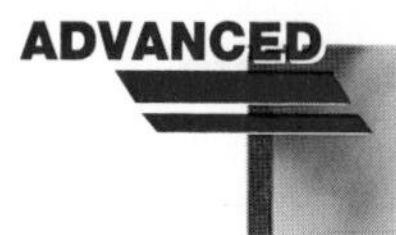

Giving a Cleansing Enema

Name: ______________________

Date: ______________________

Pre-Procedure

	S	U	Comments
• Knocked before entering the person's room.	____	____	____
• Addressed the person by name.	____	____	____
• Introduced yourself by name and title.	____	____	____
1. Followed Delegation Guidelines. Reviewed Safety Alert.	____	____	____
2. Explained the procedure to the person.	____	____	____
3. Practiced hand hygiene.	____	____	____
4. Collected the following:			
• Bedpan or commode	____	____	____
• Disposable enema kit as directed by the nurse (enema bag, tube, clamp, and waterproof pad)	____	____	____
• Bath thermometer	____	____	____
• Waterproof pad	____	____	____
• Water-soluble lubricant	____	____	____
• Gloves	____	____	____
• 3 to 5 ml (1 teaspoon) castile soap or 1 to 2 teaspoons of salt	____	____	____
• Toilet tissue	____	____	____
• Bath blanket	____	____	____
• IV pole	____	____	____
• Robe and nonskid footwear	____	____	____
• Paper towels	____	____	____
5. Identified the person. Checked the ID bracelet with the assignment sheet. Called the person by name.	____	____	____
6. Provided for privacy.	____	____	____
7. Raised the bed for body mechanics. Bed rails were up if used.	____	____	____

Procedure

	S	U	Comments
8. Lowered the bed rail near you if up.	____	____	____
9. Covered the person with a bath blanket. Fanfolded top linens to the foot of the bed.	____	____	____
10. Positioned the IV pole so the enema bag was 12 inches above the anus, or it was at a height directed by the nurse.	____	____	____
11. Raised the bed rail if used.	____	____	____
12. Prepared the enema:	____	____	____
a. Closed the clamp on the tube.	____	____	____
b. Adjusted water flow until it was lukewarm.	____	____	____

Procedure—cont'd	S	U	Comments
c. Filled the enema bag for the amount ordered.			
d. Measured water temperature with the bath thermometer.			
e. Prepared the enema solution as directed by the nurse:			
(1) Saline enema: added 1 to 2 teaspoons of salt			
(2) Soapsuds enema: added 3 to 5 ml (1 teaspoon) of castile soap			
(3) Tap-water enema: added nothing to the water			
f. Stirred the solution with the bath thermometer. Scooped off any suds (SSE).			
g. Sealed the bag.			
h. Hung the bag on the IV pole.			
13. Lowered the bed rail near you.			
14. Positioned the person in Sins' position or in a left side-lying position.			
15. Put on the gloves.			
16. Placed a waterproof pad under the buttocks.			
17. Exposed the anal area.			
18. Placed the bedpan behind the person.			
19. Positioned the enema tube in the bedpan. Removed the cap from the tubing.			
20. Opened the clamp. Let solution flow through the tube to remove air. Clamped the tube.			
21. Lubricated the tube 3 to 4 inches from the tip.			
22. Separated the buttocks to see the anus.			
23. Asked the person to take a deep breath through the mouth.			
24. Inserted the tube gently 3 to 4 inches into the adult's rectum. Did this when the person was exhaling. Stopped if the person complained of pain, resistance was felt, or bleeding occurred.			
25. Checked the amount of solution in the bag.			
26. Unclasped the tube. Gave the solution slowly.			
27. Asked the person to take slow deep breaths.			
28. Clamped the tube if the person needed to defecate, had cramping, or started to expel solution. Unclasped when symptoms subsided.			
29. Gave the amount of solution ordered. Stopped if the person could not tolerate the procedure.			
30. Clamped the tube before it was empty.			
31. Held toilet tissue around the tube and against the anus. Removed the tube.			
32. Discarded the toilet tissue into the bedpan.			
33. Wrapped the tubing tip with paper towels. Placed it inside the enema bag.			

Procedure—cont'd	S	U	Comments
34. Helped the person onto the bedpan. Raised the head of the bed, and raised the bed rail if used. Assisted the person to the bathroom or commode. The person wore a robe and nonskid footwear. The bed was in the lowest position.			
35. Placed the signal light and toilet tissue within reach. Reminded the person not to flush the toilet.			
36. Discarded disposable items.			
37. Removed the gloves. Decontaminated hands.			
38. Left the room if the person could be left alone.			
39. Returned when the person signaled. Knocked before entering.			
40. Decontaminated hands and put on gloves. Lowered the bed rail if up.			
41. Observed enema results for amount, color, consistency, and odor. Called for the nurse to observe the results.			
42. Provided perineal care as needed.			
43. Removed the bed protector.			
44. Emptied, cleaned, and disinfected the bedpan or commode. Flushed the toilet after the nurse observed the results. Returned items to their proper place.			
45. Removed the gloves. Practiced hand hygiene.			
46. Assisted with handwashing. Wore gloves if needed.			
47. Covered the person. Removed the bath blanket.			

Post-Procedure

	S	U	Comments
48. Provided for comfort.			
49. Placed the signal light within reach.			
50. Lowered the bed to its lowest position.			
51. Raised or lowered bed rails. Followed the care plan.			
52. Unscreened the person.			
53. Followed agency policy for soiled linen and used supplies. Wore gloves if necessary.			
54. Removed the gloves. Decontaminated hands.			
55. Reported and recorded observations.			

Date of Satisfactory Completion ____________ Instructor's Initials ____________

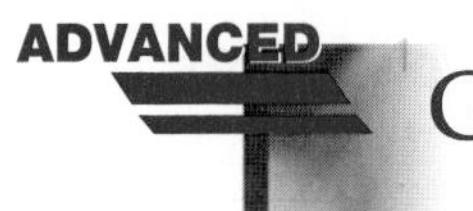

Giving a Small-Volume Enema

Name: ______________________

Date: ______________________

Pre-Procedure	S	U	Comments
• Knocked before entering the person's room.			
• Addressed the person by name.			
• Introduced yourself by name and title.			
1. Followed Delegation Guidelines. Reviewed Safety Alert.			
2. Explained the procedure to the person.			
3. Practiced hand hygiene.			
4. Collected the following:			
• Small-volume enema			
• Bedpan or commode			
• Waterproof pad			
• Toilet tissue			
• Gloves			
• Robe and nonskid footwear			
• Bath blanket			
5. Identified the person. Checked the ID bracelet against the treatment card. Called the person by name.			
6. Provided for privacy.			
7. Raised the bed for body mechanics. Bed rails were up if used.			

Procedure	S	U	Comments
8. Lowered the bed rail near you if up.			
9. Covered the person with a bath blanket. Fanfolded top linens to the foot of the bed.			
10. Positioned the person in Sins' or a left side-lying position.			
11. Put on the gloves.			
12. Placed the waterproof pad under the buttocks.			
13. Exposed the anal area.			
14. Positioned the bedpan near the person.			
15. Removed the cap from the enema.			
16. Separated the buttocks to see the anus.			
17. Asked the person to take a deep breath through the mouth.			
18. Inserted the enema tip 2 inches into the rectum. Did this when the person was exhaling. Inserted the tip gently. Stopped if the person complained of pain, resistance was felt, or bleeding occurred.			

Procedure—cont'd	S	U	Comments
19. Squeezed and rolled the bottle gently. Released pressure on the bottle after the tip was removed from the rectum.			
20. Put the bottle into the box, tip first.			
21. Helped the person onto the bedpan; raised the head of the bed. Raised or lowered bed rails according to the care plan, or assisted the person to the bathroom or commode. The person wore a robe and nonskid footwear. The bed was in the lowest position.			
22. Placed the signal light and toilet tissue within reach. Reminded the person not to flush the toilet.			
23. Discarded disposable items.			
24. Removed the gloves. Decontaminated hands.			
25. Left the room if the person could be left alone.			
26. Returned when the person signaled. Knocked before entering.			
27. Decontaminated hands. Lowered the bed rail if up.			
28. Put on gloves.			
29. Observed enema results for amount, color, consistency, and odor.			
30. Helped the person with perineal care.			
31. Removed the bed protector.			
32. Emptied, cleaned, and disinfected the bedpan or commode. Flushed the toilet after the nurse observed the results.			
33. Returned equipment to its proper place.			
34. Removed the gloves. Practiced hand hygiene.			
35. Assisted the person with hand washing. Wore gloves if necessary.			
36. Returned top linens. Removed the bath blanket.			

Post-Procedure

	S	U	Comments
37. Followed steps 48 through 55 in procedure: *Giving a Cleansing Enema.*			

Date of Satisfactory Completion ____________ Instructor's Initials ____________

ADVANCED

Giving an Oil-Retention Enema

Name: ______________________

Date: ______________________

Pre-Procedure	S	U	Comments
• Knocked before entering the person's room.	____	____	____________
• Addressed the person by name.	____	____	____________
• Introduced yourself by name and title.	____	____	____________
1. Followed Delegation Guidelines. Reviewed Safety Alert.	____	____	____________
2. Explained the procedure to the person.	____	____	____________
3. Practiced hand hygiene.	____	____	____________
4. Collected the following:			
• Oil-retention enema	____	____	____________
• Waterproof pads	____	____	____________
• Gloves	____	____	____________
• Bath blanket	____	____	____________
5. Identified the person. Checked the ID bracelet against the assignment sheet. Called the person by name.	____	____	____________
6. Provided for privacy.	____	____	____________
7. Raised the bed for body mechanics. Bed rails were up if used.	____	____	____________
Procedure			
8. Followed steps 8 through 20 in procedure: *Giving a Small-Volume Enema.*	____	____	____________
9. Covered the person. Left the person in the Sins' or side-lying position.	____	____	____________
10. Encouraged the person to retain the enema for the time ordered.	____	____	____________
11. Placed more waterproof pads on the bed if needed.	____	____	____________
12. Removed the gloves. Decontaminate hands.	____	____	____________
13. Lowered the bed to its lowest position.	____	____	____________
14. Raised or lowered bed rails. Followed the care plan.	____	____	____________
15. Provided for comfort.	____	____	____________
16. Placed the signal light within reach.	____	____	____________
17. Unscreened the person.	____	____	____________
18. Decontaminated hands.	____	____	____________
19. Checked the person often.	____	____	____________
Post-Procedure			
20. Followed steps 48 through 55 in procedure: *Giving a Cleansing Enema.*	____	____	____________

Date of Satisfactory Completion ______________ Instructor's Initials ______________

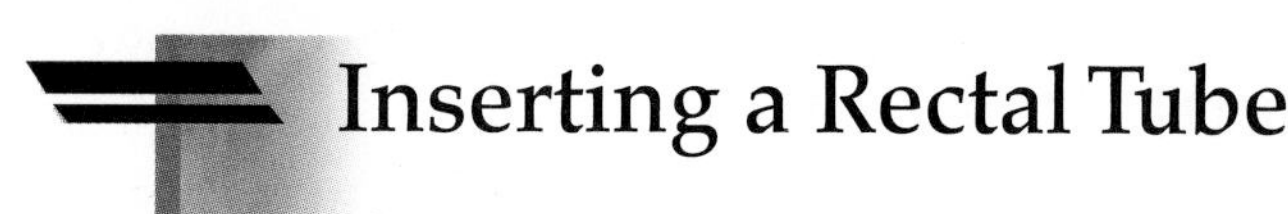

Inserting a Rectal Tube

Name: ______________________

Date: ______________________

Pre-Procedure	S	U	Comments
• Knocked before entering the person's room.			
• Addressed the person by name.			
• Introduced yourself by name and title.			
1. Followed Delegation Guidelines. Reviewed Safety Alert.			
2. Explained the procedure to the person.			
3. Practiced hand hygiene.			
4. Collected the following:			
• Disposable rectal tube with flatus bag			
• Water-soluble lubricant			
• Tape			
• Gloves			
• Waterproof pad			
5. Identified the person. Checked the ID bracelet against the assignment sheet. Called the person by name.			
6. Provided for privacy.			
7. Raised the bed for body mechanics. Bed rails were up if used.			

Procedure	S	U	Comments
8. Lowered the bed rail near you if up.			
9. Positioned the person in Sins' or a left side-lying position.			
10. Put on the gloves.			
11. Placed the waterproof pad under the buttocks.			
12. Exposed the anal area.			
13. Lubricated 4 inches from the tube tip.			
14. Separated the buttocks to see the anus.			
15. Asked the person to take a deep breath through the mouth.			
16. Inserted the tube 4 inches into the rectum. Did this when the person was exhaling. Inserted the tube gently. Stopped if person complained of pain, resistance was felt, or bleeding occurred.			
17. Taped the rectal tube to the thigh.			
18. Positioned the flatus bag so it rests on the bed protector.			
19. Covered the person.			
20. Left the tube in place for the time directed by the nurse.			
21. Lowered the bed to its lowest position.			

Procedure—cont'd

	S	U	Comments
22. Placed the signal light within reach.			
23. Raised or lowered bed rails. Followed the care plan.			
24. Removed the gloves. Decontaminated hands.			
25. Left the room. Checked the person often. Knocked before entering the room.			
26. Returned to the room when it was time to remove the tube. Knocked before entering the room.			
27. Decontaminated hands. Put on gloves.			
28. Removed the tube. Wiped the rectal area.			
29. Wrapped the rectal tube and flatus bag in the bed protector. Removed the bed protector and the gloves. Decontaminated hands.			
30. Asked the person about the amount of gas expelled.			

Post-Procedure

	S	U	Comments
31. Provided for comfort.			
32. Placed the signal light within reach.			
33. Unscreened the person.			
34. Discarded disposable items. Followed agency policy for soiled linen. Wore gloves.			
35. Removed the gloves. Decontaminated hands.			
36. Reported and recorded observations.			

Date of Satisfactory Completion ________________ Instructor's Initials ________________

ADVANCED

Changing an Ostomy Pouch

Name: ______________________

Date: ______________________

Pre-Procedure

	S	U	Comments
• Knocked before entering the person's room.	____	____	____________
• Addressed the person by name.	____	____	____________
• Introduced yourself by name and title.	____	____	____________
1. Followed Delegation Guidelines. Reviewed Safety Alert.	____	____	____________
2. Explained the procedure to the person.	____	____	____________
3. Practiced hand hygiene.	____	____	____________
4. Collected the following:			
• Clean pouch with skin barrier	____	____	____________
• Skin barrier (if not part of the pouch)	____	____	____________
• Pouch clamp, clip, or wire closure	____	____	____________
• Clean ostomy belt (if used)	____	____	____________
• Gauze squares or wash cloths	____	____	____________
• Adhesive remover	____	____	____________
• Cotton balls	____	____	____________
• Bedpan with cover	____	____	____________
• Waterproof pad	____	____	____________
• Bath blanket	____	____	____________
• Toilet tissue	____	____	____________
• Wash basin	____	____	____________
• Bath thermometer	____	____	____________
• Prescribed soap or cleansing agent	____	____	____________
• Pouch deodorant	____	____	____________
• Paper towels	____	____	____________
• Gloves	____	____	____________
• Disposable bag	____	____	____________
5. Arranged the work area.	____	____	____________
6. Identified the person. Checked the ID bracelet against the assignment sheet. Called the person by name.	____	____	____________
7. Provided for privacy.	____	____	____________
8. Raised the bed for body mechanics. Bed rails were up if used.	____	____	____________

Procedure

	S	U	Comments
9. Lowered the bed rail near you if up.	____	____	____________
10. Covered the person with a bath blanket. Fanfold linens to the foot of the bed.	____	____	____________

Procedure—cont'd

	S	U	Comments
11. Put on the gloves.			
12. Placed the waterproof pad under the buttocks.			
13. Disconnected the pouch from the belt if one was worn. Removed the belt.			
14. Removed the pouch gently. Gently pushed the skin down and away from the skin barrier. Placed the pouch in the bedpan.			
15. Wiped around the stoma with toilet tissue or a gauze square. Placed soiled tissue in the bedpan. Discarded gauze squares in the bag.			
16. Moistened a cotton ball with adhesive remover. Cleaned around the stoma to remove any remaining skin barrier. Cleaned from the stoma outward.			
17. Covered the bedpan. Took it to the bathroom. If the person used bed rails, they were up before you left the bedside.			
18. Measured the amount of feces. Noted the color, amount, consistency, and odor of the feces.			
19. Asked the nurse to observe abnormal feces. Then emptied the pouch and bedpan into the toilet. Put the pouch in the bag.			
20. Removed the gloves and practiced hand hygiene. Put on clean gloves.			
21. Filled the basin with warm water. Placed the basin on the overbed table on top of the paper towels. Lowered the bed rail near you if up.			
22. Washed the skin around the stoma. Rinsed and patted dry. Used soap or other cleansing agent as directed by the nurse.			
23. Applied the skin barrier if it was a separate device.			
24. Put a clean ostomy belt on the person (if a belt was worn).			
25. Added deodorant to the new pouch.			
26. Removed adhesive backing on the pouch.			
27. Centered the pouch over the stoma. The drain pointed downward.			
28. Pressed around the skin barrier so the pouch sealed to the skin. Applied gentle pressure from the stoma outward.			
29. Maintained pressure for 1 to 2 minutes.			
30. Connected the belt to the pouch (if a belt was worn).			
31. Removed the waterproof pad.			
32. Removed the gloves. Decontaminated hands.			
33. Covered the person. Removed the bath blanket.			

Post-Procedure

	S	U	Comments
34. Provided for comfort.			
35. Raised or lowered bed rails. Followed the care plan.			
36. Lowered the bed to its lowest position.			

Post-Procedure—cont'd	S	U	Comments
37. Placed the signal light within reach.			
38. Unscreened the person.			
39. Cleaned equipment. Wore gloves for this step.			
40. Returned equipment to its proper place.			
41. Discarded the bag according to agency policy. Followed agency policy for soiled linen.			
42. Removed the gloves. Practiced hand hygiene.			
43. Reported and recorded observations.			

Date of Satisfactory Completion ____________ Instructor's Initials ____________

Preparing the Person for Meals

Name: ______________________

Date: ______________________

Pre-Procedure	S	U	Comments
• Knocked before entering the person's room.			
• Addressed the person by name.			
• Introduced yourself by name and title.			
1. Followed Delegation Guidelines. Reviewed Safety Alert.			
2. Explained to the person that it was mealtime.			
3. Practiced hand hygiene.			
4. Collected the following:			
• Equipment for oral hygiene			
• Bedpan, urinal, or commode and toilet tissue			
• Wash basin			
• Soap			
• Washcloth			
• Towel			
• Gloves			
5. Provided for privacy.			
Procedure			
6. Made sure eyeglasses and hearing aids were in place.			
7. Assisted with oral hygiene. Made sure dentures were in place.			
8. Assisted with elimination. Made sure the incontinent person was clean and dry.			
9. Assisted the person with handwashing.			
10. Did the following if the person ate in bed:			
a. Raised the head of the bed to a comfortable position.			
b. Cleaned the overbed table. Adjusted it in front of the person.			
c. Placed the signal light within reach.			
d. Unscreened the person.			
11. Did the following if the person sat in a chair:			
a. Positioned the person in a chair or wheelchair.			
b. Removed items from the overbed table. Cleaned the table.			
c. Adjusted the overbed table in front of the person.			
d. Placed the signal light within reach.			
e. Unscreened the person.			
12. Assisted the person to the dining area (if the person ate in the dining area).			

Post-Procedure	S	U	Comments
13. Returned to the room. Knocked before entering.	______	______	____________________
14. Cleaned and returned equipment to its proper place. Wore gloves for this step.	______	______	____________________
15. Straightened the room. Eliminated unpleasant noise, odors, or equipment.	______	______	____________________
16. Removed the gloves. Decontaminated hands.	______	______	____________________

Date of Satisfactory Completion ____________________ Instructor's Initials ____________________

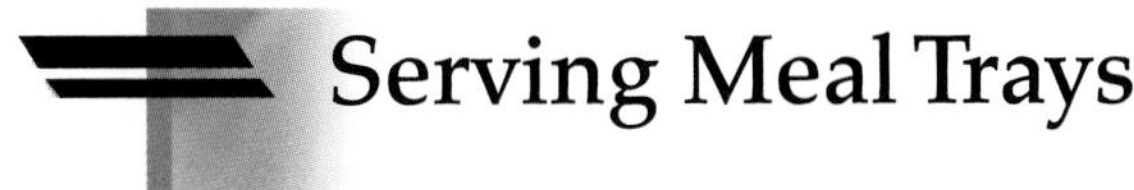

Serving Meal Trays

Name: ______________________

Date: ______________________

Pre-Procedure	S	U	Comments
• Knocked before entering the person's room.	____	____	____________
• Addressed the person by name.	____	____	____________
• Introduced yourself by name and title.	____	____	____________
1. Followed Delegation Guidelines. Reviewed Safety Alert.	____	____	____________
2. Practiced hand hygiene.	____	____	____________
Procedure			
3. Made sure the tray was complete. Checked items on the tray with the dietary card. Made sure adaptive equipment was included.	____	____	____________
4. Identified the person. Checked the ID bracelet with the dietary card. Called the person by name.	____	____	____________
5. Placed the tray within the person's reach. Adjusted the overbed table as needed.	____	____	____________
6. Removed food covers. Opened cartons, cut meat, and buttered bread as needed.	____	____	____________
7. Placed the napkin, clothes protector, adaptive equipment, and silverware within reach.	____	____	____________
8. Measured and recorded intake if ordered. Noted the amount and type of foods eaten.	____	____	____________
9. Checked for and removed any food in the mouth. Wore gloves. Decontaminated hands after removing the gloves.	____	____	____________
10. Removed the tray.	____	____	____________
11. Cleaned spills. Changed soiled linen.	____	____	____________
12. Helped the person return to bed if indicated.	____	____	____________
Post-Procedure			
13. Assisted the person with oral hygiene and handwashing. Wore gloves.	____	____	____________
14. Removed the gloves. Decontaminated hands.	____	____	____________
15. Provided for comfort.	____	____	____________
16. Placed the signal light within reach.	____	____	____________
17. Raised or lowered bed rails. Followed the care plan.	____	____	____________
18. Followed agency policy for soiled linen.	____	____	____________
19. Decontaminated hands.	____	____	____________
20. Reported and recorded observations.	____	____	____________

Date of Satisfactory Completion ______________ Instructor's Initials ______________

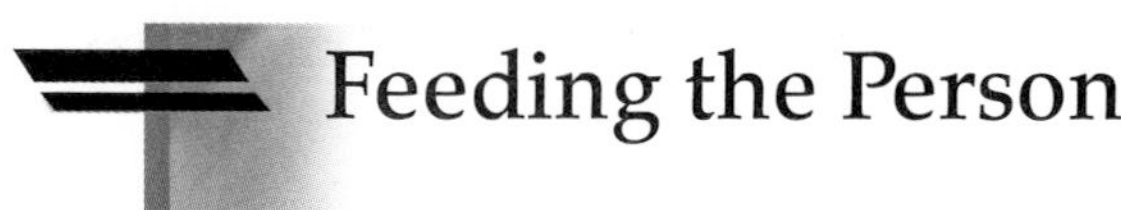

Feeding the Person

Name: ______________________

Date: ______________________

Pre-Procedure	S	U	Comments
• Knocked before entering the person's room.			
• Addressed the person by name.			
• Introduced yourself by name and title.			
1. Followed Delegation Guidelines. Reviewed Safety Alert.			
2. Explained the procedure to the person.			
3. Practiced hand hygiene.			
4. Positioned the person in a sitting position.			
5. Got the tray. Placed it on the overbed table or dining table.			
Procedure			
6. Identified the person. Checked the ID bracelet with the dietary card. Called the person by name.			
7. Draped a napkin across the person's chest and underneath the chin.			
8. Told the person what foods and fluids were on the tray.			
9. Prepared food for eating. Seasoned food as the person preferred and was allowed on the care plan.			
10. Served foods in the order the person preferred. Alternated between solid and liquid foods. Used a spoon for safety. Allowed enough time for chewing. Did not rush the person.			
11. Used straws for liquids if the person could not drink out of a glass or cup. Had one straw for each liquid. Provided short straws for weak persons.			
12. Followed the care plan if the person has dysphagia. Gave thickened liquid with a spoon.			
13. Conversed with the person in a pleasant manner.			
14. Encouraged the person to eat as much as possible.			
15. Wiped the person's mouth with a napkin.			
16. Noted how much and which foods were eaten.			
17. Measured and recorded intake if ordered.			
18. Removed the tray.			
19. Took the person back to his or her room.			
20. Assisted the person with oral hygiene and hand washing. Provided for privacy, and put on gloves. Decontaminated hands after removing the gloves.			

Post-Procedure	S	U	Comments
21. Provided for comfort.			
22. Placed the signal light within reach.			
23. Raised or lowered bed rails. Followed the care plan.			
24. Decontaminated hands.			
25. Reported and recorded observations.			

Date of Satisfactory Completion ____________________ Instructor's Initials ____________________

ADVANCED

Giving a Tube Feeding

Name: ______________________

Date: ______________________

Pre-Procedure	S	U	Comments
• Knocked before entering the person's room.			
• Addressed the person by name.			
• Introduced yourself by name and title.			
1. Followed Delegation Guidelines. Reviewed Safety Alert.			
2. Reviewed the manufacturer's instructions for the feeding pump.			
3. Asked a nurse to check tube placement. Checked and inspected the tube with the nurse. Made sure the correct tube was used.			
4. Explained the procedure to the person.			
5. Practiced hand hygiene.			
6. Collected the following:			
• Syringe or feeding bag with connecting tubing			
• Feeding pump (if used)			
• IV pole			
• Formula as directed by the nurse			
• 30 to 60 ml of water			
• Gloves			
7. Checked the date on the formula. Did not use the formula if the expiration date had passed.			
8. Let refrigerated formula warm to room temperature.			
9. Cleaned the formula container.			
10. Identified the person. Checked the ID bracelet against the assignment sheet. Called the person by name.			
11. Provided for privacy.			
12. Raised the bed for body mechanics (if using the syringe method). Bed rails were up if used.			

Procedure

13. Lowered the bed rail near you if up.			
14. Positioned the person as directed.			
15. Put on gloves.			
16. Opened the container.			
17. Syringe method:			
a. Pinched the feeding tube. Removed the clamp, cap, or plug.			
b. Removed the plunger from the syringe. Attached the syringe to the feeding tube.			

Procedure—cont'd	S	U	Comments
c. Filled the syringe with formula.	______	______	______
d. Unpinched the tube.	______	______	______
e. Kept the syringe 18 inches above stomach or intestinal level.	______	______	______
f. Let the formula slowly pass from the syringe into the feeding tube. Raised or lowered the syringe to adjust the flow rate.	______	______	______
g. Added formula as necessary. Did not let the syringe empty.	______	______	______
h. Asked the person about feelings of fullness or cramping. Pinched or clamped the tube if one or both occurred.	______	______	______
i. Gave formula over 30 minutes or as directed by the nurse.	______	______	______
j. Pinched the feeding tube as the syringe emptied.	______	______	______
k. Added water to the syringe. The nurse told you how much to use.	______	______	______
l. Released the tube. Let the water clear the tube.	______	______	______
m. Pinched or clamped the tube as the syringe emptied. Did not let air enter the tube.	______	______	______
n. Removed the syringe.	______	______	______
o. Clamped, capped, or plugged the tube.	______	______	______
18. Feeding bag method:			
a. Closed the clamp on the connecting tubing.	______	______	______
b. Filled the feeding bag with formula.	______	______	______
c. Squeezed the drip chamber so it partially filled with formula.	______	______	______
d. Opened the clamp on the connecting tubing slowly.	______	______	______
e. Let formula flow through the connecting tubing.	______	______	______
f. Clamped the connecting tubing.	______	______	______
g. Hung the feeding bag on an IV pole. Positioned the pole so that the bag was no more than 18 inches above the stomach or the intestines.	______	______	______
h. Attached the connecting tubing to the feeding tube. Unclasped the tube.	______	______	______
i. Adjusted the flow rate. Used the clamp on the connecting tubing. The nurse told you the number of drops per minute.	______	______	______
j. Clamped the connecting tubing before the bag emptied of formula.	______	______	______
k. Added water to the bag. The nurse told you how much to use.	______	______	______
l. Unclasped the connecting tubing. Let the water clear the tube.	______	______	______
m. Clamped the connecting tubing as it emptied of water. Did not let air enter the feeding tube.	______	______	______

Procedure—cont'd	S	U	Comments
n. Pinched or clamped the feeding tube.			
o. Disconnected the connecting tubing from the feeding tube.			
p. Clamped, capped, or plugged the feeding tube.			
19. Feeding pump method:			
a. Followed steps 18a through 18h.			
b. Threaded the connecting tubing through the pump. Followed the manufacturer's instructions.			
c. Set the flow rate. The nurse told you the number of drops per minute.			
d. Added ice around the bag as directed by the nurse.			
e. Told the nurse when the bag was emptying. The nurse assessed the person, checked for tube placement, and flushed the tube before adding more formula.			

Post-Procedure

	S	U	Comments
20. Removed the gloves. Decontaminated hands.			
21. Recorded the amount of formula given on the intake and output record. Also recorded the amount of water used to clear the tube.			
22. Positioned the person as the nurse directed.			
23. Provided for comfort.			
24. Placed the signal light within reach.			
25. Raised or lowered bed rails. Followed the care plan.			
26. Lowered the bed to its lowest position.			
27. Unscreened the person.			
28. Cleaned and returned equipment to its proper place. Wore gloves for this step.			
29. Removed the gloves. Decontaminated hands.			
30. Reported and recorded observations.			

Date of Satisfactory Completion ____________________ Instructor's Initials ____________________

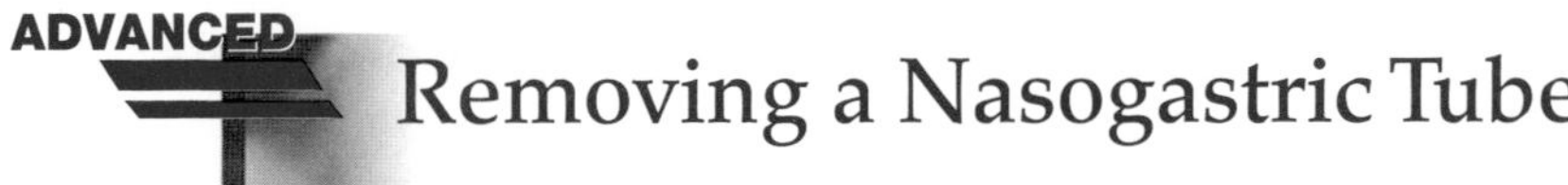

Removing a Nasogastric Tube

Name: ______________________

Date: ______________________

Pre-Procedure	S	U	Comments
• Knocked before entering the person's room.			
• Addressed the person by name.			
• Introduced yourself by name and title.			
1. Followed Delegation Guidelines. Reviewed Safety Alert.			
2. Explained the procedure to the person.			
3. Decontaminated your hands.			
4. Collected the following:			
• Disposable towel			
• Tissues			
• Gloves			
• Equipment for oral hygiene			
5. Identified the person. Checked the ID bracelet against the assignment sheet. Called the person by name.			
6. Provided for privacy.			
7. Raised the bed for body mechanics. Bed rails were up if used.			
Procedure			
8. Lowered the bed rail near you if up.			
9. Positioned the person in semi-Fowler's position.			
10. Put on the gloves.			
11. Placed the towel across the person's chest.			
12. Gave the person tissues.			
13. Unpinned or untaped the tube from the person's gown.			
14. Removed the tape or tube holder from the person's nose.			
15. Disconnected the tube if it was attached to suction.			
16. Pinched the tube shut.			
17. Asked the person to take a deep breath. Asked the person to hold the breath.			
18. Removed the tube. Used quick, smooth motions.			
19. Placed the tube and towel in a biohazard bag.			
20. Removed the gloves and decontaminated hands. Put on clean gloves.			
21. Assisted the person with oral hygiene.			
22. Removed the gloves. Decontaminated hands.			

Post-Procedure	S	U	Comments
23. Provided for comfort.			
24. Placed the signal light within reach.			
25. Raised or lowered bed rails. Followed the care plan.			
26. Lowered the bed to its lowest position.			
27. Unscreened the person.			
28. Cleaned and returned equipment to its proper place. Followed agency policy for soiled linen. Wore gloves for this step.			
29. Removed the gloves. Decontaminated hands.			
30. Reported and recorded observations.			

Date of Satisfactory Completion ____________ Instructor's Initials ____________

Measuring Intake and Output

Name: ______________________

Date: ______________________

Pre-Procedure	S	U	Comments
• Knocked before entering the person's room.	____	____	____________
• Addressed the person by name.	____	____	____________
• Introduced yourself by name and title.	____	____	____________
1. Followed Delegation Guidelines. Reviewed Safety Alert.	____	____	____________
2. Explained the procedure to the person.	____	____	____________
3. Practiced hand hygiene.	____	____	____________
4. Collected the following:			
• Intake and output (I&O) record	____	____	____________
• Graduates	____	____	____________
• Gloves	____	____	____________

Procedure

	S	U	Comments
5. Put on gloves.	____	____	____________
6. Measured intake as follows:			
a. Poured liquid remaining in a container into the graduate.	____	____	____________
b. Measured the amount at eye level. Kept the container level.	____	____	____________
c. Checked the serving amount on the I&O record.	____	____	____________
d. Subtracted the remaining amount from the full serving amount. Recorded the amount.	____	____	____________
e. Repeated steps 6a through 6d for each liquid.	____	____	____________
f. Added the amounts from each liquid together.	____	____	____________
g. Recorded the time and amount on the I&O record.	____	____	____________
7. Measured output as follows:			
a. Poured the fluid into the graduate used to measure output.	____	____	____________
b. Measured the amount at eye level. Kept the container level.	____	____	____________
8. Disposed of fluid in the toilet. Avoided splashes.	____	____	____________
9. Rinsed the graduate. Disposed of rinse into the toilet. Returned the graduate to its proper place.	____	____	____________
10. Cleaned and rinsed the bedpan, urinal, kidney basin, or other drainage container. Discarded the rinse into the toilet. Returned the item to its proper place.	____	____	____________
11. Removed the gloves. Decontaminated hands.	____	____	____________
12. Recorded the amount on the I&O record.	____	____	____________

Post-Procedure	**S**	**U**	**Comments**
13. Reported and recorded observations.	______	______	______________________

Date of Satisfactory Completion ______________________ Instructor's Initials ______________________

ADVANCED

Priming IV Tubing

Name: ______________________

Date: ______________________

Pre-Procedure	S	U	Comments
• Knocked before entering the person's room.	____	____	______________
• Addressed the person by name.	____	____	______________
• Introduced yourself by name and title.	____	____	______________
1. Followed Delegation Guidelines. Reviewed Safety Alerts.	____	____	______________
2. Practiced hand hygiene.	____	____	______________
3. Collected the following as directed by the RN:			
• IV solution bag (if it does not contain drugs)	____	____	______________
• Infusion set	____	____	______________
• IV pole	____	____	______________
• IV gown (sleeves close with snaps or Velcro)	____	____	______________
• IV label	____	____	______________
• Gloves	____	____	______________
4. Checked the expiration date on the IV bag. Did not use the bag if the expiration date had passed.	____	____	______________
5. Checked the IV bag. Made sure that:			
• The solution was clear and free of particles	____	____	______________
• The bag was not open	____	____	______________
• The bag did not leak	____	____	______________
• The bag was not cracked	____	____	______________
6. Asked the RN to check the IV bag.	____	____	______________
7. Arranged equipment on a clean work area.	____	____	______________
8. Identified the person. Checked the ID bracelet against the assignment sheet. Called the person by name.	____	____	______________
9. Explained the procedure to the person.	____	____	______________
10. Provided for privacy.	____	____	______________

Procedure

	S	U	Comments
11. Helped the person meet hygiene or elimination needs. Wore gloves. Cleaned and returned equipment to its proper place. Practiced hand hygiene.	____	____	______________
12. Helped the person change into the IV gown.	____	____	______________
13. Wrote the person's name, the date, and the time on the IV label.	____	____	______________
14. Applied the IV label to the bag. Applied it so it could be read when the bag is hanging.	____	____	______________
15. Opened the infusion set. The protective caps were on the spike and needle adapter.	____	____	______________

Procedure—cont'd	S	U	Comments
16. Opened the clamp. Moved it to the end of the drip chamber.	______	______	____________
17. Closed the clamp all the way.	______	______	____________
18. Removed the protective cap from the bag. Did not touch the opening.	______	______	____________
19. Removed the protective cap from the spike. Did not touch or let anything touch the spike.	______	______	____________
20. Inserted the spike into the bag.	______	______	____________
21. Hung the bag on the IV pole.	______	______	____________
22. Squeezed the drip chamber gently until it was about 1/2 full.	______	______	____________
23. Removed the protective cap from the needle adapter. Saved the cap for step 28. Did not touch or let anything touch the adapter.	______	______	____________
24. Held the needle end of the tubing over a sink or container.	______	______	____________
25. Opened the clamp slowly. Opened it only halfway.	______	______	____________
26. Allowed fluid to flow through the tubing until it was free of air and bubbles.	______	______	____________
27. Closed the clamp.	______	______	____________
28. Put the protective cap on the needle adapter. Did not touch the adapter.	______	______	____________
29. Checked the tube for bubbles. Gently tapped tubing at a bubble site to remove the bubble.	______	______	____________

Post-Procedure

30. Provided for comfort.	______	______	____________
31. Placed the signal light within reach.	______	______	____________
32. Raised or lowered bed rails. Followed the care plan.	______	______	____________
33. Told the person that the RN would start the IV.	______	______	____________
34. Unscreened the person.	______	______	____________
35. Told the RN that the tubing is primed. Reported any observations.	______	______	____________
36. Decontaminated hands.	______	______	____________

Date of Satisfactory Completion ____________________ Instructor's Initials ____________________

ADVANCED

Changing a Peripheral IV Dressing

Name: ______________________

Date: ______________________

Pre-Procedure	S	U	Comments
• Knocked before entering the person's room.			
• Addressed the person by name.			
• Introduced yourself by name and title.			
1. Followed Delegation Guidelines. Reviewed Safety Alerts.			
2. Explained the procedure to the person.			
3. Practiced hand hygiene.			
4. Collected the following:			
• Povidone-iodine swabs			
• Alcohol swabs			
• Transparent dressing			
• Transparent tape			
• Gloves			
• Towel			
• Leak-proof plastic bag			
5. Arranged equipment on the overbed table.			
6. Identified the person. Checked the ID bracelet against the assignment sheet. Called the person by name.			
7. Provided for privacy.			
8. Raised the bed for body mechanics. The far bed rail was up if bed rails were used.			
9. Made sure of good lighting.			

Procedure	S	U	Comments
10. Cut a strip of tape. Hung the tape from the edge of the overbed table for later use.			
11. Opened the dressing and the swabs.			
12. Exposed the IV site. Placed the towel under the person's arm.			
13. Put on the gloves.			
14. Removed the soiled dressing. Did not remove the tape securing the catheter or needle.			
a. Removed the dressing. Touched only the outer edge of the dressing.			
b. Discarded the dressing into the plastic bag.			
15. Observed the IV site for redness, swelling, and drainage. Called for the RN to assess the site.			

Procedure—cont'd	S	U	Comments
16. Held the hub of the needle or catheter to keep it in place. Used the non-dominant hand. Held the hub through step 20.	____	____	________
17. Removed any tape securing the catheter or needle. Discarded the tape into the plastic bag.	____	____	________
18. Cleaned the IV site with the alcohol swab. Used a circular motion starting at the IV site. Worked outward about 2 inches. Let the site dry. Discarded used swabs into the plastic bag.	____	____	________
19. Cleaned the IV site with the povidone-iodine swab. Cleaned the site as in step 18. Discarded used swabs into the plastic bag.	____	____	________
20. Let the site dry for 2 minutes.	____	____	________
21. Applied the dressing. Did not cover the needle adapter. Smoothed and sealed the dressing over the IV site.	____	____	________
22. Made a loop in the IV tubing over the dressing. Made sure the needle adapter was securely attached to the catheter hub.	____	____	________
23. Secured the loop to the dressing with tape. Applied the tape over the tape on the dressing.	____	____	________
24. Wrote the following on the tape:			
• The date and time of the dressing change	____	____	________
• The size of the catheter (Got this information from the RN.)	____	____	________
• Your name or initials	____	____	________
25. Removed the towel.	____	____	________
26. Removed and discarded the gloves into the plastic bag.	____	____	________
27. Decontaminated hands.	____	____	________
28. Checked the flow rate. Asked the RN to adjust the flow rate if needed.	____	____	________

Post-Procedure

29. Provided for comfort.	____	____	________
30. Placed the signal light within reach.	____	____	________
31. Raised or lowered bed rails. Followed the care plan.	____	____	________
32. Lowered the bed to its lowest position.	____	____	________
33. Unscreened the person.	____	____	________
34. Discarded the plastic bag and supplies. Followed agency policy for soiled linen. (Wore gloves if contact with blood was likely.)	____	____	________
35. Decontaminated hands.	____	____	________
36. Reported and recorded observations.	____	____	________

Date of Satisfactory Completion ________________ Instructor's Initials ________________

ADVANCED

Discontinuing a Peripheral IV

Name: ______________________

Date: ______________________

Pre-Procedure	S	U	Comments
• Knocked before entering the person's room.			
• Addressed the person by name.			
• Introduced yourself by name and title.			
1. Followed Delegation Guidelines. Reviewed Safety Alert.			
2. Explained the procedure to the person.			
3. Practiced hand hygiene.			
4. Collected the following:			
• Two sterile 2 × 2 or 4 × 4 gauze dressings			
• Alcohol swabs			
• Povidone-iodine swab			
• Tape			
• Towel			
• Gloves			
• Leak-proof plastic bag			
5. Arranged supplies on the overbed table.			
6. Identified the person. Checked the ID bracelet against the assignment sheet. Called the person by name.			
7. Provided for privacy.			
8. Raised the bed for body mechanics. The far bed rail was up if bed rails were used.			

Procedure	S	U	Comments
9. Opened the dressings and the swabs.			
10. Put on the gloves.			
11. Exposed the IV site.			
12. Put the towel under the site.			
13. Stopped the flow of IV fluids. Closed the clamp, or moved it to the OFF position.			
14. Noted the amount of fluid remaining in the IV bag.			
15. Held the hub of the catheter or needle through step 20.			
16. Removed the dressing. Discarded it into the plastic bag.			
17. Removed any adhesive. Used cotton balls moistened with adhesive remover. Discarded cotton balls into the plastic bag.			
18. Cleaned the IV site with an alcohol swab. Discarded the swab into the plastic bag.			
19. Cleaned the IV site with a povidone-iodine swab. Discarded the swab into the plastic bag.			

Procedure—cont'd	S	U	Comments
20. Placed a gauze square over the IV site. Held it in place.			
21. Removed the needle or catheter. Held the hub, slowly pulled the needle or catheter straight out of the vein.			
22. Checked the needle or catheter to make sure it was intact. Called the RN immediately if it was not.			
23. Discarded the catheter or needle into the sharps container in the room.			
24. Elevated the extremity.			
25. Applied pressure to the IV site with the gauze dressing. Applied pressure for 2 to 3 minutes.			
26. Removed the gauze dressing. Discarded it into the plastic bag.			
27. Applied a sterile gauze dressing to the IV site.			
28. Taped the dressing in place.			
29. Removed the towel.			
30. Discarded used supplies into the plastic bag.			
31. Removed the gloves. Decontaminated hands.			

Post-Procedure

	S	U	Comments
32. Provided for comfort.			
33. Placed the signal light within reach.			
34. Raised or lowered bed rails. Followed the care plan.			
35. Lowered the bed to its lowest position.			
36. Unscreened the person.			
37. Discarded used supplies, the plastic bag, the IV bag, and soiled linen according to agency policy. (Wore gloves for this step if contact with blood was likely.)			
38. Decontaminated hands.			
39. Reported and recorded the following:			
• The amount of fluid remaining in the IV bag			
• Observations of the IV site			
• Other observations or patient or resident complaints			

Date of Satisfactory Completion ____________________ Instructor's Initials ____________________

ADVANCED

Obtaining Blood From the Blood Bank

Name: ______________________

Date: ______________________

Pre-Procedure	S	U	Comments
• Knocked before entering the person's room.	______	______	______________
• Addressed the person by name.	______	______	______________
• Introduced yourself by name and title.	______	______	______________
1. Followed Delegation Guidelines. Reviewed Safety Alert.	______	______	______________
2. Practiced hand hygiene.	______	______	______________
3. Took the blood requisition form to the blood bank.	______	______	______________
4. Told the laboratory technician the following:			
• Who you were	______	______	______________
• What was wanted	______	______	______________
• That you had a requisition for blood or a blood product	______	______	______________
5. Checked the requisition form and the blood bag label with the laboratory technician. Followed agency policy. Read the following out loud:	______	______	______________
• The person's name—last name, first name, and middle initial	______	______	______________
• The person's ID number	______	______	______________
• The person's blood type—A, B, AB, or O	______	______	______________
• The person's Rh factor—Rh+ or Rh−	______	______	______________
• The blood donor number	______	______	______________
• Expiration date on the blood	______	______	______________
6. Thanked the technician for helping.	______	______	______________
7. Returned immediately to the nursing unit.	______	______	______________
8. Gave the blood to the RN.	______	______	______________
9. Practiced hand hygiene.	______	______	______________

Date of Satisfactory Completion ______________ Instructor's Initials ______________

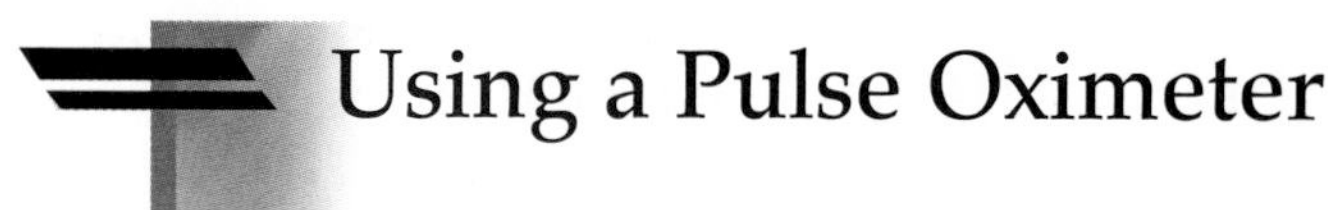

Using a Pulse Oximeter

Name: ______________________

Date: ______________________

Pre-Procedure	S	U	Comments
• Knocked before entering the person's room.			
• Addressed the person by name.			
• Introduced yourself by name and title.			
1. Followed Delegation Guidelines. Reviewed Safety Alert.			
2. Explained the procedure to the person.			
3. Practiced hand hygiene.			
4. Collected the following:			
• Oximeter and sensor			
• Nail polish remover			
• Cotton balls			
• SpO_2 flow sheet			
• Tape			
• Towel			
5. Identified the person. Checked the ID bracelet against your assignment sheet. Called the person by name.			
6. Provided for privacy.			

Procedure

	S	U	Comments
7. Provided for comfort.			
8. Removed nail polish from the finger or toenail. Used nail polish remover and a cotton ball.			
9. Dried the site with a towel.			
10. Clipped or taped the sensor to the site.			
11. Turned on the oximeter.			
12. Set the high and low alarm limits for SpO_2 and pulse rate. Turned on audio and visual alarms.			
13. Checked the person's pulse (apical or radial) with the pulse on the display. Told the nurse if the pulses were not equal.			
14. Read the SpO_2 on the display. Noted the value on the flow sheet and the assignment sheet.			
15. Left the sensor in place for continuous monitoring. Otherwise, turned off the device and removed the sensor.			

Post-Procedure

	S	U	Comments
16. Provided for comfort.			
17. Placed the signal light within the person's reach.			
18. Raised or lowered bed rails. Followed the care plan.			
19. Unscreened the person.			
20. Returned the device to its proper place unless monitoring is continuous.			
21. Decontaminated hands.			
22. Reported and recorded the SpO_2, the pulse rate, and other observations.			

Date of Satisfactory Completion ______________________ Instructor's Initials ____________________

Assisting With Coughing and Deep Breathing Exercises

Name: ______________________

Date: ______________________

Pre-Procedure	S	U	Comments
• Knocked before entering the person's room.	____	____	____________
• Addressed the person by name.	____	____	____________
• Introduced yourself by name and title.	____	____	____________
1. Followed Delegation Guidelines.	____	____	____________
2. Explained the procedure to the person.	____	____	____________
3. Practiced hand hygiene.	____	____	____________
4. Identified the person. Checked the ID bracelet against the assignment sheet. Called the person by name.	____	____	____________
5. Provided for privacy.	____	____	____________
Procedure			
6. Helped the person to a comfortable sitting position: dangling, semi-Fowler's, or Fowler's.	____	____	____________
7. Had the person deep breathe:	____	____	____________
a. Had the person place the hands over the rib cage.	____	____	____________
b. Asked the person to exhale. Explained that the ribs should move as far down as possible.	____	____	____________
c. Had the person take a deep breath. Reminded the person to inhale through the nose.	____	____	____________
d. Asked the person to hold the breath for 3 seconds.	____	____	____________
e. Asked the person to exhale slowly through pursed lips. The person exhaled until the ribs moved as far down as possible.	____	____	____________
f. Repeated this step 4 more times.	____	____	____________
8. Asked the person to cough:	____	____	____________
a. Had the person interlace the fingers over the incision. The person could also hold a pillow or folded towel over the incision.	____	____	____________
b. Had the person take in a deep breath as in step 7.	____	____	____________
c. Asked the person to cough strongly twice with the mouth open.	____	____	____________
Post-Procedure			
9. Provided for comfort.	____	____	____________
10. Raised or lowered bed rails. Followed the care plan.	____	____	____________
11. Placed the signal light within reach.	____	____	____________

Post-Procedure—cont'd	S	U	Comments
12. Unscreened the person.			
13. Decontaminated hands.			
14. Reported and recorded observations.			

Date of Satisfactory Completion ____________________ Instructor's Initials ____________________

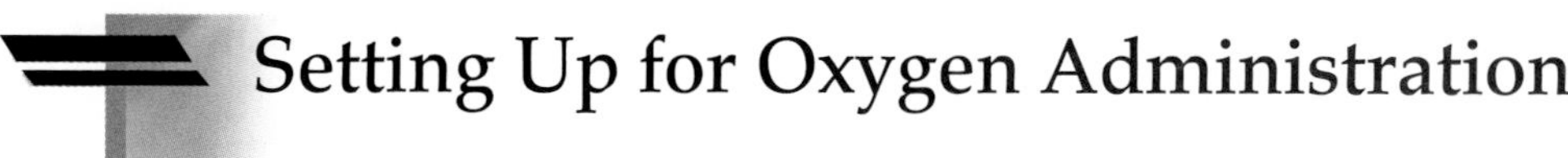

Setting Up for Oxygen Administration

Name: ______________________

Date: ______________________

Pre-Procedure	S	U	Comments
• Knocked before entering the person's room.	____	____	____________
• Addressed the person by name.	____	____	____________
• Introduced yourself by name and title.	____	____	____________
1. Followed Delegation Guidelines. Reviewed Safety Alerts.	____	____	____________
2. Practiced hand hygiene.	____	____	____________
3. Collected the following:			
• Oxygen device with connecting tubing	____	____	____________
• Flowmeter	____	____	____________
• Humidifier (if ordered)	____	____	____________
• Distilled water (if using a humidifier)	____	____	____________
4. Identified the person. Checked the ID bracelet against the assignment sheet. Called the person by name.	____	____	____________
5. Explained the procedure to the person.	____	____	____________

Procedure	S	U	Comments
6. Made sure the flowmeter was in the OFF position.	____	____	____________
7. Attached the flowmeter to the wall outlet or to the tank.	____	____	____________
8. Filled the humidifier with distilled water.	____	____	____________
9. Attached the humidifier to the bottom of the flowmeter.	____	____	____________
10. Attached the oxygen device and connecting tubing to the humidifier. Did not set the flowmeter. Did not apply the oxygen device on the person.	____	____	____________

Post-Procedure	S	U	Comments
11. Discarded packaging.	____	____	____________
12. Made sure the cap was securely on the distilled water. Stored it according to agency policy.	____	____	____________
13. Provided for comfort.	____	____	____________
14. Placed the signal light within reach.	____	____	____________
15. Decontaminated hands.	____	____	____________
16. Told the nurse when you were done.	____	____	____________

Date of Satisfactory Completion ______________ Instructor's Initials ______________

ADVANCED

Giving Tracheostomy Care

Name: ____________________

Date: ____________________

Pre-Procedure	S	U	Comments
• Knocked before entering the person's room.			
• Addressed the person by name.			
• Introduced yourself by name and title.			
1. Followed Delegation Guidelines. Reviewed Safety Alert.			
2. Asked a co-worker to help. Explained what the co-worker should do.			
3. Explained the procedure to the person.			
4. Practiced hand hygiene.			
5. Collected the following:			
• Tracheostomy suction supplies			
• Sterile tracheostomy dressing			
• 3 sterile 4 × 4 gauze square packages			
• Hydrogen peroxide			
• Sterile saline			
• 3 sterile cotton swab packages			
• Sterile basin			
• Sterile brush			
• Tracheostomy ties or Velcro collar			
• Disposable inner cannula (if used)			
• Scissors			
• Sterile gloves (2 pairs)			
• Disposable gloves			
• Cotton twill tape or Velcro collar			
• Face shield			
• Towel			
6. Arranged supplies on the overbed table.			
7. Identified the person. Checked the ID bracelet against the assignment sheet. Called the person by name.			
8. Provided for privacy.			
9. Raised the bed for body mechanics. The far bed rail was up if used.			
10. Positioned the person supine or in Fowler's position.			

Procedure

	S	U	Comments
11. Suctioned the tracheostomy tube. Wore a face shield.			

Procedure—cont'd	S	U	Comments
12. Prepared a sterile field:			
a. Opened 2 sterile 4 × 4 gauze packages.	___	___	___
b. Opened 2 sterile swab packages.	___	___	___
c. Poured sterile saline onto 1 sterile 4 × 4 gauze package and 1 sterile swab package.	___	___	___
d. Poured hydrogen peroxide onto 1 sterile 4 × 4 gauze package and 1 sterile swab package.	___	___	___
e. Opened the tracheostomy dressing package.	___	___	___
f. Opened the sterile basin. Poured hydrogen peroxide into the basin. The peroxide was about 3/4-inch deep in the basin.	___	___	___
g. Opened the sterile brush package.	___	___	___
13. Put on the sterile gloves.	___	___	___
14. Removed the inner cannula:	___	___	___
a. Unlocked the inner cannula with the non-dominant hand. Turned the lock counterclockwise.	___	___	___
b. Pulled the inner cannula toward you with the non-dominant hand.	___	___	___
c. Dropped the inner cannula into the basin with hydrogen peroxide. Discarded a disposable cannula.	___	___	___
15. Cleaned the inner cannula. Went to step 16 if using a disposable inner cannula:	___	___	___
a. Cleaned the inside and outside of the cannula with the sterile brush. Used the dominant hand.	___	___	___
b. Removed all secretions and crusts.	___	___	___
c. Picked up the bottle of sterile saline. Used the non-dominant hand.	___	___	___
d. Held the cannula over the basin with hydrogen peroxide. Used the dominant hand.	___	___	___
e. Poured sterile saline over the inner cannula.	___	___	___
f. Tapped the inner cannula against the inside of the sterile basin.	___	___	___
16. Suctioned the outer cannula if secretions were present.	___	___	___
17. Replaced the inner cannula with the dominant hand. Followed the direction of the tube's curve.	___	___	___
18. Locked the inner cannula in place. Turned the lock clockwise to an upright position.	___	___	___
19. Cleaned flange of the outer cannula with the dominant hand. Used sterile swabs and sterile 4 × 4 gauze moistened with hydrogen peroxide. Used a new swab or gauze square for each stroke. Made sure fluid did not enter the stoma.	___	___	___
20. Removed the tracheostomy dressing. Used the non-dominant hand.	___	___	___

Procedure—cont'd

Procedure—cont'd	S	U	Comments
21. Cleaned under the stoma. Cleaned in circular motions away from the stoma. Used sterile swabs and sterile 4 × 4 gauze moistened with hydrogen peroxide. Used 1 swab or gauze square for each stroke. Made sure fluid did not enter the stoma.			
22. Rinsed the flange and under the stoma. Rinsed outward from the stoma using sterile swabs and sterile 4 × 4 gauze moistened with sterile saline. Made sure fluid did not enter the stoma.			
23. Patted dry the area around the stoma and the flange. Used the dry sterile swabs and the dry sterile 4 × 4 dressing.			
24. Asked the co-worker to put on sterile gloves.			
25. Had the co-worker hold the tracheostomy tube in place. The tube was held in place for steps 26 to 28.			
26. Cut the ties or removed the Velcro collar following the manufacturer's instructions.			
27. Changed the ties or applied a new Velcro collar following the manufacturer's instructions. Changed ties as follows:			
a. Cut a length of twill tape about 24 to 30 inches long for the new ties. Cut the tape longer if the person had a large neck.			
b. Inserted one end of the tie through the eyelet on the flange of the outer cannula.			
c. Slid the ends of the tie under the person's neck.			
d. Brought the end of the tie around to the eyelet on the other side of the flange.			
e. Inserted one tie through the eyelet.			
f. Pulled both ends of the tie so they were snug but not tight.			
g. Tied each end of the ties with two square knots at the left and right side of the person's neck.			
28. Applied the sterile tracheostomy dressing under the flange and clean ties. Checked the dressing for loose gauze and lint. Got a new dressing if necessary.			
29. Asked the co-worker to let go of the outer cannula.			
30. Removed and discarded the gloves and face shield. Decontaminated hands.			

Post-Procedure

Post-Procedure	S	U	Comments
31. Provided for comfort.			
32. Placed the signal light within reach.			
33. Raised or lowered bed rails. Followed the care plan.			
34. Lowered the bed to its lowest position.			
35. Unscreened the person.			
36. Made sure that an extra tracheostomy tube was at the bedside. (It must be the correct size.)			

Post-Procedure—cont'd	S	U	Comments
37. Emptied the sterile basin.			
38. Capped the hydrogen peroxide and saline bottles. Marked the date and time on each bottle. Stored the bottles according to agency policy.			
39. Discarded used supplies and equipment. Followed agency policy. Wore disposable gloves for this step if necessary.			
40. Decontaminated hands.			
41. Reported and recorded observations.			

Date of Satisfactory Completion ______________________ Instructor's Initials ____________________

ADVANCED

Oropharyngeal Suctioning

Name: ______________________

Date: ______________________

Pre-Procedure	S	U	Comments
• Knocked before entering the person's room.			
• Addressed the person by name.			
• Introduced yourself by name and title.			
1. Followed Delegation Guidelines. Reviewed Safety Alert.			
2. Practiced hand hygiene.			
3. Collected the following:			
• Suction catheter (the nurse tells you the kind and size)			
• Connecting tubing			
• Water (about 100 ml)			
• Clean basin			
• Suction machine (if no wall outlet suction)			
• Sterile gloves			
• Disposable gloves			
• Face shield			
• Sterile towel			
4. Identified the person. Checked the ID bracelet against the assignment sheet. Called the person by name.			
5. Explained the procedure to the person.			
6. Provided for privacy.			
7. Raised the bed for body mechanics. Bed rails were up if used.			

Procedure	S	U	Comments
8. Lowered the bed rail near you if up.			
9. Positioned the person in semi-Fowler's position. Turned the person's head toward you.			
10. Placed the towel under the person's chin and across the chest.			
11. Filled the basin with water.			
12. Turned on the suction to the pressure directed.			
13. Attached the connecting tubing to the wall suction or suction machine.			
14. Opened the sterile suction catheter package. Did not let the suction catheter touch any non-sterile surface.			
15. Attached the suction catheter to the connecting tubing. Touched only the connecting end of the catheter.			
16. Put on the face shield.			
17. Decontaminated hands.			

Procedure—cont'd

	S	U	Comments
18. Put on the sterile gloves.			
19. Picked up the suction catheter with the dominant hand. Held the catheter with the thumb and forefinger.			
20. Checked equipment function. Suctioned some water out of the basin.			
21. Removed the oxygen mask if the person was using one. Used the non-dominant hand only.			
22. Inserted the suction catheter into the person's mouth along the gum line to the pharynx.			
23. Applied suction as the catheter was moved along the gum lines and around the mouth.			
24. Removed the catheter.			
25. Rinsed the catheter and connecting tubing. To rinse, suctioned a small amount of water from the basin.			
26. Repeated steps 22 through 25 no more than 2 times.			
27. Reapplied the oxygen mask.			
28. Cleared the catheter and connecting tubing of secretions. Suctioned water from the basin until the tubing was clear.			
29. Disconnected the catheter from the connecting tubing.			
30. Rolled the catheter into a ball in your hand, or wrapped it around the gloved hand.			
31. Removed the sterile glove on the hand holding the catheter. The catheter was inside the glove as the glove was pulled off.			
32. Put the glove with the catheter in the other hand.			
33. Pulled the glove over the glove in your hand.			
34. Discarded the gloves and catheter into a leak-proof bag. Decontaminated hands.			
35. Turned off the suction.			
36. Removed the towel. Discarded it into the leak-proof bag.			

Post-Procedure

	S	U	Comments
37. Provided for comfort.			
38. Placed the signal light within reach.			
39. Raised or lowered bed rails. Followed the care plan.			
40. Lowered the bed to its lowest position.			
41. Unscreened the person.			
42. Put on disposable gloves to care for supplies and equipment.			
43. Emptied the basin. Followed agency policy for reusing or discarding the basin.			
44. Discarded used supplies.			
45. Removed gloves. Decontaminated hands.			
46. Reported and recorded observations.			
47. Collected supplies used during the procedure. Replaced them at the bedside.			

Date of Satisfactory Completion ____________ Instructor's Initials ____________

ADVANCED

Suctioning a Tracheostomy

Name: ______________________

Date: ______________________

Pre-Procedure	S	U	Comments
• Knocked before entering the person's room.	_____	_____	__________
• Addressed the person by name.	_____	_____	__________
• Introduced yourself by name and title.	_____	_____	__________
1. Followed Delegation Guidelines. Reviewed Safety Alerts.	_____	_____	__________
2. Asked a nurse or respiratory therapist to perform the hyperventilation function.	_____	_____	__________
3. Decontaminated hands.	_____	_____	__________
4. Collected the following:			
• Sterile suction catheter	_____	_____	__________
• Connecting tubing	_____	_____	__________
• Sterile water or sterile saline (about 100 ml)	_____	_____	__________
• Sterile basin	_____	_____	__________
• Suction machine (if no wall outlet suction)	_____	_____	__________
• Sterile gloves	_____	_____	__________
• Disposable gloves	_____	_____	__________
• Face shield	_____	_____	__________
• Sterile drape	_____	_____	__________
• Ambu bag	_____	_____	__________
• Leak-proof bag	_____	_____	__________
5. Identified the person. Checked the ID bracelet against the assignment sheet. Called the person by name.	_____	_____	__________
6. Explained the procedure to the person.	_____	_____	__________
7. Provided for privacy.	_____	_____	__________
8. Arranged equipment on the bedside table.	_____	_____	__________
9. Raised the bed for body mechanics. Bed rails were up if used.	_____	_____	__________

Procedure

10. Lowered the bed rail near you if used.	_____	_____	__________
11. Positioned the person in semi-Fowler's position. Turned the person's head toward you.	_____	_____	__________
12. Decontaminated hands.	_____	_____	__________
13. Opened the sterile towel. Placed it across the person's chest.	_____	_____	__________
14. Opened the sterile basin.	_____	_____	__________
15. Poured the sterile water or saline into the basin.	_____	_____	__________

Procedure—cont'd	S	U	Comments
16. Turned on the suction to the pressure directed.			
17. Attached the connecting tubing to the wall suction or suction machine.			
18. Opened the sterile suction catheter package. Did not let the suction catheter touch any non-sterile surface.			
19. Attached the suction catheter to the connecting tubing. Touched only the connecting end of the catheter.			
20. Put on the face shield.			
21. Decontaminated hands.			
22. Put on the sterile gloves.			
23. Picked up the suction catheter with the dominant hand. Held the catheter with the thumb and forefinger.			
24. Checked equipment function. Suctioned some water or saline out of the basin.			
25. Asked the nurse or respiratory therapist to hyperventilate the person's lungs.			
26. Inserted the suction catheter into the tracheostomy. Inserted the catheter until the person coughed or resistance was felt. Did not apply suction.			
27. Pulled the catheter back about 1/2 inch (1 to 2 cm). Did not apply suction.			
28. Applied suction intermittently and uncovered the thumb part. Used the non-dominant hand to cover and uncover the thumb port.			
29. Rotated the catheter and slowly withdrew it while applying intermittent suction.			
30. Removed the catheter after 10 seconds. Uncovered the thumb port to release the suction.			
31. Asked the nurse or respiratory therapist to hyperventilate the person's lungs.			
32. Rinsed the catheter and connecting tubing.			
33. Waited 1 to 3 minutes before repeating steps 25 through 32. Repeated the steps no more than 2 times.			
34. Asked the nurse or respiratory therapist to connect the oxygen delivery device to the tracheostomy.			
35. Cleared the catheter and connecting tubing of secretions. Suctioned water or saline from the basin until the tubing was clear.			
36. Disconnected the catheter from the connecting tubing.			
37. Rolled the catheter into a ball in your hand, or wrapped it around the gloved hand.			
38. Removed the sterile glove on the hand holding the catheter. The catheter was inside the glove as the glove was pulled off.			
39. Put the glove with the catheter in the other hand.			
40. Pulled the glove over the glove in your hand.			
41. Discarded the gloves and catheter into a leak-proof bag.			

Procedure—cont'd	S	U	Comments
42. Turned off the suction.	______	______	____________________
43. Removed the sterile towel. Discarded it into the leak-proof bag.	______	______	____________________

Post-Procedure

	S	U	Comments
44. Followed steps 37 through 47 in procedure: *Oropharyngeal Suctioning.*	______	______	____________________

Date of Satisfactory Completion ____________________ Instructor's Initials ____________________

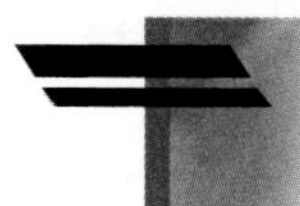

Performing Range-of-Motion Exercises

Name: ______________________

Date: ______________________

Pre-Procedure	S	U	Comments
• Knocked before entering the person's room.			
• Addressed the person by name.			
• Introduced yourself by name and title.			
1. Followed Delegation Guidelines. Reviewed Safety Alert.			
2. Identified the person. Checked the ID bracelet against the assignment sheet. Called the person by name.			
3. Explained the procedure to the person.			
4. Practiced hand hygiene.			
5. Obtained a bath blanket.			
6. Provided for privacy.			
7. Raised the bed for body mechanics. Bed rails were up if used.			

Procedure

	S	U	Comments
8. Lowered the bed rail near you if up.			
9. Positioned the person supine.			
10. Covered the person with a bath blanket. Fanfolded top linens to the foot of the bed.			
11. Exercised the neck if allowed by the agency and if the RN instructed to do so:			
a. Placed your hands over the person's ears to support the head. Supported the jaws with the fingers.			
b. Flexion—brought the head forward. The chin touched the chest.			
c. Extension—straightened the head.			
d. Hyperextension—brought the head backward until the chin pointed up.			
e. Rotation—turned the head from side to side.			
f. Lateral flexion—moved the head to the right and to the left.			
g. Repeated flexion, extension, hyperextension, rotation, and lateral flexion 5 times—or the number of times stated on the care plan.			
12. Exercised the shoulder:			
a. Grasped the wrist with one hand. Grasped the elbow with the other hand.			
b. Flexion—raised the arm straight in front and over the head.			

Procedure—cont'd	S	U	Comments
c. Extension—brought the arm down to the side.			
d. Hyperextension—moved the arm behind the body. (Did this if the person sits in a straight-backed chair or is standing.)			
e. Abduction—moved the straight arm away from the side of the body.			
f. Adduction—moved the straight arm to the side of the body.			
g. Internal rotation—bent the elbow. Placed it at the same level as the shoulder. Moved the forearm down toward the body.			
h. External rotation—moved the forearm toward the head.			
i. Repeated flexion, extension, hyperextension, abduction, adduction, and internal and external rotation 5 times—or the number of times stated on the care plan.			
13. Exercised the elbow:			
a. Grasped the person's wrist with one hand. Grasped the elbow with the other hand.			
b. Flexion—bent the arm so the same-side shoulder is touched.			
c. Extension—straightened the arm.			
d. Repeated flexion and extension 5 times—or the number of times stated on the care plan.			
14. Exercised the forearm:			
a. Pronation—turned the hand so the palm was down.			
b. Supination—turned the hand so the palm was up.			
c. Repeated pronation and supination 5 times—or the number of times stated on the care plan.			
15. Exercised the wrist:			
a. Held the wrist with both hands.			
b. Flexion—bent the hand down.			
c. Extension—straightened the hand.			
d. Hyperextension—bent the hand back.			
e. Radial flexion—turned the hand toward the thumb.			
f. Ulnar flexion—turned the hand toward the little finger.			
g. Repeated flexion, extension, hyperextension, and radial and ulnar flexion 5 times—or the number of times stated on the care plan.			
16. Exercised the thumb:			
a. Held the person's hand with one hand. Held the thumb with the other hand.			
b. Abduction—moved the thumb out from the inner part of the index finger.			
c. Adduction—moved the thumb back next to the index finger.			

Procedure—cont'd	S	U	Comments
d. Opposition—touched each fingertip with the thumb.			
e. Flexion—bent the thumb into the hand.			
f. Extension—moved the thumb out to the side of the fingers.			
g. Repeated abduction, adduction, opposition, flexion, and extension 5 times—or the number of times stated on the care plan.			
17. Exercised the fingers:			
a. Abduction—spread the fingers and the thumb apart.			
b. Adduction—brought the fingers and thumb together.			
c. Extension—straightened the fingers so the fingers, hand, and arm were straight.			
d. Flexion—made a fist.			
e. Repeated abduction, adduction, extension, and flexion 5 times—or the number of times stated on the care plan.			
18. Exercised the hip:			
a. Supported the leg. Placed one hand under the knee. Placed the other hand under the ankle.			
b. Flexion—raised the leg.			
c. Extension—straightened the leg.			
d. Abduction—moved the leg away from the body.			
e. Adduction—moved the leg toward the other leg.			
f. Internal rotation—turned the leg inward.			
g. External rotation—turned the leg outward.			
h. Repeated flexion, extension, abduction, adduction, and internal and external rotation 5 times—or the number of times stated on the care plan.			
19. Exercised the knee:			
a. Supported the knee. Placed one hand under the knee. Placed the other hand under the ankle.			
b. Flexion—bent the leg.			
c. Extension—straightened the leg.			
d. Repeated flexion and extension of the knee 5 times—or the number of times stated on the care plan.			
20. Exercised the ankle:			
a. Supported the foot and ankle. Placed one hand under the foot. Placed the other hand under the ankle.			
b. Dorsiflexion—pulled the foot forward. Pushed down on the heel at the same time.			
c. Plantar flexion—turned the foot down, or pointed the toes.			
d. Repeated dorsiflexion and plantar flexion 5 times—or the number of times stated on the care plan.			

Procedure—cont'd	S	U	Comments
21. Exercised the foot:			
a. Continued to support the foot and ankle.			
b. Pronation—turned the outside of the foot up and the inside down.			
c. Supination—turned the inside of the foot up and the outside down.			
d. Repeated pronation and supination 5 times—or the number of times stated on the care plan.			
22. Exercised the toes:			
a. Flexion—curled the toes.			
b. Extension—straightened the toes.			
c. Abduction—spread the toes apart.			
d. Adduction—pulled the toes together.			
e. Repeated flexion, extension, abduction, and adduction 5 times—or the number of times stated on the care plan.			
23. Covered the leg. Raised the bed rail if used.			
24. Went to the other side. Lowered the bed rail near you if up.			
25. Repeated steps 12 through 22.			

Post-Procedure

	S	U	Comments
26. Provided for comfort.			
27. Covered the person. Removed the bath blanket.			
28. Raised or lowered bed rails. Followed the care plan.			
29. Lowered the bed to its lowest level.			
30. Placed the signal light within reach.			
31. Unscreened the person.			
32. Returned the bath blanket to its proper place.			
33. Decontaminated hands.			
34. Reported and recorded observations.			

Date of Satisfactory Completion ______________________ Instructor's Initials ____________________

Helping the Person Walk

Name: ____________________

Date: ____________________

Pre-Procedure	**S**	**U**	**Comments**
• Knocked before entering the person's room.	____	____	____________
• Addressed the person by name.	____	____	____________
• Introduced yourself by name and title.	____	____	____________
1. Followed Delegation Guidelines. Reviewed Safety Alert.	____	____	____________
2. Explained the procedure to the person.	____	____	____________
3. Practiced hand hygiene.	____	____	____________
4. Collected the following:			
• Robe and nonskid shoes	____	____	____________
• Paper or sheet to protect bottom linens	____	____	____________
• Transfer (gait or safety) belt	____	____	____________
5. Identified the person. Checked the ID bracelet against the assignment sheet. Called the person by name.	____	____	____________
6. Provided for privacy.	____	____	____________
Procedure			
7. Lowered the bed to its lowest position. Locked the bed wheels. Lowered the bed rail if up.	____	____	____________
8. Fanfolded top linens to the foot of the bed.	____	____	____________
9. Placed the paper or sheet under the person's feet. Put the shoes on the person.	____	____	____________
10. Helped the person to dangle.	____	____	____________
11. Helped the person put on the robe.	____	____	____________
12. Applied the gait belt.	____	____	____________
13. Helped the person stand.	____	____	____________
14. Stood at the person's side while the person gained balance. Held the belt at the side and back, or had one arm around the back to support the person.	____	____	____________
15. Encouraged the person to stand erect with the head up and back straight.	____	____	____________
16. Helped the person walk. Walked to the side and slightly behind the person. Provided support with the gait belt, or had one arm around the back to support the person.	____	____	____________
17. Encouraged the person to walk normally.	____	____	____________
18. Walked the required distance if the person tolerated the activity. Did not rush the person.	____	____	____________
19. Helped the person return to bed.	____	____	____________
20. Lowered the head of the bed. Helped the person to the center of the bed.	____	____	____________

Procedure—cont'd	S	U	Comments
21. Removed the shoes. Removed the paper or sheet over the bottom sheet.	_____	_____	__________

Post-Procedure	S	U	Comments
22. Provided for comfort. Covered the person.	_____	_____	__________
23. Placed the signal light within reach.	_____	_____	__________
24. Raised or lowered bed rails. Followed the care plan.	_____	_____	__________
25. Returned the robe and shoes to their proper place.	_____	_____	__________
26. Unscreened the person.	_____	_____	__________
27. Decontaminated hands.	_____	_____	__________
28. Reported and recorded observations. • How well the person tolerated the activity. • The distance walked.	_____	_____	__________

Date of Satisfactory Completion ____________________ Instructor's Initials ____________________

Helping the Falling Person

Name: ______________________

Date: ______________________

Procedure	S	U	Comments
1. Stood with your feet apart. Kept the back straight.	____	____	____________
2. Brought the person close to your body as fast as possible. Used the gait belt, or wrapped the arms around the person's waist. The person could also be held under the arms.	____	____	____________
3. Moved your leg so the person's buttocks rested on it. Moved the leg near the person.	____	____	____________
4. Lowered the person to the floor. The person slid down the leg to the floor. Bent at the hips and knees as the person was lowered.	____	____	____________
5. Called a nurse to check the person.	____	____	____________
6. Helped the nurse return the person to bed. Got other staff to help if needed.	____	____	____________
7. Reported the following to the nurse:	____	____	____________
a. How the fall occurred	____	____	____________
b. How far the person walked	____	____	____________
c. How activity was tolerated before the fall	____	____	____________
d. Complaints before the fall	____	____	____________
e. How much help the person needed while walking	____	____	____________
8. Completed an incident report.	____	____	____________

Date of Satisfactory Completion ______________ Instructor's Initials ______________

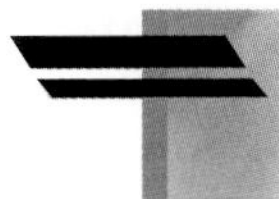

Taking a Temperature With a Glass Thermometer

Name: ____________________

Date: ____________________

Pre-Procedure	S	U	Comments
• Knocked before entering the person's room.			
• Addressed the person by name.			
• Introduced yourself by name and title.			
1. Followed Delegation Guidelines. Reviewed Safety Alerts.			
2. Explained the procedure to the person.			
3. Collected the following:			
• Oral or rectal thermometer and holder			
• Tissues			
• Plastic covers if used			
• Gloves			
• Toilet tissue (rectal temperature)			
• Water-soluble lubricant (rectal temperature)			
• Towel (axillary temperature)			
4. Practiced hand hygiene.			
5. Identified the person. Checked the ID bracelet against the assignment sheet. Called the person by name.			
6. Provided for privacy.			
Procedure			
7. Put on the gloves.			
8. Rinsed the thermometer in cold water if it was soaking in a disinfectant. Dried it with tissues.			
9. Checked for breaks, cracks, or chips.			
10. Shook down the thermometer below the lowest number.			
11. Inserted it into a plastic cover if used.			
12. For an oral temperature:			
a. Asked the person to moisten the lips.			
b. Placed the bulb end of the thermometer under the tongue.			
c. Asked the person to close the lips around the thermometer to hold it in place.			
d. Asked the person not to talk. Reminded the person not to bite down on the thermometer.			
e. Left it in place for 2 to 3 minutes or as required by agency policy.			

Procedure—cont'd	S	U	Comments
13. For a rectal temperature:			
a. Positioned the person in Sims' position.			
b. Put a small amount of lubricant on a tissue. Lubricated the bulb end of the thermometer.			
c. Folded back top linens to expose the anal area.			
d. Raised the upper buttock to expose the anus.			
e. Inserted the thermometer 1 inch into the rectum. Did not force the thermometer.			
f. Held the thermometer in place for 2 minutes or as required by agency policy. Did not let go of it while it was in the rectum.			
14. For an axillary temperature:			
a. Helped the person remove an arm from the gown. Did not expose the person.			
b. Dried the axilla with the towel.			
c. Placed the bulb end of the thermometer in the center of the axilla.			
d. Asked the person to place the arm over the chest to hold the thermometer in place. Held it and the arm in place if he or she could not help.			
e. Left the thermometer in place for 5 to 10 minutes or as required by agency policy.			
15. Removed the thermometer.			
16. Used tissues to remove the plastic cover. Wiped the thermometer with a tissue if no cover was used. Wiped from the stem to the bulb end.			
17. For a rectal temperature:			
a. Placed used toilet tissue on a paper towel or several thicknesses of toilet tissue.			
b. Placed the thermometer on clean toilet tissue.			
c. Wiped the anal area to remove excess lubricant and any feces.			
d. Covered the person.			
18. For an axillary temperature: Helped the person put the gown back on.			
19. Read the thermometer.			
20. Recorded the person's name and temperature on the note pad or assignment sheet. Wrote R for a rectal temperature. Wrote A for an axillary temperature.			
21. Shook down the thermometer.			
22. Cleaned it according to agency policy.			
23. Discarded tissue and the paper towel.			
24. Removed the gloves. Decontaminated hands.			

Post-Procedure	S	U	Comments
25. Provided for comfort.			
26. Placed the signal light within reach.			
27. Unscreened the person.			
28. Recorded the temperature in the proper place. Reported any abnormal temperature to the nurse. Noted the temperature site.			

Date of Satisfactory Completion ____________ Instructor's Initials ____________

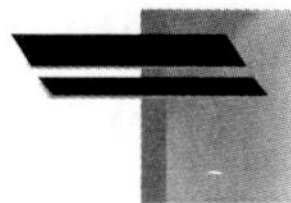

Taking a Temperature With an Electronic Thermometer

Name: ______________________

Date: ______________________

Pre-Procedure	**S**	**U**	**Comments**
• Knocked before entering the person's room.	____	____	______________
• Addressed the person by name.	____	____	______________
• Introduced yourself by name and title.	____	____	______________
1. Followed Delegation Guidelines. Reviewed Safety Alerts.	____	____	______________
2. Explained the procedure to the person. For an oral temperature, asked the person not to eat, drink, smoke, or chew gum for at least 15 to 20 minutes.	____	____	______________
3. Collected the following:			
• Thermometer—electronic or tympanic membrane	____	____	______________
• Probe (Blue for an oral or axillary temperature. Red for a rectal temperature.)	____	____	______________
• Probe covers	____	____	______________
• Toilet tissue (rectal temperature)	____	____	______________
• Water-soluble lubricant (rectal temperature)	____	____	______________
• Gloves	____	____	______________
• Towel (axillary temperature)	____	____	______________
4. Plugged the probe into the thermometer. (This is not done for a tympanic membrane thermometer.)	____	____	______________
5. Practiced hand hygiene.	____	____	______________
6. Identified the person. Checked the ID bracelet against the assignment sheet. Called the person by name.	____	____	______________

Procedure			
7. Provided for privacy. Positioned the person for an oral, rectal, axillary, or tympanic membrane temperature.	____	____	______________
8. Put on gloves if contact with blood, body fluids, secretions, or excretions was likely.	____	____	______________
9. Inserted the probe into a probe cover.	____	____	______________
10. For an oral temperature:			
a. Asked the person to open the mouth and raise the tongue.	____	____	______________
b. Placed the covered probe at the base of the tongue.	____	____	______________
c. Asked the person to lower the tongue and close the mouth.	____	____	______________

Procedure—cont'd

Procedure—cont'd	S	U	Comments
11. For a rectal temperature:			
a. Placed some lubricant on toilet tissue.			
b. Lubricated the end of the covered probe.			
c. Exposed the anal area.			
d. Raised the upper buttock.			
e. Inserted the probe 1/2 inch into the rectum.			
f. Held the probe in place.			
12. For an axillary temperature:			
a. Helped the person remove an arm from the gown. Did not expose the person.			
b. Dried the axilla with the towel.			
c. Placed the covered probe in the axilla.			
d. Placed the person's arm over the chest.			
e. Held the probe in place.			
13. For a tympanic membrane temperature:			
a. Asked the person to turn the head so the ear was in front of you.			
b. Pulled back on the ear to straighten the ear canal.			
c. Inserted the covered probe gently.			
14. Started the thermometer.			
15. Held the probe in place until a tone was heard or a flashing or steady light was seen.			
16. Read the temperature on the display.			
17. Removed the probe. Pressed the eject button to discard the cover.			
18. Recorded the person's name and temperature on the note pad or assignment sheet. Noted the temperature site.			
19. Returned the probe to the holder.			
20. Provided for comfort. Helped the person put the gown back on (axillary temperature). For a rectal temperature:			
a. Wiped the anal area with tissue to remove lubricant.			
b. Covered the person.			
c. Discarded used toilet tissue.			
d. Removed the gloves. Decontaminated hands.			

Post-Procedure

Post-Procedure	S	U	Comments
21. Provided for comfort.			
22. Placed the signal light within reach.			
23. Unscreened the person.			
24. Returned the thermometer to the charging unit.			
25. Decontaminated hands.			
26. Recorded the temperature in the proper place. Noted the temperature site. Reported any abnormal temperature.			

Date of Satisfactory Completion ______________ Instructor's Initials ______________

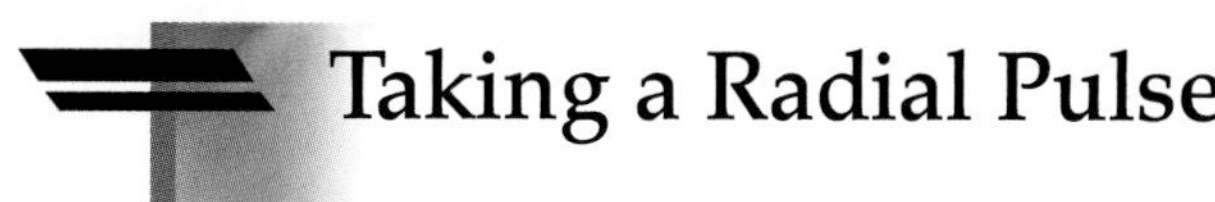

Taking a Radial Pulse

Name: ______________________

Date: ______________________

Pre-Procedure	S	U	Comments
• Knocked before entering the person's room.			
• Addressed the person by name.			
• Introduced yourself by name and title.			
1. Followed Delegation Guidelines. Reviewed Safety Alert.			
2. Practiced hand hygiene.			
3. Identified the person. Checked the ID bracelet against the assignment sheet. Called the person by name.			
4. Explained the procedure to the person.			
5. Provided for privacy.			

Procedure

	S	U	Comments
6. Had the person sit or lie down.			
7. Located the radial pulse. Used the first 2 or 3 middle fingers.			
8. Noted if the pulse was strong or weak, and regular or irregular.			
9. Counted the pulse for 30 seconds. Multiplied the number of beats by 2. Or, counted the pulse for 1 minute as directed by the nurse or if required by agency policy.			
10. Counted the pulse for 1 minute if it was irregular.			
11. Recorded the person's name and pulse on the note pad or assignment sheet. Noted the strength of the pulse. Noted if it was regular or irregular.			

Post-Procedure

	S	U	Comments
12. Provided for comfort.			
13. Placed the signal light within reach.			
14. Unscreened the person.			
15. Decontaminated hands.			
16. Reported and recorded the pulse rate and observations.			

Date of Satisfactory Completion ______________________ Instructor's Initials ______________________

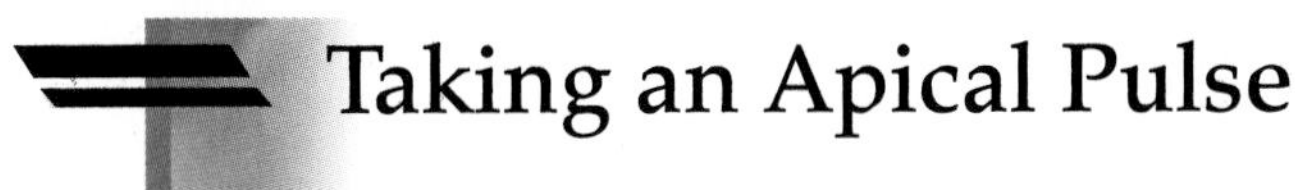

Taking an Apical Pulse

Name: ____________________

Date: ____________________

Pre-Procedure	S	U	Comments
• Knocked before entering the person's room.			
• Addressed the person by name.			
• Introduced yourself by name and title.			
1. Followed Delegation Guidelines. Reviewed Safety Alert.			
2. Collected a stethoscope and antiseptic wipes.			
3. Practiced hand hygiene.			
4. Identified the person. Checked the ID bracelet against the assignment sheet. Called the person by name.			
5. Explained the procedure to the person.			
6. Provided for privacy.			
Procedure			
7. Cleaned the earpieces and diaphragm with the wipes.			
8. Had the person sit or lie down.			
9. Exposed the nipple area of the left chest. Did not expose a woman's breasts.			
10. Warmed the diaphragm in your palm.			
11. Placed the earpieces in your ears.			
12. Found the apical pulse. Placed the diaphragm 2 to 3 inches to the left of the breastbone and below the left nipple.			
13. Counted the pulse for 1 minute. Noted if it was regular or irregular.			
14. Covered the person. Removed the earpieces.			
15. Recorded the person's name and pulse on the note pad or assignment sheet. Noted if the pulse was regular or irregular.			
Post-Procedure			
16. Provided for comfort.			
17. Placed the signal light within reach.			
18. Unscreened the person.			
19. Cleaned the earpieces and diaphragm with the wipes.			
20. Returned the stethoscope to its proper place.			
21. Decontaminated hands.			
22. Reported and recorded observations. Recorded the pulse rate with Ap for apical pulse.			

Date of Satisfactory Completion ____________________ Instructor's Initials ____________________

Taking an Apical-Radial Pulse

Name: ______________________

Date: ______________________

Pre-Procedure	S	U	Comments
• Knocked before entering the person's room.	____	____	____________
• Addressed the person by name.	____	____	____________
• Introduced yourself by name and title.	____	____	____________
1. Followed Delegation Guidelines. Reviewed Safety Alerts.	____	____	____________
2. Asked a nurse or a nursing assistant to help.	____	____	____________
3. Collected a stethoscope and antiseptic wipes.	____	____	____________
4. Practiced hand hygiene.	____	____	____________
5. Identified the person. Checked the ID bracelet against the assignment sheet. Called the person by name.	____	____	____________
6. Explained the procedure to the person.	____	____	____________
7. Provided for privacy.	____	____	____________
Procedure			
8. Wiped the earpieces and diaphragm with the wipes.	____	____	____________
9. Had the person sit or lie down.	____	____	____________
10. Warmed the diaphragm in your palm.	____	____	____________
11. Exposed the left nipple area of the chest. Did not expose a woman's breasts.	____	____	____________
12. Placed the earpieces in your ears.	____	____	____________
13. Found the apical pulse. The helper found the radial pulse.	____	____	____________
14. Gave the signal to begin counting.	____	____	____________
15. Counted the pulse for 1 minute.	____	____	____________
16. Gave the signal to stop counting.	____	____	____________
17. Covered the person. Removed the earpieces.	____	____	____________
18. Recorded the person's name and the apical and radial pulses on the note pad or assignment sheet. Subtracted the radial pulse from the apical pulse for the pulse deficit. Noted whether the pulse was regular or irregular.	____	____	____________
Post-Procedure			
19. Provided for comfort.	____	____	____________
20. Placed the signal light within reach.	____	____	____________
21. Unscreened the person.	____	____	____________
22. Cleaned the earpieces and diaphragm with the wipes.	____	____	____________
23. Returned the stethoscope to its proper place.	____	____	____________
24. Decontaminated hands.	____	____	____________

Post-Procedure—cont'd

	S	U	Comments
25. Reported and recorded observations. Included:	_____	_____	_____
• The apical and radial pulse rates	_____	_____	_____
• The pulse deficit	_____	_____	_____

Date of Satisfactory Completion _______________ Instructor's Initials _______________

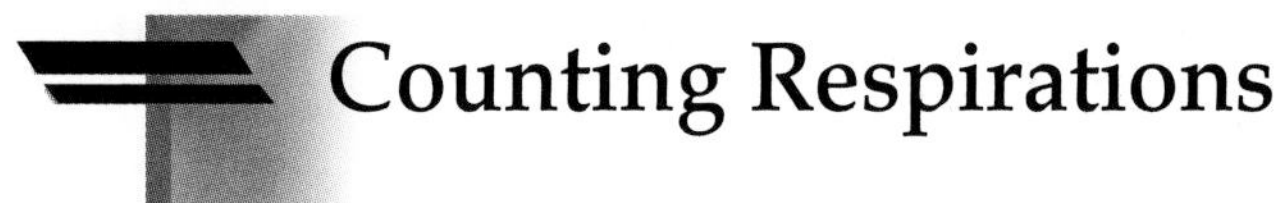

Counting Respirations

Name: ______________________

Date: ______________________

Procedure	S	U	Comments
1. Followed Delegation Guidelines.	____	____	____________
2. Kept your fingers or the stethoscope over the pulse site.	____	____	____________
3. Did not tell the person that respirations were being counted.	____	____	____________
4. Began counting when the chest rose. Counted each rise and fall of the chest as 1 respiration.	____	____	____________
5. Noted the following:			
• If respirations were regular	____	____	____________
• If both sides of the chest rose equally	____	____	____________
• The depth of respirations	____	____	____________
• If the person had any pain or difficulty breathing	____	____	____________
6. Counted respirations for 30 seconds. Multiplied the number by 2.	____	____	____________
7. Counted respirations for 1 minute if they were abnormal or irregular.	____	____	____________
8. Recorded the person's name, respiratory rate, and other observations on the note pad or assignment sheet.	____	____	____________
Post-Procedure			
9. Provided for comfort.	____	____	____________
10. Placed the signal light within reach.	____	____	____________
11. Decontaminated hands.	____	____	____________
12. Reported and recorded observations.	____	____	____________

Date of Satisfactory Completion ______________ Instructor's Initials ______________

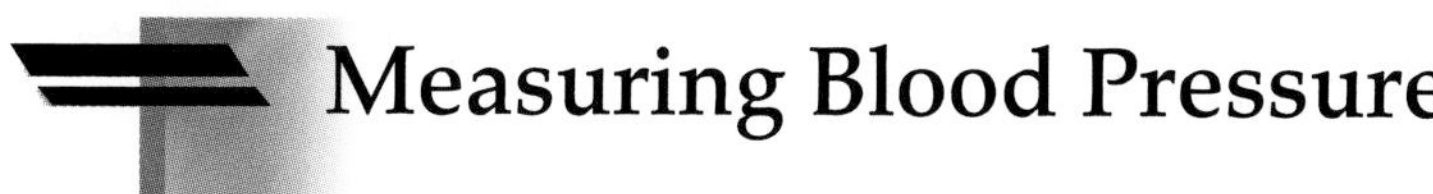

Measuring Blood Pressure

Name: ____________________

Date: ____________________

Pre-Procedure	S	U	Comments
• Knocked before entering the person's room.			
• Addressed the person by name.			
• Introduced yourself by name and title.			
1. Followed Delegation Guidelines. Reviewed Safety Alerts.			
2. Collected the following:			
• Sphygmomanometer			
• Stethoscope			
• Antiseptic wipes			
3. Practiced hand hygiene.			
4. Identified the person. Checked the ID bracelet against the assignment sheet. Called the person by name.			
5. Explained the procedure to the person.			
6. Provided for privacy.			

Procedure	S	U	Comments
7. Wiped the stethoscope earpieces and diaphragm with the wipes.			
8. Had the person sit or lie down.			
9. Positioned the person's arm level with the heart. The palm was up.			
10. Stood no more than 3 feet away from the manometer.			
11. Exposed the upper arm.			
12. Squeezed the cuff to expel any remaining air. Closed the valve on the bulb.			
13. Found the brachial artery at the inner aspect of the elbow.			
14. Placed the arrow on the cuff over the brachial artery. Wrapped the cuff around the upper arm at least 1 inch above the elbow. It was even and snug.			
15. Method 1:			
a. Placed the stethoscope earpieces in your ears.			
b. Found the radial or brachial artery.			
c. Inflated the cuff until the pulse could no longer be felt. Noted this point.			
d. Inflated the cuff 30 mm Hg beyond the point where the pulse was last felt.			

Procedure—cont'd	S	U	Comments
16. Method 2:			
a. Found the radial or brachial artery.			
b. Inflated the cuff until the pulse could no longer be felt. Noted this point.			
c. Inflated the cuff 30 mm Hg beyond the point where the pulse was last felt.			
d. Deflated the cuff slowly. Noted the point when the pulse was felt.			
e. Waited 30 seconds.			
f. Placed the stethoscope earpieces in your ears.			
g. Inflated the cuff 30 mm Hg beyond the point where you felt the pulse return.			
17. Placed the diaphragm over the brachial artery. Did not place it under the cuff.			
18. Deflated the cuff at an even rate of 2 to 4 millimeters per second. Turned the valve counterclockwise to deflate the cuff.			
19. Noted the point where the first sound was heard.			
20. Continued to deflate the cuff. Noted the point where the sound disappeared.			
21. Deflated the cuff completely. Removed it from the person's arm. Removed the stethoscope.			
22. Recorded the person's name and blood pressure on the note pad or assignment sheet.			
23. Returned the cuff to the case or wall holder.			

Post-Procedure

	S	U	Comments
24. Provided for comfort.			
25. Placed the signal light within reach.			
26. Unscreened the person.			
27. Cleaned the earpieces and diaphragm with the wipes.			
28. Returned the equipment to its proper place.			
29. Decontaminated hands.			
30. Reported and recorded the blood pressure.			

Date of Satisfactory Completion ____________________ Instructor's Initials ____________________

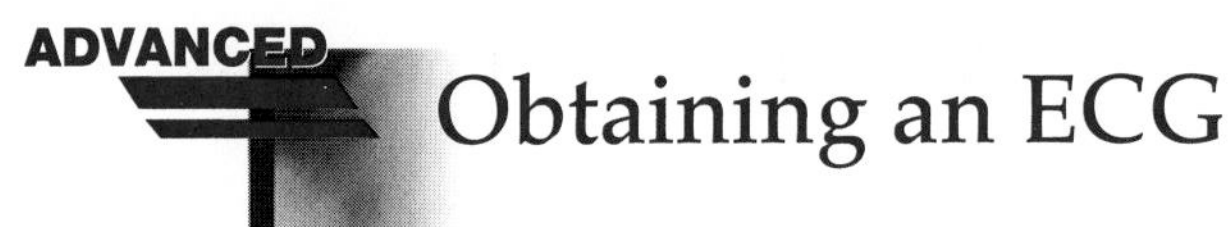

Obtaining an ECG

Name: ______________________

Date: ______________________

Pre-Procedure	**S**	**U**	**Comments**
• Knocked before entering the person's room.	____	____	______________
• Addressed the person by name.	____	____	______________
• Introduced yourself by name and title.	____	____	______________
1. Followed Delegation Guidelines. Reviewed Safety Alert.	____	____	______________
2. Explained the procedure to the person.	____	____	______________
3. Practiced hand hygiene.	____	____	______________
4. Collected the following:			
• Electrocardiograph	____	____	______________
• Electrodes	____	____	______________
• Alcohol wipes	____	____	______________
• Razor	____	____	______________
• Towel	____	____	______________
• Gloves	____	____	______________
• Requisition slip	____	____	______________
• Stethoscope	____	____	______________
• Sphygmomanometer	____	____	______________
5. Reviewed the manufacturer's instructions for the ECG machine.	____	____	______________
6. Arranged equipment in the person's room. Plugged the machine into an outlet and turned on the machine.	____	____	______________
7. Identified the person. Checked the ID bracelet against the requisition slip. Called the person by name.	____	____	______________
8. Provided for privacy.	____	____	______________
9. Raised the bed for body mechanics. The far bed rail was up if used.	____	____	______________
10. Assisted with elimination needs. Cleaned and returned equipment to its proper place. Removed gloves and decontaminated hands.	____	____	______________

Procedure

11. Measured the person's vital signs. Noted them on the assignment sheet.	____	____	______________
12. Positioned the person supine.	____	____	______________
13. Exposed only the person's chest, arms, and legs.	____	____	______________

Procedure—cont'd

	S	U	Comments
14. Shaved electrode sites as needed:			
a. Placed a towel under the site.			
b. Put on the gloves.			
c. Shaved the site.			
d. Moved the towel to the next site. Avoided getting hair on bed linens.			
e. Shaved that site.			
f. Repeated steps 14d and 14e as necessary.			
g. Removed and discarded the gloves. Decontaminated hands.			
15. Cleaned the electrode sites with the alcohol wipes. Let the sites dry.			
16. Applied the electrodes to the chest, arms, and legs.			
17. Connected the cables from the machine to the electrodes.			
18. Asked the person to lie still. Reminded the person not to talk or to cross the legs.			
19. Obtained an 8- to 12-inch tracing of each lead. Called for the nurse if any abnormal patterns were seen.			
20. Turned off the machine.			
21. Tore the tracing off the machine.			
22. Labeled the tracing with the person's identifying information: full name, ID number, room and bed number, and age. Also noted the date and time.			
23. Disconnected the cables.			
24. Removed the electrodes.			
25. Covered the person.			

Post-Procedure

	S	U	Comments
26. Provided for comfort.			
27. Placed the signal light within reach.			
28. Raised or lowered bed rails. Followed the care plan.			
29. Lowered the bed to its lowest position.			
30. Unscreened the person.			
31. Discarded used supplies. Followed agency policy for soiled linen.			
32. Unplugged and returned the ECG machine to its proper location.			
33. Showed the ECG to the nurse. Reported any observations or complaints from the person.			
34. Took or sent the ECG and requisition to the appropriate department.			
35. Decontaminated hands.			

Date of Satisfactory Completion ______________ Instructor's Initials ______________

Collecting a Random Urine Specimen

Name: ______________________

Date: ______________________

Pre-Procedure	S	U	Comments
• Knocked before entering the person's room.	_____	_____	______________
• Addressed the person by name.	_____	_____	______________
• Introduced yourself by name and title.	_____	_____	______________
1. Followed Delegation Guidelines. Reviewed Safety Alert.	_____	_____	______________
2. Explained the procedure to the person.	_____	_____	______________
3. Practiced hand hygiene.	_____	_____	______________
4. Collected the following:			
• Voiding receptacle—bedpan and cover, urinal, or specimen pan	_____	_____	______________
• Specimen container and lid	_____	_____	______________
• Label	_____	_____	______________
• Gloves	_____	_____	______________
• Plastic bag	_____	_____	______________
Procedure			
5. Labeled the container.	_____	_____	______________
6. Put the container and lid in the bathroom.	_____	_____	______________
7. Identified the person. Checked the ID bracelet against the requisition slip. Called the person by name.	_____	_____	______________
8. Provided for privacy.	_____	_____	______________
9. Put on the gloves.	_____	_____	______________
10. Asked the person to void into the receptacle. Reminded the person to put toilet tissue into the wastebasket or toilet.	_____	_____	______________
11. Took the receptacle to the bathroom.	_____	_____	______________
12. Poured about 120 ml (4 oz) of urine into the specimen container. Disposed of excess urine.	_____	_____	______________
13. Placed the lid on the specimen container. Put the container in the plastic bag.	_____	_____	______________
14. Cleaned and returned the receptacle to its proper place.	_____	_____	______________
15. Assisted the person with handwashing.	_____	_____	______________
16. Practiced hand hygiene.	_____	_____	______________
Post-Procedure			
17. Provided for comfort.	_____	_____	______________
18. Placed the signal light within reach.	_____	_____	______________

Post-Procedure—cont'd	S	U	Comments
19. Raised or lowered bed rails. Followed the care plan.			
20. Unscreened the person.			
21. Decontaminated hands.			
22. Reported and recorded observations.			
23. Took the specimen and the requisition slip to the storage area or laboratory.			

Date of Satisfactory Completion ______________________ Instructor's Initials ______________________

Collecting a Midstream Specimen

Name: ______________________

Date: ______________________

Pre-Procedure	S	U	Comments
• Knocked before entering the person's room.	______	______	______________
• Addressed the person by name.	______	______	______________
• Introduced yourself by name and title.	______	______	______________
1. Followed Delegation Guidelines. Reviewed Safety Alert.	______	______	______________
2. Explained the procedure to the person.	______	______	______________
3. Practiced hand hygiene.	______	______	______________
4. Collected the following:			
• Midstream specimen kit (with antiseptic solution)	______	______	______________
• Label	______	______	______________
• Disposable gloves	______	______	______________
• Sterile gloves (if not part of the kit)	______	______	______________
• Voiding receptacle—bedpan, urinal, or commode if needed	______	______	______________
• Plastic bag	______	______	______________
• Supplies for perineal care	______	______	______________
5. Labeled the container.	______	______	______________
6. Identified the person. Checked the ID bracelet against the requisition slip. Called the person by name.	______	______	______________
7. Provided for privacy.	______	______	______________

Procedure

8. Provided perineal care. Removed gloves and decontaminated hands.	______	______	______________
9. Opened the sterile kit. Used sterile technique.	______	______	______________
10. Put on the sterile gloves.	______	______	______________
11. Poured the antiseptic solution over the cotton balls.	______	______	______________
12. Opened the sterile specimen container. Did not touch the inside of the container or lid. Set the lid down so the inside was up.	______	______	______________
13. For a female: cleaned the perineum with cotton balls.	______	______	______________
a. Spread the labia with the thumb and index finger. Used the non-dominant hand.	______	______	______________
b. Cleaned down the urethral area from front to back. Used a clean cotton ball for each stroke.	______	______	______________
c. Kept the labia separated to collect the urine specimen (steps 16 and 17).	______	______	______________

Procedure—cont'd	S	U	Comments
14. For a male: cleaned the penis with cotton balls.			
a. Held the penis with the non-dominant hand.			
b. Cleaned the penis starting at the meatus. Used a cotton ball and cleaned in a circular motion. Started at the center and worked outward.			
c. Kept holding the penis until the specimen was collected (steps 16 and 17).			
15. Asked the person to void into the receptacle.			
16. Passed the specimen container into the stream of urine. Kept the labia separated.			
17. Collected about 30 to 60 ml of urine (1 to 2 oz).			
18. Removed the specimen container before the person stopped voiding.			
19. Released the labia or penis.			
20. Let the person finish voiding into the receptacle.			
21. Put the lid on the specimen container. Touched only the outside of the container or lid.			
22. Wiped the outside of the container.			
23. Placed the container in a plastic bag.			
24. Provided toilet tissue after the person was done voiding.			
25. Took the receptacle to the bathroom.			
26. Measured urine if intake and output was ordered. Included the amount in the specimen container.			
27. Cleaned the receptacle and other items. Returned equipment to its proper place.			
28. Removed soiled gloves. Practiced hygiene.			
29. Put on clean gloves.			
30. Assisted the person with handwashing.			
31. Removed the gloves. Decontaminated hands.			

Post-Procedure

32. Followed steps 17 through 23 in procedure: *Collecting a Random Urine Specimen.*			

Date of Satisfactory Completion ____________________ Instructor's Initials ____________________

Collecting a 24-Hour Urine Specimen

Name: ______________________

Date: ______________________

Pre-Procedure

	S	U	Comments
• Knocked before entering the person's room.			
• Addressed the person by name.			
• Introduced yourself by name and title.			
1. Followed Delegation Guidelines. Reviewed Safety Alert.			
2. Explained the procedure to the person.			
3. Practiced hand hygiene.			
4. Collected the following:			
• Urine container for a 24-hour collection			
• Preservative if needed			
• Bucket with ice if needed			
• Two 24-hour urine specimen labels			
• Funnel			
• Voiding receptacle—bedpan, urinal, commode, or specimen pan			
• Gloves			
• Graduate			
5. Labeled the urine container.			
6. Identified the person. Checked the ID bracelet against the requisition slip. Called the person by name.			
7. Arranged equipment in the person's bathroom.			
8. Placed one label in the bathroom. Placed the other near the bed.			

Procedure

	S	U	Comments
9. Put on the gloves.			
10. Offered the bedpan or urinal, or assisted the person to the bathroom or commode.			
11. Asked the person to void.			
12. Discarded the urine, and noted the time. This started the 24-hour collection period.			
13. Cleaned the bedpan, urinal, commode, or specimen pan.			
14. Removed the gloves. Practiced hand hygiene.			
15. Marked the time the test began and the time it ended on the room and bathroom labels. Also marked the urine container.			

Procedure—cont'd	S	U	Comments
16. Asked the person to use the bedpan, urinal, commode, or specimen pan when voiding during the next 24 hours. Told the person to signal after voiding. Reminded the person not to have a bowel movement at the same time and not to put toilet tissue in the receptacle.	______	______	____________
17. Put on the gloves.	______	______	____________
18. Measured all urine if I&O was ordered.	______	______	____________
19. Poured urine into the urine container using the funnel. Did not spill any urine. Restarted the test if urine was spilled or discarded.	______	______	____________
20. Cleaned the receptacle. Removed the gloves and practiced hand hygiene.	______	______	____________
21. Added ice to the bucket as needed.	______	______	____________
22. Asked the person to void at the end of the 24-hour period. Poured the urine into the urine container. Wore gloves for this step.	______	______	____________

Post-Procedure

23. Provided for comfort.	______	______	____________
24. Placed the signal light within reach.	______	______	____________
25. Raised or lowered bed rails. Followed the care plan.	______	______	____________
26. Removed the labels from the room and bathroom.	______	______	____________
27. Cleaned and returned equipment to its proper place. Discarded disposable items. Wore gloves for this step.	______	______	____________
28. Removed the gloves and decontaminated hands.	______	______	____________
29. Reported and recorded observations.	______	______	____________
30. Took the specimen and requisition slip to the laboratory.	______	______	____________

Date of Satisfactory Completion ____________________ Instructor's Initials ____________________

Collecting a Double-Voided Specimen

Name: ______________________

Date: ______________________

Pre-Procedure

	S	U	Comments
• Knocked before entering the person's room.			
• Addressed the person by name.			
• Introduced yourself by name and title.			
1. Followed Delegation Guidelines. Reviewed Safety Alert.			
2. Explained the procedure to the person.			
3. Practiced hand hygiene.			
4. Collected the following:			
• Voiding receptacle—bedpan, urinal, commode, or specimen pan			
• Two specimen containers			
• Urine testing equipment			
• Gloves			
5. Identified the person. Checked the ID bracelet against the assignment sheet. Called the person by name.			
6. Provided for privacy.			

Procedure

	S	U	Comments
7. Put on the gloves.			
8. Asked the person to void into the receptacle. Reminded the person not to put toilet tissue in the receptacle.			
9. Took the receptacle to the bathroom.			
10. Poured some urine into the specimen container.			
11. Tested the specimen in case a second specimen could not be obtained. Discarded the urine.			
12. Cleaned the receptacle and returned the receptacle to its proper place.			
13. Removed the gloves. Practiced hand hygiene.			
14. Assisted the person with handwashing. Wore gloves if needed. Decontaminated hands after removing gloves.			
15. Asked the person to drink an 8-ounce glass of water.			
16. Provided for comfort. Raised the bed rails if needed. Placed the signal light within reach.			
17. Unscreened the person.			
18. Decontaminated hands.			
19. Returned to the room in 20 to 30 minutes.			
20. Repeated steps 6 through 14.			

Post-Procedure	S	U	Comments
21. Provided for comfort.			
22. Raised the bed rails if needed. Followed the care plan.			
23. Placed the signal light within reach.			
24. Unscreened the person.			
25. Decontaminated hands.			
26. Reported the results of the second test and any other observations.			

Date of Satisfactory Completion ____________ Instructor's Initials ____________

ADVANCED

Collecting a Sterile Urine Specimen From an Indwelling Catheter

Name: ______________________

Date: ______________________

Pre-Procedure

	S	U	Comments
• Knocked before entering the person's room.	____	____	____________
• Addressed the person by name.	____	____	____________
• Introduced yourself by name and title.	____	____	____________
1. Followed Delegation Guidelines. Reviewed Safety Alert.	____	____	____________
2. Practiced hand hygiene.	____	____	____________
3. Identified the person. Checked the ID bracelet against the laboratory requisition slip. Called the person by name.	____	____	____________
4. Put on gloves.	____	____	____________
5. Clamped the drainage tube for 15 to 30 minutes as directed by the nurse. Provided privacy during this step.	____	____	____________
6. Removed the gloves. Decontaminated hands.	____	____	____________
7. Collected the following:			
• Syringe and needle as directed	____	____	____________
• Antiseptic swabs	____	____	____________
• Sterile specimen container	____	____	____________
• Label	____	____	____________
• Plastic bag	____	____	____________
• Gloves	____	____	____________
8. Returned to the room after 15 to 30 minutes. Practiced hand hygiene.	____	____	____________
9. Identified the person again.	____	____	____________
10. Provided for privacy.	____	____	____________

Procedure

	S	U	Comments
11. Labeled the specimen container.	____	____	____________
12. Put on gloves.	____	____	____________
13. Opened the specimen container. Set the lid down so the inside was up.	____	____	____________
14. Exposed the catheter site.	____	____	____________
15. Cleaned the puncture site with an antiseptic swab. Used the collection port or end of a self-sealing catheter.	____	____	____________
16. Unclamped the catheter.	____	____	____________
17. Removed the needle cap. Pulled the cap straight off the needle.	____	____	____________
18. Inserted the needle at a 90-degree angle into a collection port. Inserted the needle at a 30-degree angle into a self-sealing catheter.	____	____	____________

Procedure—cont'd	S	U	Comments
19. Pulled back on the plunger to fill the syringe with urine.			
20. Transferred syringe contents into the specimen container. Pushed down on the plunger to eject urine from the syringe. Did not let the needle touch the outside of the specimen container.			
21. Put the lid on the specimen container. Placed the container in a plastic bag.			
22. Discarded the syringe and needle into a sharps container.			
23. Unclamped the tubing. Made sure urine flowed into the drainage bag.			
24. Covered the person.			
25. Removed the gloves. Decontaminated hands.			

Post-Procedure

	S	U	Comments
26. Provided for comfort.			
27. Placed the signal light within reach.			
28. Unscreened the person.			
29. Discarded disposable supplies.			
30. Decontaminated hands.			
31. Reported and recorded observations.			
32. Took the urine specimen and requisition slip to the laboratory.			

Date of Satisfactory Completion ____________________ Instructor's Initials ____________________

Collecting a Urine Specimen From an Infant or Child

Name: ______________________

Date: ______________________

Pre-Procedure	S	U	Comments
• Knocked before entering the person's room.	____	____	____________
• Addressed the person by name.	____	____	____________
• Introduced yourself by name and title.	____	____	____________
1. Followed Delegation Guidelines. Reviewed Safety Alert.	____	____	____________
2. Explained the procedure to the child and parents.	____	____	____________
3. Practiced hand hygiene.	____	____	____________
4. Collected the following:			
• Collection bag	____	____	____________
• Wash basin	____	____	____________
• Cotton balls	____	____	____________
• Bath towel	____	____	____________
• Two diapers	____	____	____________
• Specimen container	____	____	____________
• Gloves	____	____	____________
• Plastic bag	____	____	____________
• Scissors	____	____	____________
5. Identified the child. Checked the ID bracelet against the requisition slip. Called the child by name.	____	____	____________
6. Provided for privacy.	____	____	____________

Procedure	S	U	Comments
7. Put on the gloves.	____	____	____________
8. Removed and disposed of the diaper.	____	____	____________
9. Cleaned the perineal area. Used a new cotton ball for each stroke. Rinsed and dried the area.	____	____	____________
10. Removed the gloves and practiced hand hygiene. Bed rails were up before leaving the bedside.	____	____	____________
11. Put on clean gloves.	____	____	____________
12. Positioned the child on the back. Flexed the child's knees and separated the legs.	____	____	____________
13. Removed the adhesive backing from the collection bag.	____	____	____________
14. Applied the bag to the perineum. Did not cover the anus.	____	____	____________
15. Cut a slit in the bottom of a new diaper.	____	____	____________
16. Diapered the child.	____	____	____________
17. Pulled the collection bag through the slit in the diaper.	____	____	____________
18. Removed the gloves. Decontaminated hands.	____	____	____________

Procedure—cont'd	S	U	Comments
19. Raised the head of the crib if allowed.			
20. Unscreened the child.			
21. Decontaminated hands.			
22. Checked the child often. Checked the bag for urine. Wore gloves and provided for privacy.			
23. Provided privacy if the child had voided.			
24. Removed the diaper.			
25. Removed the collection bag gently.			
26. Pressed the adhesive surfaces of the bag together, or transferred urine to the specimen container using the drainage tab.			
27. Cleaned the perineal area. Rinsed and dried well.			
28. Diapered the child.			
29. Removed the gloves. Practiced hygiene.			

Post-Procedure

	S	U	Comments
30. Provided for comfort. Raised the bed rail.			
31. Unscreened the child.			
32. Labeled the specimen container. Placed it in the plastic bag.			
33. Cleaned and returned equipment to its proper place. Discarded disposable items. Wore gloves for this step.			
34. Practiced hand hygiene.			
35. Reported and recorded observations.			
36. Took the requisition slip and the specimen to the storage area or laboratory.			

Date of Satisfactory Completion ____________________ Instructor's Initials ____________________

Testing Urine With Reagent Strips

Name: ______________________

Date: ______________________

Pre-Procedure	**S**	**U**	**Comments**
• Knocked before entering the person's room.			
• Addressed the person by name.			
• Introduced yourself by name and title.			
1. Followed Delegation Guidelines. Reviewed Safety Alerts.			
2. Explained the procedure to the person.			
3. Practiced hand hygiene.			
4. Identified the person. Checked the ID bracelet against the assignment sheet. Called the person by name.			
Procedure			
5. Put on the gloves.			
6. Collected the following:			
• Urine specimen (routine specimen for pH and occult blood; double-voided specimen for sugar and ketones)			
• Reagent strip as ordered			
• Gloves			
7. Removed a strip from the bottle. Put the cap on the bottle at once.			
8. Dipped the strip test areas into the urine.			
9. Removed the strip after the correct amount of time. Followed manufacturer's instructions.			
10. Tapped the strip gently against the container.			
11. Waited the required amount of time. Followed manufacturer's instructions.			
12. Compared the strip with the color chart on the bottle. Read the results.			
13. Discarded disposable items and the specimen.			
Post-Procedure			
14. Cleaned and returned equipment to its proper place.			
15. Removed the gloves. Practiced hand hygiene.			
16. Reported and recorded the results and other observations.			

Date of Satisfactory Completion ______________ Instructor's Initials ______________

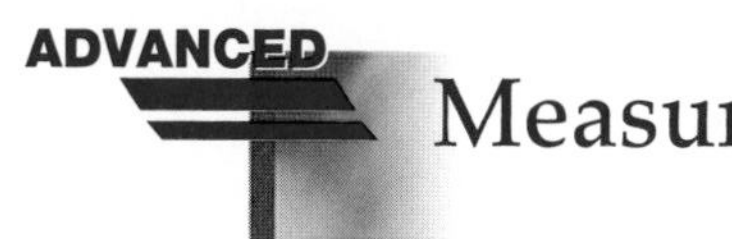

Measuring Specific Gravity

Name: ______________________

Date: ______________________

Pre-Procedure	S	U	Comments
• Knocked before entering the person's room.			
• Addressed the person by name.			
• Introduced yourself by name and title.			
1. Followed Delegation Guidelines. Reviewed Safety Alert.			
2. Practiced hand hygiene.			
3. Collected a urinometer and gloves.			
4. Identified the person. Checked the ID bracelet against the assignment sheet. Called the person by name.			
5. Provided for privacy.			
Procedure			
6. Put on the gloves.			
7. Collected a urine specimen as directed by the nurse.			
8. Filled the glass cylinder about $^1/_2$ full (about 20 ml) with urine.			
9. Placed the urinometer into the cylinder.			
10. Spun the urinometer between the thumb and index finger. Spun the device again if it stopped against the cylinder. The device floated freely.			
11. Placed the urinometer at eye level.			
12. Read the measurement at the base of the meniscus. Noted the measurement on the assignment sheet.			
13. Discarded the urine. Cleaned the urinometer.			
14. Cleaned and returned equipment to its proper place.			
15. Removed the gloves. Practiced hand hygiene.			
16. Assisted the person with handwashing.			
Post-Procedure			
17. Provided for comfort.			
18. Placed the signal light within reach.			
19. Raised or lowered bed rails. Followed the care plan.			
20. Unscreened the person.			
21. Decontaminated hands.			
22. Reported and recorded observations.			

Date of Satisfactory Completion ______________________ Instructor's Initials ______________________

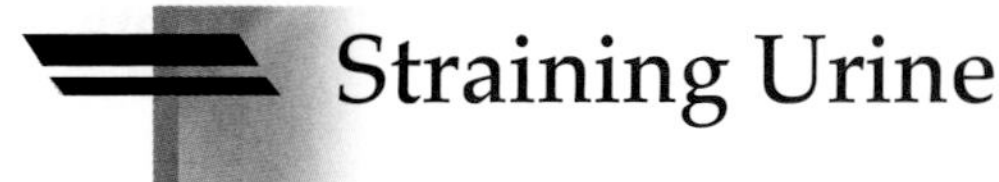

Straining Urine

Name: ______________________

Date: ______________________

Pre-Procedure	S	U	Comments
• Knocked before entering the person's room.			
• Addressed the person by name.			
• Introduced yourself by name and title.			
1. Followed Delegation Guidelines. Reviewed Safety Alert.			
2. Explained the procedure to the person. Also explained that the urinal, bedpan, commode, or specimen pan is used for voiding.			
3. Practiced hand hygiene.			
4. Collected the following:			
• Strainer or 4 × 4 gauze			
• Specimen container			
• Bedpan, urinal, commode, or specimen pan			
• Two labels stating that all urine is strained			
• Gloves			
• Plastic bag			
5. Identified the person. Checked the ID bracelet against the assignment sheet. Called the person by name.			
6. Arranged items in the person's bathroom. Placed the specimen pan in the toilet.			
7. Placed one label in the bathroom. Placed the other near the bed.			

Procedure	S	U	Comments
8. Put on the gloves.			
9. Offered the bedpan or urinal, or assisted the person to the commode or bathroom.			
10. Provided for privacy.			
11. Told the person to signal after voiding.			
12. Removed the gloves. Decontaminated hands.			
13. Returned when the person signaled. Knocked before entering the room.			
14. Decontaminated hands. Put on gloves.			
15. Placed the strainer or gauze into the specimen container.			
16. Poured urine into the specimen container. Urine passed through the strainer or gauze.			
17. Discarded the urine.			

Procedure—cont'd	S	U	Comments
18. Placed the strainer or gauze in the specimen container if any crystals, stones, or particles appeared.			
19. Provided perineal care if needed.			
20. Cleaned and returned equipment to its proper place.			
21. Removed soiled gloves. Practiced hand hygiene, and put on clean gloves.			
22. Assisted the person with handwashing.			
23. Removed the gloves. Decontaminated hands.			

Post-Procedure

	S	U	Comments
24. Provided for comfort.			
25. Placed the signal light within reach.			
26. Raised or lowered bed rails. Followed the care plan.			
27. Unscreened the person.			
28. Labeled the specimen container. Put it in the plastic bag. Wore gloves for this step.			
29. Removed the gloves. Decontaminated hands.			
30. Reported and recorded observations.			
31. Took the specimen and requisition slip to the laboratory or storage area.			

Date of Satisfactory Completion ____________ Instructor's Initials ____________

Collecting a Stool Specimen

Name: ______________________

Date: ______________________

Pre-Procedure	S	U	Comments
• Knocked before entering the person's room.			
• Addressed the person by name.			
• Introduced yourself by name and title.			
1. Followed Delegation Guidelines. Reviewed Safety Alert.			
2. Explained the procedure to the person.			
3. Practiced hand hygiene.			
4. Collected the following:			
• Bedpan and cover or commode			
• Urinal for voiding			
• Specimen pan for the toilet or commode			
• Specimen container and lid			
• Tongue blade			
• Disposable bag			
• Gloves			
• Toilet tissue			
• Laboratory requisition slip			
• Plastic bag			

Procedure	S	U	Comments
5. Labeled the container.			
6. Identified the person. Checked the ID bracelet against the requisition slip. Called the person by name.			
7. Provided for privacy.			
8. Asked the person to void. Provided the bedpan, commode, or urinal for voiding if the person did not use the bathroom. Emptied and cleaned the device.			
9. Put the specimen pan on the toilet if the person would use the bathroom. Placed it at the back of the toilet.			
10. Assisted the person onto the bedpan or to the toilet or commode. The person wore a robe and nonskid footwear.			
11. Asked the person not to put toilet tissue in the bedpan, commode, or specimen pan. Provided a bag for toilet tissue.			
12. Placed the signal light and toilet tissue within reach. Raised or lowered bed rails. Followed the care plan.			
13. Decontaminated hands. Left the room.			
14. Returned when the person signaled. Knocked before entering. Decontaminated hands.			

Procedure—cont'd	S	U	Comments
15. Lowered the bed rail near you if up.			
16. Put on the gloves. Provided perineal care if needed.			
17. Used a tongue blade to take about 2 tablespoons of stool to the specimen container. Took the sample from the middle of a formed stool. If required by agency policy, took stool from 2 different places on the specimen.			
18. Put the lid on the specimen container. Did not touch the inside of the lid or container. Placed the container in the plastic bag.			
19. Wrapped the tongue blade in toilet tissue.			
20. Discarded the tongue blade into the bag.			
21. Emptied, cleaned, and disinfected equipment.			
22. Removed the gloves. Practiced hand hygiene.			
23. Returned equipment to its proper place.			
24. Helped the person with handwashing. Wore gloves if necessary. Decontaminated hands.			

Post-Procedure	S	U	Comments
25. Provided for comfort.			
26. Placed the signal light within reach.			
27. Lowered the bed to its lowest position.			
28. Raised or lowered bed rails. Followed the care plan.			
29. Unscreened the person.			
30. Took the specimen and requisition slip to the laboratory.			
31. Decontaminated hands.			
32. Reported and recorded observations.			

Date of Satisfactory Completion ____________ Instructor's Initials ____________

Testing a Stool Specimen for Blood

Name: ______________________

Date: ______________________

Pre-Procedure	S	U	Comments
• Knocked before entering the person's room.			
• Addressed the person by name.			
• Introduced yourself by name and title.			
1. Followed Delegation Guidelines. Reviewed Safety Alert.			
2. Explained the procedure to the person.			
3. Decontaminated hands.			
Procedure			
4. Collected a stool specimen.			
5. Collected the following:			
• Paper towels			
• Hemoccult test kit			
• Tongue blades			
• Gloves			
6. Put on the gloves.			
7. Opened the test kit.			
8. Used the tongue blade to obtain a small amount of stool.			
9. Applied a thin smear of stool on box A on the test paper.			
10. Used another tongue blade to obtain stool from another part of the specimen.			
11. Applied a thin smear of stool on box B on the test paper.			
12. Closed the test packet.			
13. Turned the test packet to the other side. Opened the flap. Applied developer (from the kit) to boxes A and B. Followed the manufacturer's instructions.			
14. Waited the amount of time noted in the manufacturer's instructions.			
15. Noted and recorded the color changes.			
Post-Procedure			
16. Disposed of the test packet.			
17. Wrapped the tongue blades with toilet tissue then discarded them.			
18. Disposed of the specimen.			
19. Removed the gloves. Decontaminated hands.			
20. Reported and recorded the test results and observations.			

Date of Satisfactory Completion ______________________ Instructor's Initials ______________________

Collecting a Sputum Specimen

Name: ______________________

Date: ______________________

Pre-Procedure	S	U	Comments
• Knocked before entering the person's room.			
• Addressed the person by name.			
• Introduced yourself by name and title.			
1. Followed Delegation Guidelines. Reviewed Safety Alert.			
2. Explained the procedure to the person.			
3. Practiced hand hygiene.			
4. Collected the following:			
• Sputum specimen container and label			
• Laboratory requisition			
• Disposable bag			
• Gloves			
• Tissues			
5. Labeled the container.			
6. Identified the person. Checked the ID bracelet against the requisition slip. Called the person by name.			
7. Provided for privacy.			

Procedure

	S	U	Comments
8. Asked the person to rinse the mouth out with clear water.			
9. Put on the gloves.			
10. Had the person hold the container. Only the outside was touched.			
11. Asked the person to cover the mouth and nose with tissues when coughing.			
12. Asked the person to take 2 or 3 deep breaths and cough up the sputum.			
13. Had the person expectorate directly into the container. Sputum did not touch the outside.			
14. Collected 1 to 2 tablespoons of sputum unless told to collect more.			
15. Put the lid on the container.			
16. Placed the container in the bag. Attached the requisition to the bag.			
17. Removed the gloves. Decontaminated hands.			

Post-Procedure	S	U	Comments
18. Provided for comfort.	______	______	______
19. Placed the signal light within reach.	______	______	______
20. Unscreened the person.	______	______	______
21. Decontaminated hands.	______	______	______
22. Took the bag to the laboratory or storage area.	______	______	______
23. Decontaminated hands.	______	______	______
24. Reported and recorded observations.	______	______	______

Date of Satisfactory Completion ______________ Instructor's Initials ______________

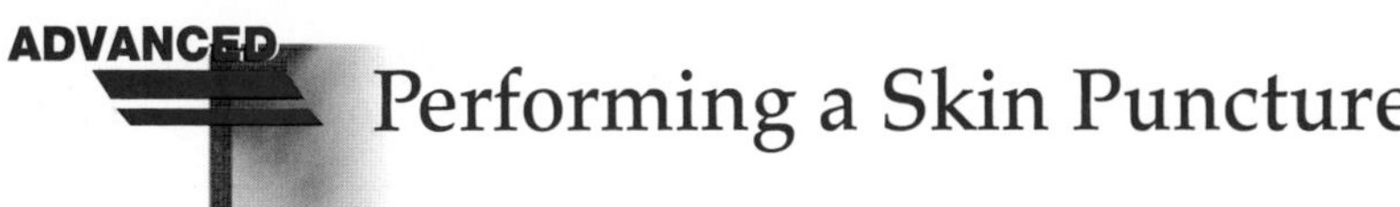

Performing a Skin Puncture

Name: ______________________

Date: ______________________

Pre-Procedure	**S**	**U**	**Comments**
• Knocked before entering the person's room.			
• Addressed the person by name.			
• Introduced yourself by name and title.			
1. Followed Delegation Guidelines. Reviewed Safety Alert.			
2. Explained the procedure to the person.			
3. Practiced hand hygiene.			
4. Collected the following:			
• Sterile lancet			
• Antiseptic wipes			
• Gloves			
• Cotton balls			
• Washcloth			
• Soap, towel, and wash basin			
5. Read the manufacturer's instructions for the lancet.			
6. Arranged the work area.			
7. Identified the person. Checked the ID bracelet against the assignment sheet or laboratory requisition form. Called the person by name.			
8. Provided for privacy.			

Procedure			
9. Helped the person to a comfortable position.			
10. Assisted the person with handwashing.			
11. Opened the lancet and antiseptic wipes.			
12. Put on the gloves.			
13. Inspected the person's fingers. Selected a skin puncture site.			
14. Warmed the finger. Rubbed it gently or applied a warm washcloth.			
15. Massaged the hand and finger toward the puncture site.			
16. Lowered the finger to below the person's waist.			
17. Held the finger with the thumb and forefinger. Used the non-dominant hand. Held the finger until step 23.			
18. Cleaned the site with an antiseptic wipe. Did not touch the site after cleaning.			
19. Let the site dry.			
20. Picked up the sterile lancet.			

Procedure—cont'd

	S	U	Comments
21. Placed the lancet against the side of the finger.			
22. Pushed the button on the lancet to puncture the skin. Followed the manufacturer's instructions.			
23. Wiped away the first blood drop. Used a cotton ball.			
24. Applied gentle pressure below the puncture site.			
25. Let a large drop of blood form.			
26. Collected and tested the specimen.			
27. Applied pressure to the puncture site until bleeding stopped. Used a cotton ball. If able, had the person apply pressure to the site.			
28. Discarded the lancet into the sharps container.			
29. Discarded the cotton balls following agency policy.			
30. Removed and discarded the gloves. Decontaminated hands.			

Post-Procedure

	S	U	Comments
31. Provided for comfort.			
32. Placed the signal light within reach.			
33. Raised or lowered bed rails. Followed the care plan.			
34. Lowered the bed to its lowest position.			
35. Unscreened the person.			
36. Discarded used supplies. Cleaned and returned the bath basin to its proper place.			
37. Followed agency policy for soiled linen.			
38. Decontaminated hands.			
39. Reported and recorded observations.			

Date of Satisfactory Completion ____________________ Instructor's Initials ____________________

ADVANCED

Collecting Blood Specimens With a Needle and Syringe

Name: ______________________

Date: ______________________

Pre-Procedure	S	U	Comments
• Knocked before entering the person's room.			
• Addressed the person by name.			
• Introduced yourself by name and title.			
1. Followed Delegation Guidelines. Reviewed Safety Alert.			
2. Explained the procedure to the person.			
3. Practiced hand hygiene.			
4. Collected the following:			
• Antiseptic wipes			
• Tourniquet			
• Sterile 2 × 2 gauze dressing			
• Band-Aid			
• Sterile needle			
• Sterile syringe			
• Color-coded vacuum test tube (checked the expiration date)			
• Laboratory requisition forms			
• Labels for the blood specimens			
• Towel			
• Gloves			
• Leak-proof plastic bag			
• Portable sharps container (optional)			
5. Completed the labels for the blood specimens.			
6. Arranged a work area on the overbed table. If a blood collection tray was used, placed it on the bedside table or the chair.			
7. Identified the person. Checked the ID bracelet against the laboratory requisition slip. Called the person by name.			
8. Provided for privacy.			
9. Raised the bed for body mechanics. The far bed rail was up if used.			

Procedure	S	U	Comments
10. Helped the person to a comfortable supine, sitting, or semi-Fowler's position.			
11. Inspected both arms for skin breaks and hematomas. Asked which arm the person preferred for the venipuncture.			

Procedure—cont'd	S	U	Comments
12. Positioned the work area so that supplies could be easily reached.			
13. Placed a rolled towel under the arm.			
14. Extended the arm with the palm side up.			
15. Prepared the supplies:			
a. Opened the antiseptic wipes.			
b. Opened the sterile gauze square.			
c. Opened the Band-Aid.			
d. Opened the needle and syringe packages.			
e. Attached the needle to the syringe.			
16. Put on the gloves.			
17. Applied the tourniquet 3 to 4 inches above the elbow:			
a. Crossed one end tightly over the other.			
b. Tucked the upper end under the band to form a half-bow.			
18. Palpated the radial pulse. If a pulse was not felt, released and reapplied the tourniquet.			
19. Asked the person to open and close the fist a few times.			
20. Looked and palpated for a vein. The fist was closed.			
21. Selected a vein. Avoided narrow, weak, sclerosed, or rolling veins.			
22. Released the tourniquet if it had been on longer than 1 minute. Waited 1 minute before reapplying the tourniquet.			
23. Reapplied the tourniquet.			
24. Palpated the vein again.			
25. Cleaned the site with an antiseptic wipe. Cleaned in a circular motion from the site outward about 2 inches. Did not touch the site after cleaning.			
26. Let the site dry.			
27. Picked up the needle and attached syringe.			
28. Pulled the needle cover straight off. Did not touch the needle.			
29. Pulled the skin over the site taut. Used the thumb or forefinger of the non-dominant hand. Held the site taut through step 32.			
30. Held the needle and syringe so that the needle bevel was up.			
31. Positioned the needle at a 15- to 30-degree angle to the person's arm.			
32. Inserted the needle into the vein gently and smoothly.			
33. Pulled back on the plunger slowly to withdraw blood. Used the non-dominant hand.			
34. Continued to pull back on the plunger until the necessary amount of blood was withdrawn. Kept the needle stable so it did not move.			

Procedure—cont'd	S	U	Comments
35. Released the tourniquet. Pulled on the half-bow.	____	____	____________
36. Held a gauze square over the puncture site. Did not apply pressure.	____	____	____________
37. Pulled the needle straight out.	____	____	____________
38. Applied pressure to the venipuncture site with the gauze square. If able, had the person apply pressure to the arm.	____	____	____________
39. Transferred blood from the syringe into the vacuum tube. Followed agency policy for tube order.	____	____	____________
a. Inserted the needle through the rubber stopper on the tube.	____	____	____________
b. Let the vacuum tube fill.	____	____	____________
c. Discarded the needle and syringe into the sharps container. Did not recap the needle.	____	____	____________
40. Identified the tubes with additives. To mix the blood and additives, gently inverted or rotated each tube back and forth. Followed the manufacturer's instructions for the number of times to invert the tube. Did not shake the tube.	____	____	____________
41. Checked the venipuncture site for bleeding.	____	____	____________
42. Removed the gauze square.	____	____	____________
43. Applied a Band-Aid.	____	____	____________
44. Discarded the syringe into the sharps container if not already done.	____	____	____________
45. Applied labels to the blood specimens.	____	____	____________
46. Put the specimens into the plastic bag (if this is your agency's policy).	____	____	____________
47. Removed the towel. Followed agency policy for soiled linen.	____	____	____________
48. Discarded cotton balls, gauze, and antiseptic wipes following agency policy.	____	____	____________
49. Removed and discarded the gloves. Decontaminated hands.	____	____	____________
Post-Procedure			
50. Provided for comfort.	____	____	____________
51. Placed the signal light within reach.	____	____	____________
52. Raised or lowered bed rails. Followed the care plan.	____	____	____________
53. Lowered the bed to its lowest position.	____	____	____________
54. Discarded any other used supplies.	____	____	____________
55. Unscreened the person.	____	____	____________
56. Took or sent the specimens to the laboratory.	____	____	____________
57. Decontaminated hands.	____	____	____________
58. Reported and recorded observations.	____	____	____________

Date of Satisfactory Completion ____________________ Instructor's Initials ____________________

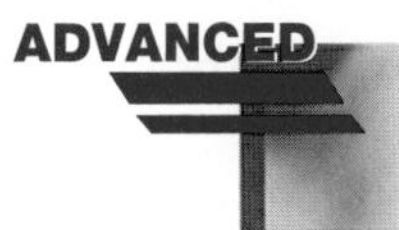

Collecting Blood Specimens Using the Vacutainer System

Name: ______________________

Date: ______________________

Pre-Procedure	S	U	Comments
• Knocked before entering the person's room.	___	___	___
• Addressed the person by name.	___	___	___
• Introduced yourself by name and title.	___	___	___
1. Followed Delegation Guidelines. Reviewed Safety Alert.	___	___	___
2. Explained the procedure to the person.	___	___	___
3. Practiced hand hygiene.	___	___	___
4. Collected the following:			
• Antiseptic wipes	___	___	___
• Tourniquet	___	___	___
• Sterile 2 × 2 gauze dressing	___	___	___
• Band-Aid	___	___	___
• Vacutainer tube holder	___	___	___
• Sterile double-ended Vacutainer needle	___	___	___
• Vacutainer tubes (checked the expiration date)	___	___	___
• Laboratory requisition slips	___	___	___
• Labels for the blood specimens	___	___	___
• Towel	___	___	___
• Gloves	___	___	___
• Leak-proof plastic bag	___	___	___
5. Completed the labels for the blood specimens.	___	___	___
6. Arranged a work area.	___	___	___
7. Identified the person. Checked the ID bracelet against the laboratory requisition slips. Called the person by name.	___	___	___
8. Provided for privacy.	___	___	___
9. Raised the bed for body mechanics. The far bed rail was up if used.	___	___	___
Procedure			
10. Followed steps 10 through 14 in procedure: *Collecting Blood Specimens With a Needle and Syringe.*	___	___	___
11. Prepared the supplies:	___	___	___
a. Opened the antiseptic wipes.	___	___	___
b. Opened the sterile gauze squares.	___	___	___
c. Opened the Band-Aid.	___	___	___
d. Opened the double-ended needle.	___	___	___
e. Attached the needle to the Vacutainer tube holder.	___	___	___

Procedure—cont'd	S	U	Comments
f. Placed the first tube to be used inside the holder. Did not attach it to the needle.			
g. Arranged tubes in order of use. Followed agency policy.			
12. Followed steps 16 through 26 in procedure: *Collecting a Blood Specimen With a Needle and Syringe.*			
13. Picked up the Vacutainer needle and tube holder.			
14. Removed the needle cover. Pulled it straight off. Did not touch the needle.			
15. Pulled the skin over the site taut. Used the thumb or forefinger of the non-dominant hand. Held the site taut through step 18.			
16. Held the needle so that the needle bevel was up.			
17. Positioned the needle at a 15- to 30-degree angle to the person's arm.			
18. Inserted the needle into the vein gently and slowly.			
19. Pushed the Vacutainer tube forward onto the end of the needle in the holder. Pushed gently.			
20. Let the tube fill with blood.			
21. Removed the filled tube from the holder. Grasped it firmly.			
22. Inserted the next tube. Repeated steps 19 through 22 for the other tubes.			
23. Released the tourniquet after the last tube filled.			
24. Held a gauze square over the puncture site. Did not apply pressure.			
25. Pulled the needle straight out.			
26. Applied pressure to the venipuncture site with the gauze square. Asked the person to apply pressure to the arm.			
27. Removed the last tube from the tube holder. Did not recap the needle. Followed steps 41 through 49 in procedure: *Collecting a Blood Specimen With a Needle and a Syringe.*			

Post-Procedure

	S	U	Comments
28. Followed steps 50 through 58 in procedure: *Collecting a Blood Specimen With a Needle and Syringe.*			

Date of Satisfactory Completion ____________ Instructor's Initials ____________

ADVANCED

Measuring Blood Glucose

Name: ______________________

Date: ______________________

Pre-Procedure	S	U	Comments
• Knocked before entering the person's room.	___	___	___
• Addressed the person by name.	___	___	___
• Introduced yourself by name and title.	___	___	___
1. Followed Delegation Guidelines. Reviewed Safety Alerts.	___	___	___
2. Explained the procedure to the person.	___	___	___
3. Practiced hand hygiene.	___	___	___
4. Collected the following:			
• Sterile lancet	___	___	___
• Antiseptic wipe	___	___	___
• Cotton balls	___	___	___
• Glucose testing meter	___	___	___
• Reagent strips (Used the correct ones for the meter. Checked the expiration date.)	___	___	___
• Gloves	___	___	___
• Paper towel	___	___	___
• Soap, towel, and wash basin	___	___	___
5. Arranged the work area.	___	___	___
6. Identified the person. Checked the ID bracelet against the assignment sheet. Called the person by name.	___	___	___
7. Raised the bed for body mechanics. The far bed rail was up if used.	___	___	___

Procedure

	S	U	Comments
8. Assisted the person with handwashing.	___	___	___
9. Helped the person to a comfortable position.	___	___	___
10. Prepared the supplies:			
a. Opened the antiseptic wipes.	___	___	___
b. Removed a reagent strip from the bottle. Placed it on the paper towel. Placed the cap securely on the bottle.	___	___	___
c. Prepared the lancet.	___	___	___
d. Turned on the glucose meter.	___	___	___
11. Put on the gloves.	___	___	___
12. Performed a skin puncture to obtain a drop of blood.	___	___	___
13. Wiped off the first drop of blood with a cotton ball.	___	___	___
14. Applied gentle pressure below the puncture site.	___	___	___
15. Let a large drop of blood form.	___	___	___

Procedure—cont'd	S	U	Comments
16. Held the test area of the reagent strip close to the drop of blood.			
17. Lightly touched the reagent strip to the blood drop. Did not smear the blood.			
18. Set the timer on the glucose meter.			
19. Set the reagent strip on the paper towel, or followed the manufacturer's instructions.			
20. Waited the length of time required by the manufacturer.			
21. Applied pressure to the puncture site until bleeding stopped. Used a cotton ball. If able, had the person continue to apply pressure to the site.			
22. Treated the reagent strip as required by the manufacturer.			
23. Inserted the reagent strip into the glucose meter. Followed the manufacturer's instructions.			
24. Read the result on the display. Wrote down the result, and told the person the result.			
25. Turned off the glucose meter.			
26. Discarded the lancet into the sharps container.			
27. Discarded the cotton balls following agency policy.			
28. Removed and discarded the gloves. Decontaminated hands.			

Post-Procedure

	S	U	Comments
29. Provided for comfort.			
30. Placed the signal light within reach.			
31. Raised or lowered bed rails. Followed the care plan.			
32. Lowered the bed to its lowest position.			
33. Unscreened the person.			
34. Discarded used supplies. Cleaned and returned equipment to its proper place.			
35. Followed agency policy for soiled linen.			
36. Decontaminated hands.			
37. Reported and recorded the test results and other observations.			

Date of Satisfactory Completion ____________________ Instructor's Initials ____________________

Preparing the Person for an Examination

Name: ______________________

Date: ______________________

Pre-Procedure	S	U	Comments
• Knocked before entering the person's room.			
• Addressed the person by name.			
• Introduced yourself by name and title.			
1. Followed Delegation Guidelines. Reviewed Safety Alert.			
2. Explained the procedure to the person.			
3. Practiced hand hygiene.			
4. Collected the following:			
• Flashlight			
• Sphygmomanometer			
• Stethoscope			
• Thermometer			
• Tongue depressors (blades)			
• Laryngeal mirror			
• Ophthalmoscope			
• Otoscope			
• Nasal speculum			
• Percussion (reflex) hammer			
• Tuning fork			
• Tape measure			
• Gloves			
• Water-soluble lubricant			
• Vaginal speculum			
• Cotton-tipped applicators			
• Specimen containers and labels			
• Disposable bag			
• Kidney basin			
• Towel			
• Bath blanket			
• Tissues			
• Drape (sheet, bath blanket, drawsheet, or paper drape)			
• Paper towels			
• Cotton balls			
• Waterproof bed protector			
• Eye chart (Snellen chart)			
• Slides			
• Gown			

Pre-Procedure—cont'd	S	U	Comments
• Antiseptic wipes			
• Wastebasket			
• Container for soiled instruments			
• Marking pencils or pens			
5. Identified the person. Checked the ID bracelet against the assignment sheet. Called the person by name.			
6. Provided for privacy.			

Procedure

	S	U	Comments
7. Had the person put on the gown. Told the person to remove all clothes. Assisted as needed.			
8. Asked the person to void. Offered the bedpan, commode, or urinal if necessary. Provided for privacy.			
9. Transported the person to the exam room. (This was not done for an exam in the person's room.)			
10. Weighed and measured the person. Recorded the measurements on the exam form.			
11. Helped the person on to the exam table. Provided a step stool if necessary. (Omitted this step for an exam in the person's room.)			
12. Measured vital signs. Recorded them on the exam form.			
13. Raised the bed to its highest level. Raised the far bed rail (if used). (This was not done if an exam table was used.)			
14. Positioned the person as directed.			
15. Draped the person.			
16. Placed a bed protector under the buttocks.			
17. Raised the bed rail near you (if used).			
18. Provided adequate lighting.			
19. Put the signal light on for the examiner. Did not leave the person alone.			

Date of Satisfactory Completion ____________________ Instructor's Initials ____________________

Measuring Height and Weight

Name: ______________________

Date: ______________________

Pre-Procedure	**S**	**U**	**Comments**
• Knocked before entering the person's room.	____	____	____________
• Addressed the person by name.	____	____	____________
• Introduced yourself by name and title.	____	____	____________
1. Followed Delegation Guidelines. Reviewed Safety Alert.	____	____	____________
2. Explained the procedure to the person.	____	____	____________
3. Asked the person to void.	____	____	____________
4. Practiced hand hygiene.	____	____	____________
5. Brought the balance or lift scale and paper towels to the person's room.	____	____	____________
6. Identified the person. Checked the ID bracelet against the assignment sheet. Called the person by name.	____	____	____________
7. Provided for privacy.	____	____	____________
Procedure			
8. Balance scale:			
a. Placed the paper towels on the scale platform.	____	____	____________
b. Raised the height rod.	____	____	____________
c. Moved the weights to zero (0). The pointer was in the middle.	____	____	____________
d. Had the person remove the robe and footwear. Assisted the person onto the scale.	____	____	____________
e. Moved the weights until the balance pointer was in the middle.	____	____	____________
f. Recorded the weight on the note pad or assignment sheet.	____	____	____________
g. Asked the person to stand very straight.	____	____	____________
h. Lowered the height rod until it rested on the person's head.	____	____	____________
i. Recorded the height on the note pad or assignment sheet.	____	____	____________
9. Chair scale.	____	____	____________
a. Placed both weights on zero (0). Balanced the scale following the manufacturer's instructions.	____	____	____________
b. Helped the person transfer from the wheelchair to the chair scale.	____	____	____________
c. Placed the person's feet on the foot platform.	____	____	____________
d. Moved the weights until the balance pointer was in the middle, or noted the digital display.	____	____	____________

Procedure—cont'd	S	U	Comments
e. Recorded the weight on the notepad or assignment sheet.	______	______	____________
10. Lift scale:			
a. Attached the sling to the lift.	______	______	____________
b. Placed both weights on zero (0).	______	______	____________
c. Leveled and balanced the scale. Followed the manufacturer's instructions.	______	______	____________
d. Removed the sling from the scale.	______	______	____________
e. Placed the person on the sling and attached it to the lift. Raised the person about 4 inches off the bed.	______	______	____________
f. Moved the weights until the balance pointer was in the middle, or noted the digital display.	______	______	____________
g. Recorded the weight on the notepad or assignment sheet.	______	______	____________
h. Lowered the person to the bed.	______	______	____________
i. Removed the sling.	______	______	____________
11. Helped the person onto the examination table or back to bed.	______	______	____________

Post-Procedure

12. Provided for comfort.	______	______	____________
13. Placed the signal light within reach.	______	______	____________
14. Raised or lowered bed rails. Followed the care plan.	______	______	____________
15. Unscreened the person.	______	______	____________
16. Discarded the paper towels.	______	______	____________
17. Returned the scale to its proper place.	______	______	____________
18. Decontaminated hands.	______	______	____________
19. Reported and recorded the measurements.	______	______	____________

Date of Satisfactory Completion ____________ Instructor's Initials ____________

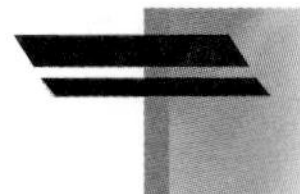

Measuring Height: The Person Is in Bed

Name: ______________________

Date: ______________________

Pre-Procedure	S	U	Comments
• Knocked before entering the person's room.			
• Addressed the person by name.			
• Introduced yourself by name and title.			
1. Followed Delegation Guidelines. Reviewed Safety Alert.			
2. Explained the procedure to the person.			
3. Practiced hand hygiene.			
4. Collected a measuring tape and ruler.			
5. Asked a co-worker to help.			
6. Identified the person. Checked the ID bracelet against the assignment sheet. Called the person by name.			
7. Provided for privacy.			

Procedure

	S	U	Comments
8. Positioned the person supine if this position was allowed.			
9. Had the co-worker hold the end of the measuring tape at the person's heel.			
10. Pulled the measuring tape along the person's body until it extended past the head.			
11. Placed the ruler flat across the top of the person's head. It extended from the person's head to the measuring tape. Made sure the ruler was level.			
12. Recorded the height on the notepad or assignment sheet.			

Post-Procedure

	S	U	Comments
13. Provided for comfort.			
14. Raised or lowered bed rails. Followed the care plan.			
15. Placed the signal light within reach.			
16. Unscreened the person.			
17. Returned equipment to its proper location.			
18. Decontaminated hands.			
19. Reported and recorded the height.			

Date of Satisfactory Completion ______________________ Instructor's Initials ______________

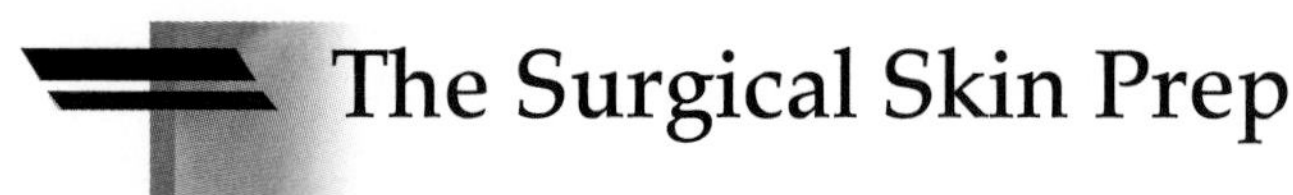

The Surgical Skin Prep

Name: ______________________

Date: ______________________

Pre-Procedure	S	U	Comments
• Knocked before entering the person's room.			
• Addressed the person by name.			
• Introduced yourself by name and title.			
1. Followed Delegation Guidelines. Reviewed Safety Alert.			
2. Explained the procedure to the person.			
3. Practiced hand hygiene.			
4. Collected the following:			
• Skin prep kit			
• Bath blanket			
• Warm water			
• Gloves			
• Waterproof pad			
• Bath towel			
5. Identified the person. Checked the ID bracelet against the assignment sheet. Called the person by name.			
6. Provided for privacy.			

Procedure	S	U	Comments
7. Made sure there was good lighting.			
8. Raised the bed for body mechanics. Lowered the bed rail near you (if up).			
9. Covered the person with a bath blanket. Fanfolded top linens to the foot of the bed.			
10. Placed the waterproof pad under the area to be shaved.			
11. Opened the skin prep kit.			
12. Positioned the person for the skin prep.			
13. Draped the person with the drape.			
14. Added warm water to the basin. Bed rails (if used) were up before leaving the bedside.			
15. Put on the gloves.			
16. Lathered the skin with the sponge.			
17. Held the skin taut. Shaved in the direction of hair growth.			
18. Shaved outward from the center using short strokes.			
19. Rinsed the razor often.			
20. Made sure the entire area was free of hair. Checked for cuts, scratches, or nicks.			

Procedure—cont'd	S	U	Comments
21. Rinsed the skin thoroughly. Patted dry.			
22. Removed the drape and waterproof pad.			
23. Removed the gloves. Decontaminated hands.			
24. Returned top linens. Removed the bath blanket.			

Post-Procedure

	S	U	Comments
25. Provided for comfort.			
26. Raised or lowered bed rails. Followed the care plan.			
27. Lowered the bed to its lowest position.			
28. Placed the signal light within reach.			
29. Unscreened the person.			
30. Returned equipment to its proper place.			
31. Discarded supplies. Followed agency policy for soiled linen.			
32. Decontaminated hands.			
33. Reported and recorded observations.			

Date of Satisfactory Completion ____________________ Instructor's Initials ____________________

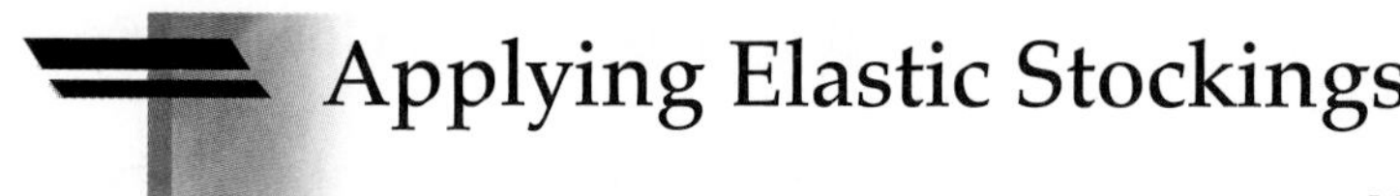

Applying Elastic Stockings

Name: ______________________

Date: ______________________

Pre-Procedure	**S**	**U**	**Comments**
• Knocked before entering the person's room.	____	____	____
• Addressed the person by name.	____	____	____
• Introduced yourself by name and title.	____	____	____
1. Followed Delegation Guidelines. Reviewed Safety Alert.	____	____	____
2. Explained the procedure to the person.	____	____	____
3. Practiced hand hygiene.	____	____	____
4. Obtained elastic stockings in the correct size and length.	____	____	____
5. Identified the person. Checked the ID bracelet against the assignment sheet. Called the person by name.	____	____	____
6. Provided for privacy.	____	____	____
7. Raised the bed for body mechanics. Bed rails were up if used.	____	____	____
Procedure			
8. Lowered the bed rail near you if up.	____	____	____
9. Positioned the person supine.	____	____	____
10. Exposed the legs. Fanfolded top linens toward the thighs.	____	____	____
11. Turned the stocking inside out down to the heel.	____	____	____
12. Slipped the foot of the stocking over the toes, foot, and heel.	____	____	____
13. Grasped the stocking top. Slipped it over the foot and heel. Pulled it up the leg. The stocking was even and snug.	____	____	____
14. Removed twists, creases, or wrinkles.	____	____	____
15. Repeated steps 11 through 14 for the other leg.	____	____	____
Post-Procedure			
16. Covered the person.	____	____	____
17. Provided for comfort.	____	____	____
18. Lowered the bed.	____	____	____
19. Raised or lowered bed rails. Followed the care plan.	____	____	____
20. Placed the signal light within reach.	____	____	____
21. Unscreened the person.	____	____	____
22. Decontaminated hands.	____	____	____
23. Reported and recorded observations.	____	____	____

Date of Satisfactory Completion ______________ Instructor's Initials ______________

Applying Elastic Bandages

Name: ______________________

Date: ______________________

Pre-Procedure	S	U	Comments
• Knocked before entering the person's room.	____	____	____________
• Addressed the person by name.	____	____	____________
• Introduced yourself by name and title.	____	____	____________
1. Followed Delegation Guidelines. Reviewed Safety Alert.	____	____	____________
2. Explained the procedure to the person.	____	____	____________
3. Practiced hand hygiene.	____	____	____________
4. Collected the following:			
• Elastic bandage as directed by the nurse	____	____	____________
• Tape or metal clips (unless the bandage had Velcro)	____	____	____________
5. Identified the person. Checked the ID bracelet against the assignment sheet. Called the person by name.	____	____	____________
6. Provided for privacy.	____	____	____________
7. Raised the bed for body mechanics. Bed rails were up if used.	____	____	____________

Procedure	S	U	Comments
8. Lowered the bed rail near you if up.	____	____	____________
9. Helped the person to a comfortable position. Exposed the part to be bandaged.	____	____	____________
10. Made sure the area was clean and dry.	____	____	____________
11. Held the bandage so the roll was up. The loose end was on the bottom.	____	____	____________
12. Applied the bandage to the smallest part of the wrist, foot, ankle, or knee.	____	____	____________
13. Made two circular turns around the part.	____	____	____________
14. Made overlapping spiral turns in an upward direction. Each turn overlapped about $^2/_3$ of the previous turn.	____	____	____________
15. Applied the bandage smoothly with firm, even pressure. It was not tight.	____	____	____________
16. Secured the bandage in place with Velcro, tape, or clips. The clips were not under the body part.	____	____	____________
17. Checked the fingers or toes for coldness or cyanosis. Asked about pain, itching, numbness, or tingling. Removed the bandage if any were noted. Reported observations to the nurse.	____	____	____________

Post-Procedure	S	U	Comments
18. Provided for comfort.			
19. Placed the signal light within reach.			
20. Lowered the bed.			
21. Raised or lowered bed rails. Followed the care plan.			
22. Unscreened the person.			
23. Decontaminated hands.			
24. Reported and recorded observations.			

Date of Satisfactory Completion ____________ Instructor's Initials ____________

ADVANCED

Applying a Dry Sterile Dressing

Name: ______________________

Date: ______________________

Pre-Procedure	S	U	Comments
• Knocked before entering the person's room.	____	____	____________
• Addressed the person by name.	____	____	____________
• Introduced yourself by name and title.	____	____	____________
1. Followed Delegation Guidelines. Reviewed Safety Alert.	____	____	____________
2. Explained the procedure to the person.	____	____	____________
3. Allowed time for pain relief drugs to take effect.	____	____	____________
4. Provided for fluid and elimination needs.	____	____	____________
5. Practiced hand hygiene.	____	____	____________
6. Collected needed supplies and equipment:			
• Disposable gloves	____	____	____________
• Sterile gloves	____	____	____________
• Personal protective equipment as needed	____	____	____________
• Sterile cleaning solution	____	____	____________
• Sterile dressing set (with sterile scissors and forceps)	____	____	____________
• Sterile basin	____	____	____________
• Sterile drape	____	____	____________
• Tape or Montgomery ties	____	____	____________
• Sterile dressings as directed by the nurse	____	____	____________
• A package of sterile 4 × 4 gauze squares	____	____	____________
• Adhesive remover	____	____	____________
• Plastic bag	____	____	____________
• Bath blanket	____	____	____________
7. Identified the person. Checked the ID bracelet against the assignment sheet. Called the person by name.	____	____	____________
8. Provided for privacy.	____	____	____________
9. Arranged the work area.	____	____	____________
10. Raised the bed for body mechanics. Bed rails were up if used.	____	____	____________
Procedure			
11. Lowered the bed rail near you if up.	____	____	____________
12. Helped the person to a comfortable position.	____	____	____________
13. Covered the person with a bath blanket. Fanfolded top linens to the foot of the bed.	____	____	____________
14. Exposed the affected body part.	____	____	____________

Procedure—cont'd	S	U	Comments
15. Made a cuff on the plastic bag. Placed it within reach.	______	______	______________
16. Put on a gown and mask if needed.	______	______	______________
17. Decontaminated hands. Put on disposable gloves.	______	______	______________
18. Undid Montgomery ties or removed tape.	______	______	______________
a. Montgomery ties: folded ties away from the wound.	______	______	______________
b. Tape: held the skin down. Gently pulled the tape toward the wound.	______	______	______________
19. Removed adhesive from the skin if necessary. Wet a 4 × 4 gauze dressing with the adhesive remover. Cleaned away from the wound.	______	______	______________
20. Removed the dressings. Started with the top dressing. The soiled side was away from the person's sight. Put dressings in the bag. They did not touch the outside of the bag.	______	______	______________
21. Removed the dressing directly over the wound very gently.	______	______	______________
22. Observed the wound, drain site, and wound drainage.	______	______	______________
23. Removed the gloves and put them into the bag. Decontaminated hands.	______	______	______________
24. Set up the sterile field:			
a. Placed the sterile drape over the work surface.	______	______	______________
b. Opened the sterile dressing set. Dropped the contents onto the sterile field.	______	______	______________
c. Opened the sterile dressings. Dropped them onto the sterile field.	______	______	______________
d. Opened the sterile bowl. Placed it on the sterile field.	______	______	______________
e. Opened the sterile 4 × 4 gauze squares. Dropped them onto the sterile field.	______	______	______________
f. Opened the sterile cleaning solution. Poured the solution into the bowl. Placed the cap and bottle outside the sterile field.	______	______	______________
25. Put on the sterile gloves.	______	______	______________
26. Picked up the sterile 4 × 4 gauze with the sterile forceps. Placed some in the cleaning solution. Saved the others for drying the skin around the wound and drain site.	______	______	______________
27. Cleaned the wound. Cleaned from the wound outward. Used a new 4 × 4 gauze for each stroke. Dropped used gauze into the plastic bag. Did not let the forceps touch the bag.	______	______	______________
28. Cleaned the area around the drain site. Cleaned from the wound outward. Used a new 4 × 4 gauze for each circular motion. Dropped used gauze into the plastic bag. Did not let the forceps touch the bag.	______	______	______________
29. Dried the skin around the wound and drain site. Used the dry gauze squares. Discarded them into the plastic bag.	______	______	______________
30. Applied a 4 × 4 gauze to the drain site. Used a pre-cut 4 × 4 gauze, or cut halfway through a 4 × 4 gauze using the sterile scissors.	______	______	______________

Procedure—cont'd	S	U	Comments
31. Applied dressings over the wound and drain site. Followed the nurse's directions.			
32. Secured the dressings in place. Used tape or Montgomery ties.			
33. Removed and discarded the gloves. Decontaminated hands.			

Post-Procedure

	S	U	Comments
34. Provided for comfort.			
35. Covered the person. Removed the bath blanket.			
36. Placed the signal light within reach.			
37. Lowered the bed to its lowest position.			
38. Raised or lowered bed rails. Followed the care plan.			
39. Unscreened the person.			
40. Discarded supplies into the bag. Tied the bag closed. Discarded the bag according to agency policy.			
41. Cleaned the work surface. Followed the Bloodborne Pathogen Standard.			
42. Decontaminated hands.			
43. Reported and recorded observations.			

Date of Satisfactory Completion ______________________ Instructor's Initials ____________________

ADVANCED

Applying Hot Compresses

Name: ______________________

Date: ______________________

Pre-Procedure	S	U	Comments
• Knocked before entering the person's room.			
• Addressed the person by name.			
• Introduced yourself by name and title.			
1. Followed Delegation Guidelines. Reviewed Safety Alert.			
2. Explained the procedure to the person.			
3. Practiced hand hygiene.			
4. Collected the following:			
• Basin			
• Bath thermometer			
• Small towel, washcloth, or gauze squares			
• Plastic wrap or aquathermia pad			
• Ties, tape, or rolled gauze			
• Bath towel			
• Waterproof pad			
5. Identified the person. Checked the ID bracelet against the assignment sheet. Called the person by name.			
6. Provided for privacy.			
Procedure			
7. Placed the waterproof pad under the body part.			
8. Filled the basin 1/2 to 2/3 full with hot water as directed by the nurse. Measured water temperature.			
9. Placed the compress in the water.			
10. Wrung out the compress.			
11. Applied the compress to the area. Noted the time.			
12. Covered the compress quickly. Used one of the following as directed by the nurse:			
a. Applied plastic wrap and then a bath towel. Secured the towel in place with ties, tape, or rolled gauze.			
b. Applied an aquathermia pad.			
13. Placed the signal light within reach.			
14. Raised or lowered bed rails. Followed the care plan.			
15. Checked the area every 5 minutes. Checked for redness and complaints of pain, discomfort, or numbness. Removed the compress if any occurred. Told the nurse at once.			
16. Changed the compress if cooling occurred.			

Procedure—cont'd	S	U	Comments
17. Removed the compress after 20 minutes or as directed by the nurse. Patted dry the area. (If the bed rail was up, lowered it for this step.)			

Post-Procedure	S	U	Comments
18. Provided for comfort.			
19. Unscreened the person.			
20. Raised or lowered bed rails. Followed the care plan.			
21. Placed the signal light within reach.			
22. Cleaned equipment. Discarded disposable items. Wore gloves for this step.			
23. Followed agency policy for soiled linen.			
24. Decontaminated hands.			
25. Reported and recorded observations.			

Date of Satisfactory Completion ______________________ Instructor's Initials ____________________

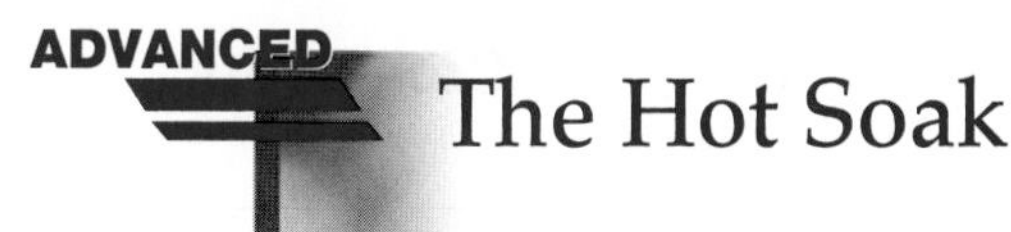

The Hot Soak

Name: ______________________

Date: ______________________

Pre-Procedure	S	U	Comments
• Knocked before entering the person's room.	____	____	______________
• Addressed the person by name.	____	____	______________
• Introduced yourself by name and title.	____	____	______________
1. Followed Delegation Guidelines. Reviewed Safety Alert.	____	____	______________
2. Explained the procedure to the person.	____	____	______________
3. Practiced hand hygiene.	____	____	______________
4. Collected the following:			
• Water basin or an arm or foot bath	____	____	______________
• Bath thermometer	____	____	______________
• Bath blanket	____	____	______________
• Waterproof pads	____	____	______________
5. Identified the person. Checked the ID bracelet against the assignment sheet. Called the person by name.	____	____	______________
6. Provided for privacy.	____	____	______________
Procedure			
7. Positioned the person for the procedure. Placed the signal light within reach.	____	____	______________
8. Placed a waterproof pad under the area.	____	____	______________
9. Filled the container 1/2 full with hot water as directed by the nurse. Measured water temperature.	____	____	______________
10. Exposed the area. Avoided unnecessary exposure.	____	____	______________
11. Placed the part into the water. Padded the edge of the container with a towel. Noted the time.	____	____	______________
12. Covered the person with a bath blanket for extra warmth.	____	____	______________
13. Checked the area every 5 minutes. Checked for redness and complaints of pain, numbness, or discomfort. Discontinued the soak if any of these occurred. Wrapped the part in a towel and told the nurse at once.	____	____	______________
14. Checked water temperature every 5 minutes. Changed water as necessary. Wrapped the part in a towel while changing the water.	____	____	______________
15. Removed the part from the water in 15 to 20 minutes. Patted dry.	____	____	______________
Post-Procedure			
16. Followed steps 18 through 25 in procedure: *Applying Hot Compresses.*	____	____	______________

Date of Satisfactory Completion ______________________ Instructor's Initials ______________________

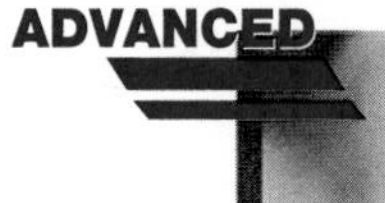

Assisting the Person With a Sitz Bath

Name: ______________________

Date: ______________________

Pre-Procedure	S	U	Comments
• Knocked before entering the person's room.	_____	_____	__________
• Addressed the person by name.	_____	_____	__________
• Introduced yourself by name and title.	_____	_____	__________
1. Followed Delegation Guidelines. Reviewed Safety Alert.	_____	_____	__________
2. Explained the procedure to the person.	_____	_____	__________
3. Practiced hand hygiene.	_____	_____	__________
4. Collected the following:			
• Disposable sitz bath if used	_____	_____	__________
• Wheelchair if the built-in sitz bath was used	_____	_____	__________
• Bath thermometer	_____	_____	__________
• Two bath blankets, bath towels, and a clean gown	_____	_____	__________
• Footstool if the person is short	_____	_____	__________
• Disinfectant solution	_____	_____	__________
• Utility gloves	_____	_____	__________
5. Identified the person. Checked the ID bracelet against the assignment sheet. Called the person by name.	_____	_____	__________
6. Provided for privacy.	_____	_____	__________
Procedure			
7. Did one of the following:			
a. Placed the disposable sitz bath on the toilet seat.	_____	_____	__________
b. Transported the person by wheelchair to the sitz bath room.	_____	_____	__________
8. Filled the sitz bath 2/3 full with water as directed by the nurse. Measured water temperature.	_____	_____	__________
9. Padded the metal part of the sitz bath with towels. Padded the part in contact with the person.	_____	_____	__________
10. Secured the gown above the waist.	_____	_____	__________
11. Helped the person sit in the sitz bath.	_____	_____	__________
12. Placed a bath blanket around the shoulders. Placed another over the legs for warmth.	_____	_____	__________
13. Provided a footstool if the edge of the sitz bath caused pressure under the knees.	_____	_____	__________
14. Placed the signal light within reach. Provided for comfort.	_____	_____	__________
15. Stayed with a person who was weak or unsteady.	_____	_____	__________

Procedure—cont'd	S	U	Comments
16. Checked the person every 5 minutes for complaints of weakness, faintness, and drowsiness. Checked for a rapid pulse. If any occurred, called for the nurse. Assisted the person back to bed.			
17. Helped the person out of the sitz bath after 20 minutes or as directed by the nurse.			
18. Assisted the person with drying and dressing.			
19. Assisted the person back to bed.			

Post-Procedure

	S	U	Comments
20. Provided for comfort.			
21. Unscreened the person.			
22. Placed the signal light within reach.			
23. Raised or lowered bed rails. Followed the care plan.			
24. Cleaned the sitz bath with disinfectant solution. Wore utility gloves.			
25. Cleaned and returned reusable items to their proper place. Followed agency policy for soiled linen. Wore gloves for this step.			
26. Decontaminated hands.			
27. Reported and recorded observations.			

Date of Satisfactory Completion ______________ Instructor's Initials ______________

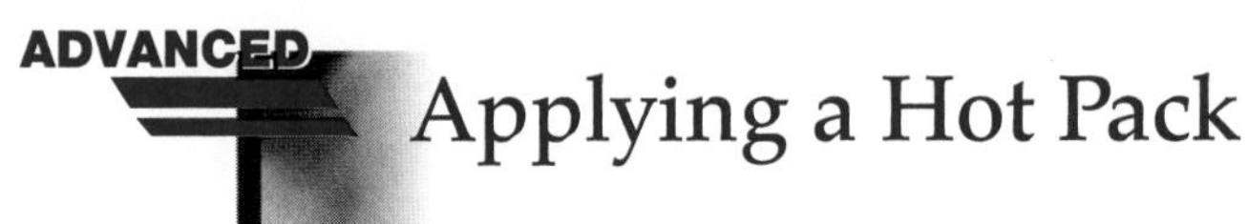

Applying a Hot Pack

Name: ______________________

Date: ______________________

Pre-Procedure	S	U	Comments
• Knocked before entering the person's room.	____	____	________
• Addressed the person by name.	____	____	________
• Introduced yourself by name and title.	____	____	________
1. Followed Delegation Guidelines. Reviewed Safety Alert.	____	____	________
2. Explained the procedure to the person.	____	____	________
3. Practiced hand hygiene.	____	____	________
4. Collected the following:			
• Commercial pack	____	____	________
• Towel	____	____	________
• Pack cover	____	____	________
• Ties, tape, or rolled gauze (if needed)	____	____	________
• Waterproof pad	____	____	________
5. Heated the pack. Followed the manufacturer's instructions.	____	____	________
6. Put the pack in the cover.	____	____	________
7. Identified the person. Checked the ID bracelet against the assignment sheet. Called the person by name.	____	____	________
8. Provided for privacy.	____	____	________

Procedure

	S	U	Comments
9. Placed the waterproof pad under the body part.	____	____	________
10. Applied the pack quickly. Noted the time.	____	____	________
11. Secured the pack in place with ties, tape, Velcro straps, or rolled gauze.	____	____	________
12. Placed the signal light within reach.	____	____	________
13. Raised or lowered bed rails. Followed the care plan.	____	____	________
14. Checked the area every 5 minutes. Checked for redness and complaints of pain, discomfort, or numbness. Removed the pack if any occurred. Told the nurse at once.	____	____	________
15. Changed the pack if cooling occurred.	____	____	________
16. Removed the pack after 20 minutes or as directed by the nurse. Patted the area dry. (If the bed rail was up, lowered it for this step.)	____	____	________

Post-Procedure	S	U	Comments
17. Followed steps 18 through 25 in procedure: *Applying Hot Compresses.*	______	______	______________________
18. Cleaned a reusable pack. Followed agency policy and the manufacturer's instructions.	______	______	______________________

Date of Satisfactory Completion ______________________ Instructor's Initials ____________________

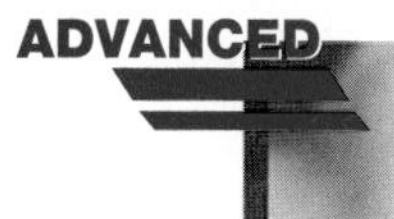

Applying an Aquathermia Pad

Name: ______________________

Date: ______________________

Pre-Procedure	S	U	Comments
• Knocked before entering the person's room.	____	____	________
• Addressed the person by name.	____	____	________
• Introduced yourself by name and title.	____	____	________
1. Followed Delegation Guidelines. Reviewed Safety Alerts.	____	____	________
2. Explained the procedure to the person.	____	____	________
3. Practiced hand hygiene.	____	____	________
4. Collected the following:			
• Aquathermia pad and heating unit	____	____	________
• Distilled water	____	____	________
• Flannel cover, pillowcase, or towel	____	____	________
• Ties, tape, or rolled gauze	____	____	________
5. Identified the person. Checked the ID bracelet against the assignment sheet. Called the person by name.	____	____	________
6. Provided for privacy.	____	____	________

Procedure			
7. Filled the heating unit to the fill line with distilled water.	____	____	________
8. Removed bubbles. Placed the pad and tubing below the heating unit. Tilted the heating unit from side to side.	____	____	________
9. Set the temperature as the nurse directed. Removed the key. (Gave the key to the nurse after the procedure.)	____	____	________
10. Placed the pad in the cover.	____	____	________
11. Plugged in the unit. Let water warm to the desired temperature.	____	____	________
12. Set the heating unit on the bedside stand. Kept the pad and connecting hoses level with the unit. Hoses did not have kinks.	____	____	________
13. Applied the pad to the part. Noted the time.	____	____	________
14. Secured the pad in place with ties, tape, or rolled gauze. Did not use pins.	____	____	________
15. Unscreened the person. Placed the signal light within reach.	____	____	________
16. Raised or lowered bed rails. Followed the care plan.	____	____	________
17. Checked the person every 5 minutes. Checked the skin for redness, swelling, and blisters. Asked about pain, discomfort, or decreased sensation. Removed the pad if any occurred. Told the nurse at once.	____	____	________

Procedure—cont'd

	S	U	Comments
18. Removed the pad at the specified time. (If bed rails were up, lowered the near one for this step.)	______	______	____________________

Post-Procedure

	S	U	Comments
19. Followed steps 18 through 25 in procedure: *Applying Hot Compresses.*	______	______	____________________

Date of Satisfactory Completion ____________________ Instructor's Initials ____________________

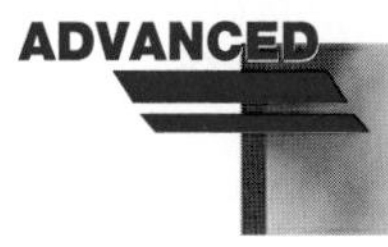

Applying an Ice Bag, Ice Collar, Ice Glove, or Dry Cold Pack

Name: ______________________

Date: ______________________

Pre-Procedure	S	U	Comments
• Knocked before entering the person's room.			
• Addressed the person by name.			
• Introduced yourself by name and title.			
1. Followed Delegation Guidelines. Reviewed Safety Alerts.			
2. Explained the procedure to the person.			
3. Practiced hand hygiene.			
4. Collected a cold pack or the following:			
• Ice bag, collar, or glove			
• Crushed ice			
• Flannel cover, towel, or pillowcase			
• Paper towels			
5. Applied an ice bag, collar, or glove:			
a. Filled it with water. Put in the stopper. Turned the device upside down to check for leaks.			
b. Emptied the device.			
c. Filled the device 1/2 to 2/3 full with crushed ice or ice chips.			
d. Removed excess air. Bent, twisted, or squeezed the device, or pressed it against a firm surface.			
e. Placed the cap or stopper on securely.			
f. Dried the device with the paper towels.			
g. Placed the device in the cover.			
6. Applied a cold pack:			
a. Squeezed, kneaded, or struck the cold pack as directed by the manufacturer.			
b. Placed the pack in the cover.			
7. Identified the person. Checked the ID bracelet against the assignment sheet. Called the person by name.			
8. Provided for privacy.			

Procedure

Procedure	S	U	Comments
9. Applied the device. Secured it in place with ties, tape, or rolled gauze. Noted the time.			
10. Placed the signal light within reach. Raised or lowered bed rails. Followed the care plan.			
11. Checked the skin every 5 minutes. Checked for blisters; pale, white, or gray skin; cyanosis; and shivering. Asked about numbness, pain, or burning. Removed the device if any occurred. Told the nurse at once.			

Procedure—cont'd	S	U	Comments
12. Removed the device after 20 minutes or as directed by the nurse.	______	______	______________________
Post-Procedure			
13. Followed steps 18 through 25 in procedure: *Applying Hot Compresses.*	______	______	______________________
14. Cleaned a reusable cold pack. Followed agency policy and the manufacturer's instructions.	______	______	______________________

Date of Satisfactory Completion ______________________ Instructor's Initials ______________________

ADVANCED

Applying Cold Compresses

Name: ______________________

Date: ______________________

Pre-Procedure	S	U	Comments
• Knocked before entering the person's room.	____	____	______________
• Addressed the person by name.	____	____	______________
• Introduced yourself by name and title.	____	____	______________
1. Followed Delegation Guidelines. Reviewed Safety Alert.	____	____	______________
2. Explained the procedure to the person.	____	____	______________
3. Practiced hand hygiene.	____	____	______________
4. Collected the following:			
• Large basin with ice	____	____	______________
• Small basin with cold water	____	____	______________
• Gauze squares, washcloths, or small towels	____	____	______________
• Waterproof pad	____	____	______________
• Bath towel	____	____	______________
5. Identified the person. Checked the ID bracelet against the assignment sheet. Called the person by name.	____	____	______________
6. Provided for privacy.	____	____	______________
Procedure			
7. Placed the waterproof pad under the affected body part. Exposed the area.	____	____	______________
8. Placed the small basin with cold water into the large basin with ice.	____	____	______________
9. Placed the compresses into the cold water.	____	____	______________
10. Wrung out a compress.	____	____	______________
11. Applied the compress to the part. Noted the time.	____	____	______________
12. Checked the area every 5 minutes. Checked for blisters; pale, white, or gray skin; cyanosis; or shivering. Asked about numbness, pain, or burning. Removed the compress if any occurred. Told the nurse at once.	____	____	______________
13. Changed the compress when it warmed.	____	____	______________
14. Removed the compress after 20 minutes or as directed by the nurse.	____	____	______________
15. Patted the area dry.	____	____	______________
Post-Procedure			
16. Followed steps 18 through 25 in procedure: *Applying Hot Compresses.*	____	____	______________

Date of Satisfactory Completion ______________ Instructor's Initials ______________

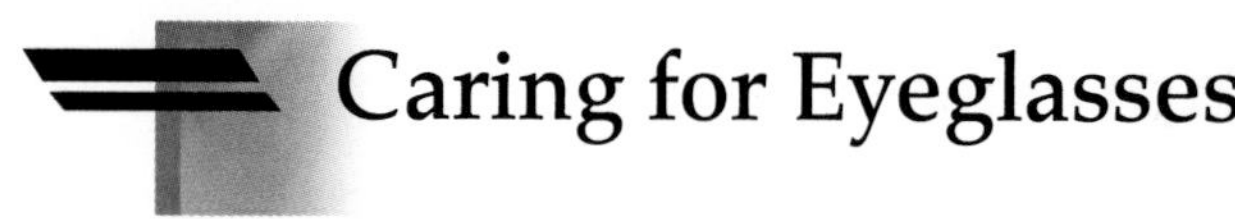

Caring for Eyeglasses

Name: ______________________

Date: ______________________

Pre-Procedure	S	U	Comments
• Knocked before entering the person's room.	_____	_____	__________
• Addressed the person by name.	_____	_____	__________
• Introduced yourself by name and title.	_____	_____	__________
1. Followed Delegation Guidelines. Reviewed Safety Alert.	_____	_____	__________
2. Explained the procedure to the person.	_____	_____	__________
3. Practiced hand hygiene.	_____	_____	__________
4. Collected the following:			
• Eyeglass case	_____	_____	__________
• Cleaning solution or warm water	_____	_____	__________
• Tissues or cloth	_____	_____	__________

Procedure	S	U	Comments
5. Removed the glasses:			
a. Held the frames in front of the ear on both sides.	_____	_____	__________
b. Lifted the frames from the ears. Brought the glasses down away from the face.	_____	_____	__________
6. Cleaned the glass with the cleaning solution or warm water. Dried the lenses with tissues.	_____	_____	__________
7. Opened the eyeglass case.	_____	_____	__________
8. Folded the glasses. Put them in the case. Did not touch the clean lenses.	_____	_____	__________
9. Placed the glasses case in the top drawer of the bedside stand or in the drawer of the overbed table. Or, put the glasses back on the person as follows:	_____	_____	__________
a. Unfolded the glasses.	_____	_____	__________
b. Held the frame at each side. Placed them over the ears.	_____	_____	__________
c. Adjusted the glasses so the nosepiece rested on the nose.	_____	_____	__________
d. Returned the glasses case to the drawer in the bedside stand.	_____	_____	__________
10. Decontaminated hands.	_____	_____	__________

Date of Satisfactory Completion ______________ Instructor's Initials ______________

Cleaning Baby Bottles

Name: ______________________

Date: ______________________

Pre-Procedure	S	U	Comments
1. Reviewed Safety Alert.	____	____	____________
2. Practiced hand hygiene.	____	____	____________
3. Collected the following:			
• Bottles, nipples, and caps	____	____	____________
• Funnel	____	____	____________
• Can opener	____	____	____________
• Bottle brush	____	____	____________
• Dishwashing soap	____	____	____________
• Other items used to prepare formula	____	____	____________
• Towel	____	____	____________

Procedure	S	U	Comments
4. Washed the bottles, nipples, caps, funnel, and can opener in hot, soapy water. Washed other items used to prepare formula.	____	____	____________
5. Cleaned inside baby bottles with the bottle brush.	____	____	____________
6. Squeezed hot, soapy water through the nipples.	____	____	____________
7. Rinsed all items thoroughly in hot water. Squeezed hot water through the nipples to remove soap.	____	____	____________
8. Laid a clean towel on the counter.	____	____	____________
9. Stood bottles upside down to drain. Placed nipples, caps, and other items on the towel. Let the items air-dry.	____	____	____________

Date of Satisfactory Completion ______________ Instructor's Initials ______________

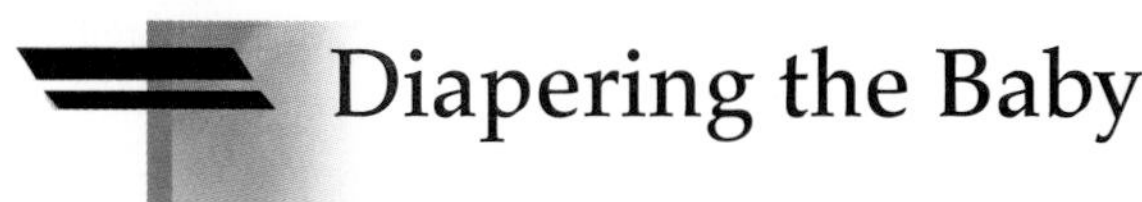

Diapering the Baby

Name: ______________________

Date: ______________________

Pre-Procedure	S	U	Comments
1. Followed Delegation Guidelines. Reviewed Safety Alert.			
2. Practiced hand hygiene.			
3. Collected the following:			
• Gloves			
• Clean diaper			
• Waterproof changing pad			
• Washcloth			
• Disposable wipes or cotton balls			
• Basin of warm water			
• Baby soap			
• Baby lotion or cream			
4. Placed the changing pad under the baby.			

Procedure	S	U	Comments
5. Put on the gloves.			
6. Unfastened the dirty diaper. Placed diaper pins out of the baby's reach.			
7. Wiped the genital area with the front of the diaper. Wiped from the front to the back.			
8. Folded the diaper so urine and feces were inside. Set the diaper aside.			
9. Cleaned the genital area from front to back. Used a wet washcloth, disposable wipes, or cotton balls. Washed with mild soap and water for a large amount of feces or if the baby had a rash. Rinsed thoroughly and patted the area dry.			
10. Gave cord care and cleaned the circumcision at this time.			
11. Applied cream or lotion to the genital area and buttocks. Did not use too much.			
12. Raised the baby's legs. Slid a clean diaper under the buttocks.			
13. Folded a cloth diaper so extra thickness was in the front for a boy. For girls, folded the diaper so the extra thickness was at the back.			
14. Brought the diaper between the baby's legs.			
15. Made sure the diaper was snug around the hips and abdomen. It was loose near the penis if the circumcision had not healed. It was below the umbilicus if the cord stump had not healed.			

Procedure—cont'd	S	U	Comments
16. Secured the diaper in place. Used the tape strips or Velcro on disposable diapers. Made sure the tabs stuck in place. Used baby pins or Velcro for cloth diapers. Pins pointed away from the abdomen.	______	______	______________
17. Applied plastic pants if cloth diapers were worn. Did not use plastic pants with disposable diapers.	______	______	______________
18. Put the baby in the crib, infant seat, or other safe location.	______	______	______________

Post-Procedure

19. Rinsed feces from the cloth diaper in the toilet.	______	______	______________
20. Stored used cloth diapers in a covered pail. Put a disposable diaper in the trash.	______	______	______________
21. Removed the gloves. Practiced hygiene.	______	______	______________
22. Reported and recorded observations.	______	______	______________

Date of Satisfactory Completion ______________ Instructor's Initials ______________

Giving the Baby a Sponge Bath

Name: ______________________

Date: ______________________

Pre-Procedure	S	U	Comments
1. Followed Delegation Guidelines. Reviewed Safety Alert.	____	____	____________
2. Practiced hand hygiene.	____	____	____________
3. Place the following items in the work area:			
• Bath basin	____	____	____________
• Bath thermometer	____	____	____________
• Bath towel	____	____	____________
• Two hand towels	____	____	____________
• Receiving blanket	____	____	____________
• Washcloth	____	____	____________
• Clean diaper	____	____	____________
• Clean clothing for the baby	____	____	____________
• Cotton balls	____	____	____________
• Baby soap	____	____	____________
• Baby shampoo	____	____	____________
• Baby lotion	____	____	____________
• Gloves	____	____	____________

Procedure	S	U	Comments
4. Filled the bath basin with warm water. Water temperature was at 100° to 105° F (37.7° to 40.5° C). Measured water temperature with the bath thermometer or used the inside of the wrist.	____	____	____________
5. Provided for privacy.	____	____	____________
6. Identified the baby according to agency policy.	____	____	____________
7. Put on gloves.	____	____	____________
8. Undressed the baby. Left the diaper on.	____	____	____________
9. Washed the baby's eyelids:			
a. Dipped a cotton ball into the water.	____	____	____________
b. Squeezed out excess water.	____	____	____________
c. Washed one eyelid from the inner part to the outer part.	____	____	____________
d. Repeated this step for the other eye with a new cotton ball.	____	____	____________
10. Moistened the washcloth and made a mitt. Cleaned the outside of the ear and then behind the ear. Repeated this step for the other ear. Was gentle.	____	____	____________
11. Rinsed and squeezed out the washcloth. Made a mitt with the washcloth.	____	____	____________

Procedure—cont'd	S	U	Comments
12. Washed the baby's face. Cleaned inside the nostrils with the washcloth. Did not use cotton swabs to clean inside the nose. Patted the face dry.	______	______	____________
13. Picked up the baby. Held the baby over the bath basin using the football hold. Supported the baby's head and neck with the wrist and hand.	______	______	____________
14. Washed the baby's head:			
a. Squeezed a small amount of water from the washcloth onto the baby's head.	______	______	____________
b. Applied a small amount of baby shampoo to the head.	______	______	____________
c. Washed the head with circular motions.	______	______	____________
d. Rinsed the head by squeezing water from a washcloth over the baby's head. Rinsed thoroughly. Did not get soap in the baby's eyes.	______	______	____________
e. Used a small hand towel to dry the head.	______	______	____________
15. Laid the baby on the table.	______	______	____________
16. Removed the diaper.	______	______	____________
17. Washed the front of the body. Used a soapy washcloth, or applied soap to hands, and washed the baby with the hands. Did not get the cord wet. Rinsed thoroughly. Patted dry. Was sure to wash and dry all creases and folds.	______	______	____________
18. Turned the baby to the prone position. Repeated step 17 for the back and buttocks.	______	______	____________
19. Gave cord care. Cleaned the circumcision.	______	______	____________
20. Applied baby lotion to the baby's body as directed by the nurse.	______	______	____________
21. Put a clean diaper and clean clothes on the baby.	______	______	____________
22. Wrapped the baby in the receiving blanket. Put the baby in the crib or other safe area.	______	______	____________

Post-Procedure

	S	U	Comments
23. Cleaned and returned equipment and supplies to the proper place.	______	______	____________
24. Removed the gloves. Practiced hand hygiene.	______	______	____________
25. Reported and recorded observations.	______	______	____________

Date of Satisfactory Completion ____________________ Instructor's Initials ________________

Giving the Baby a Tub Bath

Name: ______________________

Date: ______________________

Procedure	S	U	Comments
1. Followed steps 1 through 16 in procedure: *Giving the Baby a Sponge Bath.*	_____	_____	____________
2. Held the baby:			
a. Placed one hand under the baby's shoulders. The thumb was over the baby's shoulder. The fingers were under the arm.	_____	_____	____________
b. Supported the buttocks with the other hand. Slid the hand under the thighs. Held the far thigh with the other hand.	_____	_____	____________
3. Lowered the baby into the water feet first.	_____	_____	____________
4. Washed the front of the baby's body. Washed all folds and creases. Rinsed thoroughly.	_____	_____	____________
5. Reversed your hold. Used the other hand to hold the baby.	_____	_____	____________
6. Washed the baby's back. Rinsed thoroughly.	_____	_____	____________
7. Reversed your hold again. Held the baby with the other hand.	_____	_____	____________
8. Washed the genital area.	_____	_____	____________
9. Lifted the baby out of the water and onto a towel.	_____	_____	____________
10. Wrapped the baby in the towel. Also covered the baby's head.	_____	_____	____________
11. Patted the baby dry. Dried all folds and creases.	_____	_____	____________
12. Followed steps 20 through 25 in procedure: *Giving the Baby a Sponge Bath.*	_____	_____	____________

Date of Satisfactory Completion ______________________ Instructor's Initials ______________________

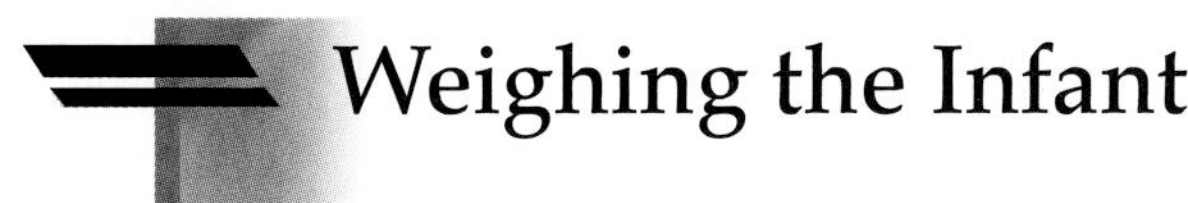

Weighing the Infant

Name: ______________________

Date: ______________________

Pre-Procedure	S	U	Comments
1. Followed Delegation Guidelines.	____	____	______________
2. Practiced hand hygiene.	____	____	______________
3. Collected the following:			
• Baby scale	____	____	______________
• Paper for the scale	____	____	______________
• Items for diaper changing	____	____	______________
• Gloves	____	____	______________
Procedure			
4. Identified the baby following agency policy.	____	____	______________
5. Placed the paper on the scale. Adjusted the scale to zero (0).	____	____	______________
6. Put on the gloves.	____	____	______________
7. Undressed the baby and removed the diaper. Cleaned the genital area.	____	____	______________
8. Laid the baby on the scale. Kept one hand over the baby to prevent falling.	____	____	______________
9. Read the digital display or moved the pointer until the scale was balanced.	____	____	______________
10. Noted the measurement.	____	____	______________
11. Diapered and dressed the baby. Laid the baby in the crib.	____	____	______________
12. Removed and discarded the gloves. Practiced hand hygiene.	____	____	______________
Post-Procedure			
13. Returned the scale to its proper place.	____	____	______________
14. Decontaminated hands.	____	____	______________
15. Reported and recorded observations.	____	____	______________

Date of Satisfactory Completion ______________ Instructor's Initials ______________

Adult CPR—One Rescuer

Name: ______________________

Date: ______________________

Procedure	S	U	Comments
1. Checked if the person was responding. Tapped or gently shook the person, called the person by name, and shouted "Are you OK?"	___	___	___
2. Called for help. Activated the EMS system or the agency's emergency response system.	___	___	___
3. Positioned the person supine. Logrolled the person so there was no twisting of the spine. The person was on a hard, flat surface. Placed the person's arms alongside the body.	___	___	___
4. Opened the airway. Used the head-tilt/chin-lift method.	___	___	___
5. Checked for breathing. Looked to see if the chest rose and fell. Listened for the escape of air. Felt for the flow of air on your cheek.	___	___	___
6. Gave 2 slow breaths if the person was not breathing or was not breathing adequately. Each breath took 2 seconds. Let the person's chest deflate between breaths.	___	___	___
7. Checked for a carotid pulse and for breathing, coughing, and moving. This took 5 to 10 seconds. Used your other hand to keep the airway open with the head-tilt/chin-lift method. Started chest compressions if there were no signs of circulation.	___	___	___
8. Gave chest compressions at a rate of 100 per minute. Gave 15 compressions and then 2 slow breaths.	___	___	___
a. Established a rhythm and counted out loud. (Try: "1 and, 2 and, 3 and, 4 and, 5 and, 6 and, 7 and, 8 and, 9 and, 10 and, 11 and, 12 and, 13 and, 14 and, 15.")	___	___	___
b. Opened the airway, and gave 2 slow breaths.	___	___	___
c. Repeated this step until 4 cycles of 15 compressions and 2 breaths were given.	___	___	___
9. Checked for a carotid pulse. Also checked for breathing, coughing, and moving.	___	___	___
10. Continued CPR if the person had no signs of circulation. Began with chest compressions. Continued the cycle of 15 compressions and 2 breaths. Checked for circulation every few minutes.	___	___	___
11. Did the following if the person had signs of circulation:			
a. Checked for breathing.	___	___	___
b. Positioned the person in the recovery position if the person was breathing.	___	___	___
c. Monitored breathing and circulation.	___	___	___

Procedure—cont'd	S	U	Comments
12. Did the following if the person had signs of circulation but breathing was absent.	______	______	______________________
a. Gave 1 rescue breath every 5 seconds.	______	______	______________________
b. Monitored circulation.	______	______	______________________

Date of Satisfactory Completion ______________________ Instructor's Initials ____________________

Adult CPR—Two Rescuers

Name: ______________________

Date: ______________________

Procedure	S	U	Comments
1. Checked if the person was responding. Tapped or gently shook the person, called the person by name, and shouted "Are you OK?" One rescuer activated the EMS system or the agency's emergency response system.	____	____	____________
2. Opened the airway and checked for breathing. Used the head-tilt/chin-lift method.	____	____	____________
3. Gave 2 slow rescue breaths if the person was not breathing or if breathing was inadequate. Let the lungs deflate between breaths.	____	____	____________
4. Checked for a pulse using the carotid artery. Also checked for breathing, coughing, and moving.	____	____	____________
5. Performed 2-person CPR if there were no signs of circulation.	____	____	____________
a. One rescuer gave chest compressions at a rate of 100 per minute. Counted out loud in a rhythm. (Try: "1 and, 2 and, 3 and, 4 and, 5 and, 6 and, 7 and, 8 and, 9 and, 10 and, 11 and, 12 and, 13 and, 14 and, 15.")	____	____	____________
b. The other rescuer gave 2 slow breaths after every 15 compressions. Paused for the breaths. Continued chest compressions after the breaths.	____	____	____________
6. One rescuer did the following after 4 cycles of 15 compressions and 2 breaths:			
a. Gave 2 slow breaths.	____	____	____________
b. Checked for circulation—carotid pulse, breathing, coughing, and moving.	____	____	____________
7. Continued with 15 compressions and 2 slow breaths if the person had no signs of circulation. Started with chest compressions.	____	____	____________

Date of Satisfactory Completion ______________ Instructor's Initials ______________

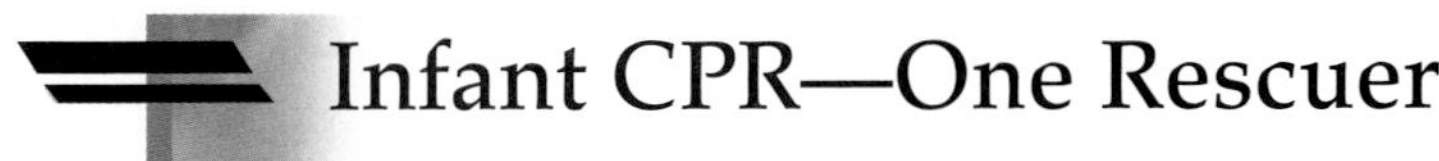

Infant CPR—One Rescuer

Name: ______________________

Date: ______________________

Procedure	S	U	Comments
1. Checked if the infant was responding. Shouted at the infant. Gently tapped an arm or leg.	____	____	____________
2. Activated the EMS system or the agency's emergency response system if help was available.	____	____	____________
3. Knelt at the infant's side near the head.	____	____	____________
4. Logrolled the infant onto his or her back. Kept the head, neck, and spine straight. Positioned the infant supine on a hard, flat surface.	____	____	____________
5. Opened the airway. Used the head-tilt/chin-lift method if injury was not suspected. Used the jaw-thrust method if injury was suspected.	____	____	____________
6. Checked for breathing. Looked to see if the chest rose and fell. Listened for the escape of air. Felt for the flow of air on the cheek.	____	____	____________
7. Covered the infant's nose and mouth with your mouth for rescue breathing.	____	____	____________
8. Gave 2 slow rescue breaths. Used enough force to make the chest rise. Took 1 to $1\frac{1}{2}$ seconds for each breath. Let the chest deflate between breaths.	____	____	____________
9. Checked for circulation. Used the brachial pulse. Also checked for breathing, coughing, and moving.	____	____	____________
10. Located hand position for chest compressions. (Kept the airway open with one hand.)	____	____	____________
a. Drew an imaginary line between the nipples. Found the sternum (breastbone).	____	____	____________
b. Placed 2 fingers on the sternum about 1 finger-width below the imaginary line.	____	____	____________
11. Gave 5 chest compressions followed by 1 slow breath. Gave 100 chest compressions per minute and 20 rescue breaths per minute.	____	____	____________
a. Used the 2 fingers on the sternum for chest compressions. Pressed the sternum down about $1/3$ to $1/2$ the depth of the chest (about $1/2$ to 1 inch).	____	____	____________
b. Released pressure after each compression. Kept the fingers on the chest.	____	____	____________
c. Counted out loud in a rhythm. (Try: "1, 2, 3, 4, 5.")	____	____	____________
d. Gave 1 breath after every 5 chest compressions.	____	____	____________
12. Checked for circulation after 1 minute.	____	____	____________
13. Did the following if there were no signs of circulation:			
a. Activated the EMS system or emergency response system.	____	____	____________
b. Continued CPR.	____	____	____________

Procedure—cont'd	S	U	Comments
14. Gave 1 rescue breath every 3 seconds if there were signs of circulation but breathing was absent or inadequate. Gave 20 rescue breaths per minute.	______	______	____________________

Date of Satisfactory Completion ____________________ Instructor's Initials ____________________

Child CPR—One Rescuer

Name: ______________________

Date: ______________________

Procedure	S	U	Comments
1. Checked if the child was responding. Shouted at the child. Gently tapped an arm or leg.	____	____	____________
2. Activated the EMS system or the agency's emergency response system if help was available.	____	____	____________
3. Knelt at the child's side near the head.	____	____	____________
4. Logrolled the child onto his or her back. Kept the head, neck, and spine straight. Positioned the child supine on a hard, flat surface.	____	____	____________
5. Opened the airway. Used the head-tilt/chin-lift method if injury was not suspected. Used the jaw-thrust method if injury was suspected.	____	____	____________
6. Checked for breathing. Looked to see if the chest rose and fell. Listened for the escape of air. Felt for the flow of air on the cheek.	____	____	____________
7. Covered the child's mouth with your mouth. Pinched the nostrils shut.	____	____	____________
8. Gave 2 slow rescue breaths. Used enough force to make the chest rise. Took 1 to 1$^1/_2$ seconds for each breath. Let the chest deflate between breaths.	____	____	____________
9. Checked for circulation. Used the carotid pulse. Checked for breathing, coughing, or moving.	____	____	____________
10. Located hand position for chest compressions. (Kept the airway open with one hand.)	____	____	____________
a. Found the middle of the sternum (breastbone).	____	____	____________
b. Placed the heel of one hand over the lower half of the sternum. Kept the fingers off the chest.	____	____	____________
11. Gave 5 chest compressions followed by 1 slow breath. Gave 100 chest compressions per minute and 20 rescue breaths per minute.	____	____	____________
a. Used the heel of the hand on the sternum for chest compressions. Pressed the sternum down about $^1/_3$ to $^1/_2$ the depth of the chest (about 1 to 1$^1/_2$ inches).	____	____	____________
b. Released pressure after each compression. Kept the heel of the hand on the chest.	____	____	____________
c. Counted out loud in a rhythm. (Try: "1, 2, 3, 4, 5.")	____	____	____________
d. Gave 1 breath after every 5 chest compressions.	____	____	____________
12. Checked for circulation after 1 minute.	____	____	____________

Procedure—cont'd	S	U	Comments
13. Did the following if there were no signs of circulation:			
a. Activated the EMS system or emergency response system.	______	______	______
b. Continued CPR.	______	______	______
14. Gave 1 rescue breath every 3 seconds if there were signs of circulation but breathing was absent or inadequate. Gave 20 rescue breaths per minute.	______	______	______

Date of Satisfactory Completion ______________________ Instructor's Initials ______________________

FBAO—The Responsive Adult

Name: ____________________

Date: ____________________

Procedure	S	U	Comments
1. Asked the person if he or she was choking.	____	____	____________
2. Asked if the person could cough or speak.	____	____	____________
3. Gave abdominal thrusts:			
a. Stood behind the person.	____	____	____________
b. Wrapped your arms around the person's waist.	____	____	____________
c. Made a fist with one hand.	____	____	____________
d. Placed the thumb side of the fist against the abdomen. The fist was in the middle above the navel and below the end of the sternum (breastbone).	____	____	____________
e. Grasped the fist with the other hand.	____	____	____________
f. Pressed the fist and hand into the person's abdomen with a quick, upward thrust.	____	____	____________
g. Repeated thrusts until the object was expelled or the person lost consciousness.	____	____	____________
4. Lowered the unresponsive person to the floor or ground. Positioned the person supine.	____	____	____________
5. Activated the EMS system or the agency's emergency response system.	____	____	____________
6. Did a finger sweep to check for a foreign object:			
a. Opened the person's mouth. Used the tongue-jaw lift method.	____	____	____________
(1) Grasped the person's tongue and lower jaw with the thumb and fingers.	____	____	____________
(2) Lifted the lower jaw upward.	____	____	____________
b. Inserted the other index finger into the mouth along the side of the cheek and deep into the throat. The finger was at the base of the tongue.	____	____	____________
c. Formed a hook with the index finger.	____	____	____________
d. Tried to dislodge and remove the object. Did not push it deeper into the throat.	____	____	____________
e. Grasped and removed the object if it was within reach.	____	____	____________
7. Opened the airway with the head-tilt/chin-lift method.	____	____	____________
8. Gave 1 or 2 rescue breaths.	____	____	____________
9. Repositioned the person's head if the chest did not rise. Gave 1 or 2 rescue breaths.	____	____	____________
10. Gave up to 5 abdominal thrusts.	____	____	____________
11. Repeated steps 6 through 10 (finger sweeps, rescue breathing, and abdominal thrusts) until rescue breathing was effective. Started CPR if necessary.	____	____	____________

Date of Satisfactory Completion ____________________ Instructor's Initials ____________________

FBAO—The Unresponsive Adult

Name: ____________________

Date: ____________________

Procedure	S	U	Comments
1. Checked to see if the person was responding.	____	____	____________
2. Called for help. Activated the EMS system or the agency's emergency response system.	____	____	____________
3. Logrolled the person to the supine position with the face up. Arms were at the sides.	____	____	____________
4. Opened the airway. Used the head-tilt/chin-lift method.	____	____	____________
5. Checked for breathing.	____	____	____________
6. Gave 1 or 2 slow rescue breaths. Repositioned the person's head and opened the airway if the chest did not rise. Gave 1 or 2 rescue breaths.	____	____	____________
7. Gave 5 abdominal thrusts if the person could not be ventilated.	____	____	____________
a. Straddled the person's thighs.	____	____	____________
b. Placed the heel of one hand against the abdomen. It was in the middle above the navel and below the end of the sternum (breastbone).	____	____	____________
c. Placed the second hand on top of the first hand.	____	____	____________
d. Pressed both hands into the abdomen with a quick, upward thrust. Gave 5 thrusts.	____	____	____________
8. Did a finger sweep to check for a foreign object.	____	____	____________
9. Repeated steps 6 through 8 until rescue breathing was effective. Started CPR if necessary.	____	____	____________

Date of Satisfactory Completion ____________________ Instructor's Initials ____________________

FBAO—The Responsive Infant

Name: ______________________

Date: ______________________

Procedure	S	U	Comments
1. Held the infant face down over your forearm. Knelt or sat to support the arm on your thigh. The infant's head was lower than the trunk. Held the infant's jaw to support the head.	____	____	____________
2. Gave up to 5 back blows. Used the heel of the hand. Gave the back blows between the shoulder blades. (Stopped the back blows if the object was expelled.)	____	____	____________
3. Turned the infant as a unit:			
a. Supported the infant's head, neck, jaw, and chest with one hand.	____	____	____________
b. Supported the infant's back with the other hand.	____	____	____________
c. Turned the infant as a unit. The infant was in the back-lying position on your forearm.	____	____	____________
4. Gave up to 5 chest thrusts:			
a. Located hand position as for chest compressions.	____	____	____________
b. Compressed the chest upward toward the head. Used 2 or 3 fingers.	____	____	____________
c. Stopped chest thrusts if the object was expelled.	____	____	____________
5. Gave 5 back blows followed by 5 chest thrusts until the object was expelled or the child became unresponsive.	____	____	____________
6. Did the following if the infant became unresponsive:			
a. Activated the EMS system or the agency's emergency response system if help was available.	____	____	____________
b. Opened the airway with the tongue-jaw lift method. Gave a rescue breath.	____	____	____________
7. Looked in the throat for an object. If an object was seen, removed it with a fingersweep.	____	____	____________
8. Repeated rescue breathing, back blows, chest thrusts, the tongue-jaw lift maneuver, and the finger sweep for a visible object until one of the following occurred:			
a. The object was expelled.	____	____	____________
b. The infant started breathing.	____	____	____________
c. CPR was needed.	____	____	____________
9. Activated the EMS system or the agency's emergency response system after following the procedure for 1 minute.	____	____	____________
10. Continued the FBAO procedure or CPR until emergency personnel arrived.	____	____	____________

Date of Satisfactory Completion ______________ Instructor's Initials ______________

FBAO—The Responsive Child

Name: ______________________

Date: ______________________

Procedure	S	U	Comments
1. Determined if the child was choking. Asked if the child was choking and if the child could speak. Told the child that you were going to help.	_____	_____	__________
2. Stood behind the child.	_____	_____	__________
3. Wrapped your arms under the child's underarms and around the chest.	_____	_____	__________
4. Made a fist with one hand. Placed the thumb side of the fist on the child's abdomen. The fist was in the middle above the navel and below the sternum (breastbone).	_____	_____	__________
5. Grabbed the fist with the other hand.	_____	_____	__________
6. Gave a quick inward and upward thrust.	_____	_____	__________
7. Repeated abdominal thrusts until the object was expelled or the child became unresponsive.	_____	_____	__________
8. Did the following if the child became unresponsive:			
a. Activated the EMS system or the agency's emergency response system if help was available.	_____	_____	__________
b. Opened the airway with the tongue-jaw lift method. Gave a rescue breath.	_____	_____	__________
9. Looked in the throat for an object. If an object was seen, removed it with a fingersweep.	_____	_____	__________
10. Repeated rescue breathing, abdominal thrusts, the tongue-jaw lift maneuver, and the finger sweep for a visible object until one of the following occurred:	_____	_____	__________
a. The object was expelled.	_____	_____	__________
b. The child started breathing.	_____	_____	__________
c. CPR was needed.	_____	_____	__________
11. Activated the EMS system or the agency's emergency response system after following the procedure for 1 minute.	_____	_____	__________
12. Continued the FBAO procedure or CPR until emergency personnel arrived.	_____	_____	__________

Date of Satisfactory Completion ______________________ Instructor's Initials ______________________

FBAO—The Unresponsive Infant or Child

Name: ______________________

Date: ______________________

Procedure	S	U	Comments
1. Checked if the infant or child was responding.	____	____	____________
2. Activated the EMS system or the agency's emergency response system if help was available.	____	____	____________
3. Opened the airway.	____	____	____________
4. Checked for breathing. Looked to see if the chest rose and fell. Listened for the escape of air. Felt for the flow of air on the cheek.	____	____	____________
5. Gave a rescue breath. Repositioned the head if the chest did not rise. Opened the airway, and gave a rescue breath.	____	____	____________
6. Did one of the following:			
a. For an infant—gave up to 5 back blows and 5 chest thrusts.	____	____	____________
b. For a child—gave up to 5 abdominal thrusts.	____	____	____________
7. Opened the airway with the tongue-jaw lift maneuver. Gave a rescue breath.	____	____	____________
8. Looked in the throat for an object. If an object was seen, removed it with a fingersweep.	____	____	____________
9. Repeated rescue breathing, abdominal thrusts (back blows and chest thrusts for an infant), the tongue-jaw lift maneuver, and the finger sweep for a visible object until one of the following occurred:	____	____	____________
a. The object was expelled.	____	____	____________
b. The infant or child started breathing.	____	____	____________
c. CPR was needed.	____	____	____________
10. Activated the EMS system or the agency's emergency response system after following the procedure for 1 minute.	____	____	____________
11. Continued the FBAO procedure or CPR until emergency personnel arrived.	____	____	____________

Date of Satisfactory Completion ______________ Instructor's Initials ______________

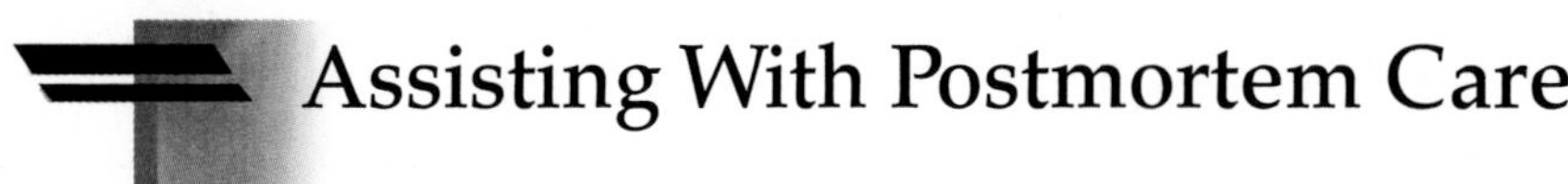

Assisting With Postmortem Care

Name: ______________________

Date: ______________________

Pre-Procedure	S	U	Comments
1. Followed Delegation Guidelines. Reviewed Safety Alert.	____	____	____________
2. Practiced hand hygiene.	____	____	____________
3. Collected the following:			
• Postmortem kit (shroud or body bag, gown, ID tags, gauze squares, safety pins)	____	____	____________
• Bed protectors	____	____	____________
• Washbasin	____	____	____________
• Bath towels and washcloths	____	____	____________
• Tape	____	____	____________
• Dressings	____	____	____________
• Gloves	____	____	____________
• Cotton balls	____	____	____________
• Gown	____	____	____________
• Valuables envelope	____	____	____________
4. Provided for privacy.	____	____	____________
5. Raised the bed for body mechanics.	____	____	____________
6. Made sure the bed was flat.	____	____	____________

Procedure	S	U	Comments
7. Put on the gloves.	____	____	____________
8. Positioned the body supine. Arms and legs were straight. A pillow was under the head and shoulders.	____	____	____________
9. Closed the eyes. Gently pulled the eyelids over the eyes. Applied moist cotton balls gently over the eyelids if the eyes would not stay closed.	____	____	____________
10. Inserted dentures if it was agency policy. If not, put them in a labeled denture container.	____	____	____________
11. Closed the mouth. If necessary, placed a rolled towel under the chin to keep the mouth closed.	____	____	____________
12. Followed agency policy about jewelry. Removed all jewelry, except for wedding rings if this was agency policy. Described the jewelry that was removed. Placed the jewelry and the list in a valuables envelope.	____	____	____________
13. Placed a cotton ball over the rings. Taped them in place.	____	____	____________
14. Removed drainage containers. Left tubes and catheters in place if there would be an autopsy. Asked the nurse about removing tubes.	____	____	____________
15. Bathed soiled areas with plain water. Dried thoroughly.	____	____	____________

Procedure—cont'd	S	U	Comments
16. Placed a bed protector under the buttocks.			
17. Removed soiled dressings. Replaced them with clean ones.			
18. Put a clean gown on the body. Positioned the body as in step 8.			
19. Brushed and combed the hair if necessary.			
20. Covered the body to the shoulders with a sheet if the family would view the body.			
21. Gathered the person's belongings. Put them in a bag labeled with the person's name.			
22. Removed supplies, equipment, and linen. Straightened the room. Provided soft lighting.			
23. Removed the gloves. Decontaminated hands.			
24. Let the family view the body. Provided for privacy. Returned to the room after they left.			
25. Decontaminated hands. Put on gloves.			
26. Filled out the ID tags. Tied one to the ankle or to the right big toe.			
27. Placed the body in the body bag or covered it with a sheet, or applied the shroud.			
a. Brought the top down over the head.			
b. Folded the bottom up over the feet.			
c. Folded the sides over the body.			
d. Pinned or taped the shroud in place.			
28. Attached the second ID tag to the shroud, sheet, or body bag.			
29. Left the denture cup with the body.			
30. Pulled the privacy curtain around the bed or closed the door.			

Post-Procedure

	S	U	Comments
31. Removed the gloves. Decontaminated hands.			
32. Stripped the unit after the body was removed. Wore gloves for this step.			
33. Removed the gloves. Decontaminated hands.			
34. Reported the following to the nurse:			
• The time the body was taken by the funeral director			
• What was done with jewelry and personal items			
• What was done with dentures			

Date of Satisfactory Completion ______________________ Instructor's Initials ____________________